T0226551

Head and Neck Cancer

Editor

JOHN A. RIDGE

SURGICAL ONCOLOGY CLINICS OF NORTH AMERICA

www.surgonc.theclinics.com

Consulting Editor
NICHOLAS J. PETRELLI

July 2015 • Volume 24 • Number 3

ELSEVIER

1600 John F. Kennedy Boulevard • Suite 1800 • Philadelphia, Pennsylvania, 19103-2899

http://www.theclinics.com

SURGICAL ONCOLOGY CLINICS OF NORTH AMERICA Volume 24, Number 3
July 2015 ISSN 1055-3207, ISBN-13: 978-0-323-39121-4

Editor: Jessica McCool
Developmental Editor: Meredith Clinton

Surgical Oncology Clinics of North America (ISSN 1055-3207) is published quarterly by Elsevier Inc., 360 Park Avenue South, New York, NY 10010-1710. Months of publication are January, April, July, and October. Business and Editorial Offices: 1600 John F. Kennedy Blvd., Ste. 1800, Philadelphia, PA 19103-2899. Customer Service Office: 3251 Riverport Lane, Maryland Heights, MO 63043. Periodicals postage paid at New York, NY and additional mailing offices. Subscription prices are $290.00 per year (US individuals), $421.00 (US institutions) $140.00 (US student/resident), $330.00 (Canadian individuals), $533.00 (Canadian institutions), $205.00 (Canadian student/resident), $410.00 (foreign individuals), $533.00 (foreign institutions), and $205.00 (foreign student/resident). Foreign air speed delivery is included in all *Clinics* subscription prices. All prices are subject to change without notice. **POSTMASTER**: Send address changes to *Surgical Oncology Clinics of North America,* Elsevier Health Science Division, Subscription Customer Service, 3251 Riverport Lane, Maryland Heights, MO 63043. **Customer Service: 1-800-654-2452 (US and Canada). 314-447-8871 (outside US and Canada). Fax: 314-447-8029. E-mail: journalscustomerservice-usa@elsevier.com** (for print support); **journalsonline support-usa@elsevier.com** (for online support).

Reprints. For copies of 100 or more, of articles in this publication, please contact the Commercial Reprints Department, Elsevier Inc., 360 Park Avenue South, New York, New York 10010-1710. Tel. 212-633-3874; Fax: 212-633-3820; E-mail: reprints@elsevier.com.

Surgical Oncology Clinics of North America is covered in *MEDLINE/PubMed (Index Medicus)* and *EMBASE/ Excerpta Medica, Current Contents/Clinical Medicine,* and *ISI/BIOMED*.

Contributors

CONSULTING EDITOR

NICHOLAS J. PETRELLI, MD, FACS
Bank of America Endowed Medical Director, Helen F. Graham Cancer Center and Research Institute, Christiana Care Health System, Newark, Delaware; Professor of Surgery, Thomas Jefferson University, Philadelphia, Pennsylvania

EDITOR

JOHN A. RIDGE, MD, PhD, FACS
Louis Della Penna Family Professor of Head and Neck Oncology, Chief, Head and Surgery Division, Vice-Chair, Department of Surgical Oncology, Fox Chase Cancer Center, Philadelphia, Pennsylvania

AUTHORS

JESTY ABRAHAM, DO
Department of Radiology, Fox Chase Cancer Center, Philadelphia, Pennsylvania

VICTORIA BANUCHI, MD, MPH
Assistant Professor, Weill Cornell Medical College, New York City, New York

JULIE E. BAUMAN, MD
Division of Hematology/Oncology, Department of Internal Medicine, University of Pittsburgh Cancer Institute, Pittsburgh, Pennsylvania

JOSEPH A. CALIFANO, MD
Department of Otolaryngology, Head and Neck Surgery, Johns Hopkins Medical Institutions, Baltimore, Maryland

ERIC I. CHANG, MD
Assistant Clinical Professor, Division of Plastic and Reconstructive Surgery, Department of Surgical Oncology, Fox Chase Cancer Center, Philadelphia, Pennsylvania

DAVID A. CLUMP, MD, PhD
Department of Radiation Oncology, University of Pittsburgh Cancer Institute, Pittsburgh, Pennsylvania

GYPSYAMBER D'SOUZA, PhD, MPH
Johns Hopkins Bloomberg School of Public Health, Baltimore, Maryland

ROBERT L. FERRIS, MD, PhD, FACS
Department of Radiation Oncology, University of Pittsburgh Cancer Institute; Department of Otolaryngology/Head and Neck Surgery, University of Pittsburgh Eye and Ear Institute, Pittsburgh, Pennsylvania

THOMAS J. GALLOWAY, MD
Assistant Professor; Director of Clinical Research, Department of Radiation Oncology, Fox Chase Cancer Center, Philadelphia, Pennsylvania

RACHEL GEORGOPOULOS, MD
Department of Otolaryngology, Temple University School of Medicine, Philadelphia, Pennsylvania

THERESA GUO, MD
Department of Otolaryngology, Head and Neck Surgery, Johns Hopkins Medical Institutions, Baltimore, Maryland

SOPHIA C. KAMRAN, MD
Harvard Radiation Oncology Residency Program, Boston, Massachusetts

JESSICA A. KOZEL, MD
Department of Pathology and Microbiology, University of Nebraska Medical Center, Omaha, Nebraska

DENNIS KRAUS, MD, FACS
Director, The Center for Head and Neck Oncology, New York Head and Neck Institute, North Shore-LIJ Cancer Institute; Co-Director, The Center for Thyroid and Parathyroid Surgery, New York Head and Neck Institute, New York, New York

MICHAEL E. KUPFERMAN, MD
Associate Professor, Department of Head and Neck Surgery, The University of Texas M. D. Anderson Cancer Center, Houston, Texas

NANCY LEE, MD
Department of Radiation Oncology, Memorial Sloan Kettering Cancer Center, New York, New York

JEFFREY C. LIU, MD, FACS
Head and Neck Section, Department of Otolaryngology, Fox Chase Cancer Center, Temple University School of Medicine, Philadelphia, Pennsylvania

WILLIAM M. LYDIATT, MD
Division of Head and Neck Surgery, Nebraska Methodist Hospital, University of Nebraska Medical Center, Omaha, Nebraska

JONATHAN MALLEN, BA
Hofstra North Shore-LIJ School of Medicine, Hempstead, New York

JEFFREY M. MARTIN, MD
Department of Radiation Oncology, Fox Chase Cancer Center, Philadelphia, Pennsylvania

CAITLIN P. MCMULLEN, MD
Administrative Chief Resident, Department of Otorhinolaryngology–Head and Neck Surgery, Montefiore Medical Center, Albert Einstein College of Medicine, Bronx, New York

RANEE MEHRA, MD
Assistant Professor, Department of Medical Oncology; Co-Leader, Head and Neck Program, Fox Chase Cancer Center, Philadelphia, Pennsylvania

PABLO H. MONTERO, MD
Head and Neck Surgery Service, Department of Surgery, Memorial Sloan Kettering Cancer Center, New York, New York

WOJCIECH K. MYDLARZ, MD
Clinical Specialist, Department of Head and Neck Surgery, The University of Texas M. D. Anderson Cancer Center, Houston, Texas

PHILIP PANCARI, MD
Fox Chase Cancer Center, Philadelphia, Pennsylvania

ARU PANWAR, MD
Division of Head and Neck Surgery, Nebraska Methodist Hospital, University of Nebraska Medical Center, Omaha, Nebraska

SAMEER A. PATEL, MD, FACS
Assistant Clinical Professor, Division of Plastic and Reconstructive Surgery, Department of Surgical Oncology, Fox Chase Cancer Center, Philadelphia, Pennsylvania

SNEHAL G. PATEL, MD
Head and Neck Surgery Service, Department of Surgery, Memorial Sloan Kettering Cancer Center, New York, New York

ELENI M. RETTIG, MD
Johns Hopkins Medical Institutions, Department of Otolaryngology-Head and Neck Surgery, Baltimore, Maryland

NADEEM RIAZ, MD
Department of Radiation Oncology, Memorial Sloan Kettering Cancer Center, New York, New York

RICHARD V. SMITH, MD, FACS
Professor and Vice-Chair, Department of Otorhinolaryngology–Head and Neck Surgery, Montefiore Medical Center, Albert Einstein College of Medicine, Bronx, New York

RANDAL S. WEBER, MD
Professor and Chairman, Department of Head and Neck Surgery, The University of Texas M. D. Anderson Cancer Center, Houston, Texas

SUE S. YOM, MD, PhD
Associate Professor, Department of Radiation Oncology, Helen Diller Family Comprehensive Cancer Center, University of California, San Francisco, San Francisco, California

Contents

This article discusses risk factors, incidence trends, and prognostic considerations for head and neck cancer (HNC). The primary causes of HNC are tobacco and alcohol use, and human papillomavirus (HPV). Tobacco-related HNC incidence rates are decreasing in countries where tobacco use has declined. HPV-HNC, which occurs primarily in the oropharynx and is associated with sexual behaviors, has been increasing over the past several decades, among white men in particular. The prognosis for HNC overall has improved slightly since the 1990s, and is influenced by site, stage, and HPV status. Prognosis for HPV-HNC is significantly better than for HPV-negative disease.

In recent years, our knowledge and understanding of head and neck squamous cell carcinoma (HNSCC) has expanded dramatically. New high-throughput sequencing technologies have accelerated these discoveries since the first reports of whole-exome sequencing of HNSCC tumors in 2011. In addition, the discovery of human papillomavirus in relationship with oropharyngeal squamous cell carcinoma has shifted our molecular understanding of the disease. New investigation into the role of immune evasion in HNSCC has also led to potential novel therapies based on immune-specific systemic therapies.

Head and neck cancer typically refers to epithelial malignancies of the upper aerodigestive tract and may include neoplasms of the thyroid, salivary glands, and soft tissue, bone sarcomas, and skin cancers. Two-thirds of patients present with advanced disease involving regional lymph nodes at the time of diagnosis. A thorough history and detailed examination are integral to oncologic staging and treatment planning. This article begins with an overview of the head and neck examination (with special attention to detailed findings with clinical implications), followed by a discussion of the major head and neck subsites, and clinical pearls surrounding the examination.

Radiation therapy plays a central and continuously evolving role in the treatment of head and neck cancer. In this review, some basic principles of radiation oncology are explained and common clinical scenarios are addressed in which radiation therapy forms part of the treatment course, with a focus on issues most pertinent to the interaction of radiation oncology with surgical treatment. These issues include refinement of the indications guiding the choice of adjuvant radiation therapy or chemoradiotherapy, sequencing and timing of therapies before or after definitive surgical management, and scientific and technical advances with the potential to reduce radiation-related toxicity.

The use of systemic therapy as part of curative treatment and palliation is an evolving paradigm for squamous cell cancer of the head and neck (SCCHN), which historically has been treated with local modalities. At present, the treatment armamentarium includes traditional cytotoxic therapy, targeted biological agents, and emerging immunotherapeutics. This article discusses the use of all of these systemic approaches for the curative and palliative treatment of SCCHN.

Imaging is an essential tool in the management of head and neck cancer. Oral, oropharyngeal, laryngeal, and hypopharyngeal lesions are initially imaged with computed tomography (CT) because it allows rapid image acquisition and reduces artifacts related to respiration and swallowing, which can degrade image quality and limit evaluation. Sinonasal, nasopharyngeal, and salivary gland tumors are better approached with MRI because it allows for better delineation of tumor extent. PET/CT is usually reserved for advanced disease to evaluate for distant metastatic disease and posttreatment residual and recurrent disease. Imaging is best used in combination with expert clinical and physical examination.

Reconstruction after surgical treatment of head and neck cancers can be challenging. Goals for reconstruction include restoration of appearance as well as function when appropriate. Commonly encountered sites requiring reconstruction include the soft tissues of the face (including the critical areas of the eyes, ears, nose, and lips), scalp, tongue and oral cavity, maxilla, mandible, and pharynx. Advanced reconstructive techniques using microsurgery may be preferable to simpler techniques to obtain optimal outcomes. In this article, techniques for reconstruction in these areas as well as anticipated outcomes are discussed.

SURGICAL ONCOLOGY
CLINICS OF NORTH AMERICA

RELATED INTEREST

Surgical Clinics of North America, February 2015 (Vol. 95, Issue 1)
Caring for the Geriatric Surgical Patient
Fred A. Luchette, *Editor*
Available at: http://www.surgical.theclinics.com/

THE CLINICS ARE AVAILABLE ONLINE!
Access your subscription at:
www.theclinics.com

Foreword

A Long Overdue Discussion of Head and Neck Cancer

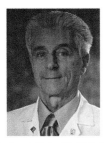

Nicholas J. Petrelli, MD, FACS
Consulting Editor

This issue of the *Surgical Oncology Clinics of North America* is devoted to head and neck cancer. The guest editor is John A. Ridge, MD, PhD, FACS, who is the Louis Della Penna Family Professor of Head and Neck Oncology, Chief of Head and Neck Surgery Division, and Vice Chair of the Department of Surgical Oncology at the Fox Chase Cancer Center in Philadelphia. Dr Ridge has gathered an outstanding group of clinicians and investigators on a very timely topic in cancer care.

The American Cancer Society estimates that there will be 45,780 oral cavity and pharynx cancers in 2015. These estimated new cancer cases in the head and neck will occur in 32,670 men and 13,110 women. The most common head and neck cancer will be pharynx with 15,522 cases followed by tongue cancer with 14,320 cases. The American Cancer Society estimates that, in 2015, there will be 8650 deaths from head and neck cancer.

As stated by Dr Ridge in his preface, "our understanding of the epidemiology, molecular biology, and immunology of head and neck cancers is increasing rapidly." In view of this statement, Dr Ridge has accumulated an outstanding group of authors in all of these areas. This is captured in the articles of Epidemiology of Head and Neck Cancer by authors Rettig and D'Souza, and Molecular Biology and Immunology of Head and Neck Cancer by authors Guo and Califano. The second half of this issue of the *Surgical Oncology Clinics of North America* is disease-site oriented with a discussion of cancers of the oral pharynx, larynx, and hypopharynx; nasopharyngeal carcinoma; and cancers of the nose, sinus, and skull base. An interesting article on head and neck squamous cell carcinoma of unknown primary by authors Martin and Galloway is also included.

Surg Oncol Clin N Am 24 (2015) xiii–xiv
http://dx.doi.org/10.1016/j.soc.2015.04.002
1055-3207/15/$ – see front matter © 2015 Published by Elsevier Inc.

surgonc.theclinics.com

It has been some time since the *Surgical Oncology Clinics of North America* has tackled head and neck cancer. I would like to thank Dr John Ridge and his collaborators for updating our readers on present-day issues for the diagnosis and treatment of head and neck cancer.

Nicholas J. Petrelli, MD, FACS
Helen F. Graham Cancer Center
and Research Institute
Christiana Care Health System
4701 Ogletown-Stanton Road
Newark, DE 19713, USA

Professor of Surgery
Thomas Jefferson University

E-mail address:
npetrelli@christianacare.org

Preface

Why "Head and Neck Cancer"?

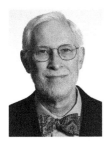

John A. Ridge, MD, PhD, FACS
Editor

The term "head and neck cancer" describes a diverse group of tumors arising in the upper aerodigestive tract. The overwhelming majority are squamous cell carcinomas caused by substance abuse, although viral causes are increasingly recognized. In aggregate, they constitute the seventh most common malignancy worldwide (more than half a million will be diagnosed this year) and the ninth most common cancer in North America. Some 60,000 Americans will develop head and neck cancers during the coming year, and perhaps 12,000 will succumb to the disease. Though not commonly considered "head and neck cancers," salivary gland tumors and cutaneous malignancies (including melanoma) also represent significant clinical problems.

To a great degree, squamous carcinomas arising from the mucosal surfaces of the head and neck ("head and neck cancers"), salivary gland tumors, and cutaneous malignancies are properly Halstedian cancers. They are largely characterized by an orderly progression from the primary site, through regional nodal involvement, to distant metastases. Seldom "systemic" at presentation, the diseases described in this issue of *Surgical Oncology Clinics of North America* are curable through local and regional therapy alone. The treatment regimens, whether surgical or radiation-based, are satisfying to deliver, and many patients survive their disease.

As with most diseases, our understanding of the epidemiology, molecular biology, and immunology of head and neck tumors is increasing rapidly. Considerable excitement surrounds the characterization of a new disease (oropharyngeal cancer induced by human papilloma virus) and the application of newly developed immunotherapeutic agents. Performance of a head and neck examination is essential in evaluating any patient suspected of harboring a cancer arising between the dura and the pleura, as is an appropriate selection of imaging studies. A multidisciplinary approach is necessary for all but the smallest and most indolent of these lesions, and a close working relationship between all oncologists (surgical, medical, reconstructive, and radiation) is indispensible.

Surg Oncol Clin N Am 24 (2015) xv–xvi
http://dx.doi.org/10.1016/j.soc.2015.04.001
1055-3207/15/$ – see front matter © 2015 Published by Elsevier Inc.

surgonc.theclinics.com

This issue provides a thorough background in the topics introduced above before addressing in detail individual diseases, including cancers of the oral cavity, oropharynx, unknown primary, larynx and hypopharynx, nasopharynx, nose and sinuses, skin cancers, and salivary gland tumors. There is something for everyone.

My distinguished coauthors and I could not have prepared this issue of *Surgical Oncology Clinics of North America* without the dedicated assistance of Meredith Clinton and the team at Elsevier. I would like to thank them for their commitment to the endeavor, and Nicholas Petrelli for inviting me to participate.

John A. Ridge, MD, PhD, FACS
Head and Surgery Division
Department of Surgical Oncology
Fox Chase Cancer Center
333 Cottman Avenue
Philadelphia, PA 19111, USA

E-mail address:
drew.ridge@fccc.edu

Epidemiology of Head and Neck Cancer

Eleni M. Rettig, MD[a], Gypsyamber D'Souza, PhD, MPH[b],*

KEYWORDS

- Head and neck cancer • Tobacco • Human papillomavirus • Alcohol • Epidemiology

KEY POINTS

- The two major causes of head and neck cancer (HNC) are (1) tobacco and alcohol, and (2) human papillomavirus (HPV).
- HPV-HNC is strongly tied to oral sexual behaviors and is most common in middle-aged white men.
- The epidemiology of HPV-HNC can be explained in part by variations in oral sexual behaviors by race and age cohort.
- Globally, incidence of HPV-negative HNC is associated with patterns of tobacco use, and is falling in countries with declining rates of tobacco smoking.
- Prognosis for HNC is determined by anatomic site, stage, and HPV tumor status. HPV-positive HNC has better survival than HPV-negative disease.

INTRODUCTION

Head and neck cancer (HNC) encompasses a heterogeneous group of upper aerodigestive tract malignancies that together comprise the seventh most common cancer worldwide,[1] and ninth most common cancer in the United States.[2] The vast majority of HNCs are squamous cell carcinomas (SCCs).[3] More than 54,000 new cases of HNC were projected in the United States in 2014, resulting in an annual incidence of 15.0 per 100,000, with 12,000 deaths attributable to the disease.[2]

There are two primary causes of HNC: (1) tobacco and alcohol use, and (2) human papillomavirus (HPV), a sexually transmitted infection. Historically, most HNCs have been caused by tobacco and alcohol, but over the past decade, HPV has been recognized as another important cause of HNC. Both HPV-negative and HPV-positive HNC have a higher incidence among men than women and increasing incidence with age; however, they have otherwise unique risk factor profiles, prognostic considerations,

The authors have nothing to disclose.
[a] Department of Otolaryngology-Head and Neck Surgery, Johns Hopkins University School of Medicine, 601 North Caroline Street, Baltimore, MD 21287, USA; [b] Department of Epidemiology, Johns Hopkins Bloomberg School of Public Health, 615 North Wolfe Street, Baltimore, MD 21205, USA
* Corresponding author.
E-mail address: gdsouza2@jhu.edu

surgonc.theclinics.com

and incidence trends (**Table 1**).[4–6] HPV-HNC patients are more likely to be white, have a higher socioeconomic status (SES), and are diagnosed at a younger age than HPV-negative HNC patients.[4,7] HPV-HNC patients also have significantly improved prognosis compared with those diagnosed with HPV-negative HNC.[8,9] In the United States, the epidemiologic landscape of HNC is changing dramatically as the incidence of HPV-HNC is rising, and declining tobacco-smoking prevalence rates are paralleled by a decreasing incidence of HPV-negative HNC.[10,11] Globally, HNC incidence trends vary widely by country, reflecting differing trends in tobacco use, alcohol use, and sexual norms across countries.[12]

This article discusses trends in risk factors, incidence, and prognosis of both HPV-negative and HPV-positive HNC. Although HNC epidemiology literature from before 2005 did not distinguish between HPV-negative and HPV-positive HNC, limiting interpretation of epidemiologic trends across that time frame, recent research has greatly broadened our understanding of the role of HPV in HNC.

RISK FACTORS FOR HEAD AND NECK CANCER

The risk factors for HNC include some common risk factors associated with both HPV-positive and HPV-negative HNC, as well as other distinct causative factors. This section reviews risk factors for HNC overall, followed by a discussion of those specific to HPV-HNC.

Noninfectious Risk Factors for Head and Neck Cancer

Although the primary risk factors for HNC are tobacco, alcohol, and HPV, HNC etiology is multifactorial and many additional causes have been identified (**Box 1**).

Tobacco
Tobacco causes most HNC, and alcohol synergistically increases the risk of HNC conferred by tobacco use.[13,14] Historically, approximately 90% of patients with HNC have a history of tobacco use,[14] with a four-fold to five-fold increase in risk of developing oral cavity, oropharynx, and hypopharynx cancers, and a 10-fold increased risk of laryngeal cancer, among tobacco users.[15] The carcinogenic effects of tobacco are dose-dependent, with the risk of HNC closely related to the frequency, duration, and intensity of cigarette smoking (P_{trend}<.001 for each parameter).[13,14] Conversely, smoking cessation may reduce the risk of HNC, with evidence that risk of HNC decreases with increasing time since smoking cessation.[16,17]

Smokeless tobacco, such as snuff or chewing tobacco, is also an important HNC risk factor, in particular for cancers of the oral cavity.[18] There is an estimated 80% increase in risk of oral cavity cancer for individuals who have ever used smokeless tobacco,[19] with a fourfold increase in odds of HNC among individuals who have used smokeless tobacco for at least 10 years compared with never-users.[20] Although approximately 7% of oral cavity cancers in the United States are attributable to chewing tobacco, the attributable fraction is as high as 53% in India and 68% in Sudan, where the use of smokeless tobacco, including betel quid or areca nut with added tobacco, is popular.[19]

Alcohol
Alcohol use independently increases the risk of HNC, with an estimated 1% to 4% of cases attributable to alcohol alone[14,21] and a twofold increase in odds of HNC for drinkers who are never-users of tobacco.[22] In particular, alcohol use increases risk of hypopharyngeal cancer when compared with other sites.[23,24] However, the larger impact of alcohol is observed in the interaction of alcohol with tobacco use. The combined effects of alcohol and tobacco use have a greater than multiplicative impact in

Table 1
HPV-negative compared with HPV-positive head and neck cancer

Parameter	HPV-Negative	HPV-Positive
Gender	2–3-fold more common in men than women	4–5-fold more common in men than women
Age	Median age late 50s and 60s	Median age early-mid 50s, with increasing incidence among younger cohorts
Race	Worse prognosis in blacks	Higher incidence in whites
Smoking	>90% have smoking history; risk increases with increasing tobacco use	50%–65% have smoking history
Alcohol use	Synergistic with tobacco in increasing risk	Not a significant risk factor
Sexual history	Not a significant risk factor	Number of oral sex partners is a strong risk factor
Site	Larynx and oral cavity most common; others include oropharynx, hypopharynx, nasopharynx, nasal cavity and paranasal sinuses	Oropharynx, specifically lymphoid tissue of tonsils and tongue base; <20% HPV-positivity at other HNC sites
Presentation	Varies	Enlarged cervical lymph nodes common; also oropharyngeal pain, dysphagia, referred otalgia
Incidence trends	Decreasing	Increasing
Prognosis	All sites: 5-year survival 65%, 5-year recurrence 50% Oropharynx: 5-year survival 20%–25%, 5-year recurrence 50%	Oropharynx: 5-year survival 60%–90%, 5-year recurrence 10%–15%

Box 1
Risk factors for head and neck cancer

Major risk factors

   Tobacco use

   Alcohol

   Human papillomavirus

   Male gender

   Older age

   Betel quid

Other risk factors

   Premalignant lesions, including leukoplakia and erythroplakia

   Human immunodeficiency virus and/or immune suppression

   Diet, including poor nutrition, low folate

   Poor oral hygiene

   Occupational exposures, including wood dust, asbestos, others

   Epstein-Barr virus (nasopharynx; high incidence in Southeast Asia)

   Sun exposure

   Plummer-Vinson syndrome

   Fanconi anemia

   Li Fraumeni syndrome

   Dyskeratosis congenita

---

increasing the risk of cancer.[13,21,25] Among individuals who smoke two or more packs of cigarettes and also drink more than four alcoholic drinks per day, the risk of HNC is increased greater than 35-fold.[13]

Gender, age, and race

HNC overall is approximately twofold to threefold more common among men than women in the United States[26] and although this ratio varies by geographic region globally, men in most countries have a twofold to fivefold greater risk of HNC than women.[12] This difference is likely related to higher rates of substance abuse, particularly tobacco use, among men than women.[12,27] The risk of HNC also increases with age, with the median age of diagnosis for most anatomic sites in the late sixth and seventh decades of life.[26]

HNC incidence patterns by race have changed in the United States. Although the incidence of HNC has historically been higher among blacks than whites in the United States, HNC incidence among blacks has been declining since the 1990s and is currently lower than in whites (age-adjusted incidence rate of all HNCs is 14.8 per 100,000 for blacks compared with 15.5 per 100,000 for whites).[26] This change is in part explained by the rising incidence of HPV-HNC among whites in the United States, which has not been observed among blacks.[11,28]

Socioeconomic status

Indicators of low SES, such as low educational attainment and income, are strongly associated with increased risk of HNC globally.[29–31] In a recent pooled analysis of

23,964 HNC cases and 31,954 controls across 27 countries, the lowest socioeconomic stratum experienced more than twofold higher risk of HNC than the highest socioeconomic stratum (education: odds ratio [OR] 2.50, 95% confidence interval [CI] 2.02–3.09, and income: OR 2.44, 95% CI 1.62–3.67).[32] Although this risk was attenuated after adjustment for tobacco smoking and alcohol use, which are associated with low SES,[33,34] approximately one-third of the risk associated with low SES remained unexplained by known risk behaviors. Even among never-users of tobacco and never-drinkers, individuals with low education had significantly increased risk of HNC (OR 1.61, 95% CI 1.13–2.31).[32] These associations vary by country, with greater effect of SES observed in South and Central America than in North America and Europe.[32] Reasons for the increased risk of HNC associated with low SES are unclear, but may include occupational exposures,[29,30] psychosocial variables, and other unrecognized behavioral factors.[32]

Immune suppression

Immune suppression secondary to solid organ transplantation or HIV infection is associated with an increased risk of HNC. After solid organ transplantation, incidence of lip cancer increases by 10-fold or more, with more modest 2-fold to 5-fold increases at other head and neck sites.[35–38] HIV-infected patients are similarly at a twofold to five-fold increased risk for HNC, which has risen in the post-HAART (highly active antiretroviral therapy) era as patients survive longer and have the "opportunity" to develop non-AIDS–defining malignancies, including HNC.[39]

Risk Factors for Human Papillomavirus-Positive Head and Neck Cancer

Human papillomavirus

HPV is a sexually transmitted infection that causes HPV-positive HNC (HPV-HNC), a distinct subset of HNCs that occur primarily in the oropharynx and arise from the lymphoid tissues of the palatine and lingual tonsils.[40,41] The proportion of oropharyngeal cancers caused by HPV is growing, with current prevalence estimates in the United States near 80%.[4,8,9,11,42–46] In contrast, HPV is detected in fewer than 20% of tumors at other anatomic sites of the head and neck, with no apparent increase in prevalence over time.[45,47] Before widespread testing of oropharyngeal cancers for HPV, the oropharyngeal predominance of HPV-HNC allowed for early epidemiologic studies to use an oropharyngeal site as a surrogate for HPV-positive tumor status.[10]

Oral HPV infection is the putative precursor to HPV-HNC. Although there are more than 100 types of HPV, only a small number of these are considered high risk or carcinogenic.[48] One type, HPV16, is responsible for the vast majority (more than 90%) of HPV-HNCs.[49,50] In the United States, the prevalence of oral HPV infection of any type in the general population is approximately 7%, and the prevalence of oral HPV16 infection is 1%.[51] Although the natural history of progression from oral HPV infection to HPV-HNC is not well understood, it is clear that the vast majority of infections do not progress to cancer. The amount of time from first oral HPV infection to the development of cancer is unknown but is believed to be more than a decade.[52,53]

Although HPV is the clear cause of HPV-HNC, other risk factors influence odds of exposure to oral HPV, as well as persistence of HPV infection after it is acquired.

Sexual behaviors and head and neck cancer

Sexual behaviors are a proxy for exposure to oral HPV infection, and as such are strongly associated with odds of HPV-HNC.[7] In contrast, sexual behaviors are not associated with HPV-negative HNC, reflecting the distinct etiology of these 2 diseases.[4] As sexual behaviors are highly correlated, not only higher number of oral sex partners, but also other measures of sexual behavior, such as higher number of vaginal sex partners, younger age at sexual debut, and history of genital warts, have been associated with HPV-HNC.[4,7,50,54] Generational changes in sexual behavior, including the "sexual revolution" of the 1960s in the United States, are thought to have contributed to the increased incidence of HPV-HNC now observed.[55–58]

Oral HPV infection has likewise been associated with various measures of sexual exposure, including number of oral and vaginal sex partners, number of rimming partners, anogenital warts, herpes simplex virus-2 seropositivity, and possibly deep kissing.[51,59–65]

Although it is difficult to delineate which specific behaviors confer the greatest risk of oral HPV infection and HPV-HNC, oral sexual behaviors are believed to be the primary mode of transmission.

Tobacco

Individuals with HPV-HNC are significantly less likely than their HPV-negative counterparts to be smokers,[4] however tobacco exposure remains common among patients with HPV-HNC. Indeed, one-half to two-thirds of patients with HPV-HNC report a history of tobacco use.[4,8,9,66,67] Furthermore, tobacco smoking is associated with significantly higher oral HPV prevalence, and oral HPV16 prevalence increases in a dose-dependent fashion with higher measures of tobacco-smoking intensity.[68] In addition to being carcinogenic in its own right, tobacco smoking is hypothesized to increase either chances of oral HPV infection when exposed, or HPV persistence, or both, and therefore may increase risk of HPV-HNC.

Demographic risk factors

HPV-HNC patients are predominantly male (85%–90%) and white (92%–95%), with a median age of 50 to 56 years.[4,9,11,44,69,70] Compared with HPV-negative HNC, patients with HPV-HNC are more likely to be male and white, have higher SES, and be married (see **Table 1**).[4,11,70,71] The median age of patients with HPV-positive HNC is lower than that of patients with HPV-negative HNC by 4 to 10 years in most studies.[9,70,72–76] Furthermore, the incidence of HPV-HNC among younger individuals ages 36 to 44 years continues to increase.[77] Initial research suggests differences in HPV-HNC and oral HPV infection by gender, race, and age cohort are explained by patterns of oral sexual behaviors in these groups.[56,78]

Oropharyngeal cancer is nearly 5 times more common among men than women (age-adjusted incidence ratio 4.71, 95% CI 4.42–5.02), and oral HPV16 infection is 7 times more common among men than women in the United States (prevalence ratio 6.79, 95% CI 2.07–22.26).[56] These gender differences are not entirely explained by differences in measures of oral sexual behavior, and may be due to higher risk of oral HPV infection when performing oral sex on a woman than a man.[78]

The proportion of oropharyngeal cancers caused by HPV is higher among whites than blacks. This racial discrepancy may be explained both by a higher rate of tobacco use and thus tobacco-related oropharyngeal cancer among blacks, as well as differences in oral sexual behavior patterns by race.[56] For example, whites are more likely to perform oral sex, and to do so at a younger age, than blacks.[56,79]

TRENDS IN HEAD AND NECK CANCER INCIDENCE
Head and Neck Cancer Incidence in the United States and Globally

Although HNC as whole is the seventh most common cancer worldwide,[1] the incidence varies considerably by anatomic tumor site (**Table 2**) and geographic region.[12]

Table 2
Incidence and mortality rates for head and neck cancers by site, United States and worldwide

Site	Incidence: Age-Adjusted Standardized Incidence Rate per 100,000	Mortality: Age-Adjusted Standardized Death Rate per 100,000	5-year Survival,[a] %
United States			
Larynx	3.3	1.1	60.0
Tongue	3.2	0.6	62.7
Tonsil	1.8	0.2	70.8
Lip	0.7	0.0	89.5
Gum and other oral cavity	1.5	0.4	59.7
Nasopharynx	0.7	0.2	59.2
Floor of mouth	0.6	0.0	51.4
Hypopharynx	0.6	0.1	31.9
Oropharynx	0.4	0.2	41.7
Other oral cavity and pharynx	0.2	0.5	35.4
Worldwide			
Lip and oral cavity	3.9	1.9	
Larynx	2.3	1.2	
Other pharynx	2.0	1.4	
Nasopharynx	1.2	0.8	

[a] Five-year relative survival. Only available for US statistics.
Data from Ferlay J, Shin HR, Bray F, et al. Estimates of worldwide burden of cancer in 2008: GLOBOCAN 2008. Int J Cancer 2010;127(12):2893–917; and Howlander N, Noone AM, Krapcho M, et al. SEER Cancer Statistics Review (CSR) 1975–2011. Bethesda (MD): National Cancer Institute; 2014.

Oral cavity and laryngeal SCC are the most common HNCs worldwide (age-adjusted standardized incidence rate [SIR] 3.9 per 100,000 and 2.3 per 100,000, respectively), with nasopharynx and other pharynx cancers less common (SIR 1.2 and 2.0 per 100,000, respectively).[1] Notably, currently available HNC incidence statistics are limited by inconsistencies in categorization by site, with broad and/or ill-defined categories used in many cancer registries. Many registries do not currently categorize by sites that would be useful in distinguishing HPV-positive compared with HPV-negative disease (eg, oropharynx compared with nonoropharynx). Therefore, interpretation of incidence and mortality rates must be approached with caution.

HNC incidence trends over time and across countries are strongly influenced by patterns of tobacco use.[80] As a general rule, tobacco use in most countries rises first among men, followed by an increase in smoking among women.[27] In the United States, tobacco use prevalence peaked in the 1940s to 1960s, first in men and then in women, before declining after the 1964 Surgeon General's report identifying tobacco as a causative agent in lung cancer. Because of a concerted public health effort, from 1965 to 2011 smoking prevalence declined from 51.9% to 19.0% among men, and from 33.9% to 17.3% among women.[81] The impact of these trends on HNC incidence became clear when, after years of increasing numbers of HNCs per year, the incidence rate for HNCs overall and those that are particularly tied to tobacco began a slow decline in the 1990s.[80] For example, the age-adjusted annual percentage change from 1992 to 2005 was −1.4 for oral cavity and pharynx cancer, and from 1992 to 2009 was −2.8 for larynx cancer.[82]

Although tobacco use has declined in the United States, global patterns of tobacco use are more heterogeneous. Several economically developed countries, such as Canada and Australia, have observed decreased smoking prevalence rates over the past several decades, similar to the United States, first among men and then among women, and are experiencing significant decreases in HNC incidence.[12,80,83] However, other countries, including many that are less economically developed, appear to be in earlier stages of the tobacco epidemic, with high smoking prevalence rates that have not yet substantially decreased.[27,84] For example, Eastern Europe has some of the highest cigarette consumption rates in the world among both men and women,[85] and in many Eastern European countries, HNC incidence is on the rise.[12,86,87] In China, smoking prevalence among men is greater than 50%, and smoking prevalence in Thailand is 40% to 50%, whereas prevalence among women in these countries is at least 10 times lower than among men[27,85,88]; a dramatic rise in HNC has not yet been observed in these countries but may be anticipated, along with a rise in other tobacco-related diseases.[12,85,89–91]

Risk for HPV-negative HNC is not limited to tobacco smoking, reflected by a variety of incidence trends in different countries and for different anatomic sites that do not follow smoking prevalence patterns.[12] For example, France has much higher incidence of HNC among men than neighboring countries, which has been attributed to patterns of combined cigarette and alcohol use.[12,87] The United Kingdom has had falling smoking prevalence rates among both men and women[27]; however, oral cavity incidence rates are significantly rising in the United Kingdom in all age groups. It is unclear whether this increase may be explained by trends in nutrition and socioeconomic factors.[87,89,92] In the United States, although oral cavity cancers as a whole are decreasing in incidence, oral tongue cancers are increasing in a specific subset of the population, that is, young white women ages 18 to 44.[93] Many of these individuals are also never-smokers and never-drinkers.[94] The cause of this trend remains unknown, and no viral etiology has been described.[95]

Increasing Incidence of Human Papillomavirus-Positive Head and Neck Cancers

In contrast with decreases in incidence of HPV-negative HNC, which is primarily tobacco-related, the incidence of HPV-HNC has risen dramatically in the United States since the 1970s, primarily oropharyngeal cancer among early middle-aged white men.[10,77,80] Analysis of the Surveillance, Epidemiology and End Results database and tissue repository demonstrated a 225% increase in HPV-positive oropharyngeal cancer incidence from 0.8 per 100,000 in 1988 to 1990, to 2.6 per 100,000 in 2003 to 2004, compared with a 50% decrease in HPV-negative oropharyngeal cancer incidence from 2.0 to 1.0 per 100,000 in the same time period.[11] Concurrently, the proportion of oropharyngeal cancers attributable to HPV rose from 16% in the 1980s to near 80% in the past decade.[4,8,9,11,42–45,69] HPV-HNC incidence is now expected to exceed cervical cancer incidence by 2020.

Several other developed countries have observed a similar rise in HPV-related HNCs in men. The incidence of oropharyngeal cancer significantly increased among men from 1983 to 2002 in Australia, Canada, and Slovakia despite stable or decreasing rates of oral cavity cancers.[89] As in the United States, this increase was primarily among men younger than 60 years.[89] In Sweden, there was a 2.8-fold increase in the incidence of tonsil cancer from 1970 to 2002, with a parallel rise in proportion of HPV-positive cases from 23.3% to 68.0%.[96] In Europe overall, the estimated prevalence of HPV in HNC has increased from 35% before 2000 to 73% after 2005 ($P = .004$).[45] Similar trends have not yet been observed in low-income countries.

PROGNOSIS

Survival after HNC is predicted primarily by anatomic site, stage, and HPV status, with other pathologic and clinical factors influencing prognosis to a lesser degree. The American Joint Committee on Cancer (AJCC) staging system for each tumor site is the primary parameter used to predict prognosis and guide treatment.[97] This system incorporates information about tumor size, cervical lymph node metastases, and distant metastases.[98] Overall, 5-year survival after a diagnosis of HNC in the United States is approximately 65.0%,[99] with a range of 31.9% for hypopharyngeal cancer to 89.5% for lip cancer (see **Table 2**).[26] Five-year survival has significantly increased for all sites over the past 20 years from 54.7% in 1992 to 1996, to 65.9% in 2002 to 2006.[99] This survival improvement is largest for tonsil cancer, where 5-year survival increased from 39.7% to 69.8%.[99] Increasing survival has been attributed to advances in treatment, and for HPV-related subsites to the remarkable improvement in survival conferred by HPV-positive tumor status.[8,11,99]

Human Papillomavirus-Positive Tumor Status Improves Prognosis

In addition to stage, HPV tumor status is increasingly a critical determinant of prognosis for oropharyngeal cancer, and is indeed the strongest independent prognostic factor for oropharyngeal cancer.[100,101] Individuals with HPV-positive oropharyngeal cancer have better response to treatment, and both overall survival and disease-specific survival are improved by greater than 50% even after adjustment for the younger age and fewer comorbidities among HPV-positive patients.[8,9,11,69,102–104] However, the favorable prognosis conferred by HPV-positive tumor status is tempered by tobacco smoking, so that patients with HPV-positive oropharyngeal cancer who smoke have an intermediate prognosis.[9] Multiple clinical trials are under way to determine the potential for risk stratification by HPV tumor status and tobacco use when selecting treatment regimens.[104] Although a small subset of nonoropharyngeal HNCs are HPV-positive, the clinical significance of HPV tumor status at these sites, if any, remains unknown.[105]

Pathologic and Clinical Determinants of Survival

Several pathologic characteristics are considered prognostic indicators for HNC but not currently included in AJCC staging. Extracapsular spread of cervical lymph node metastases is associated with a 50% reduction in survival among patients with lymph node metastases[106] and is an important component in planning for adjuvant treatment after primary surgery.[107] Microscopic disease at surgical margins and perineural invasion both are associated with worse prognosis.[108–110] Specific molecular alterations, such as TP53 disruptive mutation and EGFR overexpression, are unfavorable prognostic features but are not at present routinely evaluated in practice.[111–113]

Numerous clinical parameters modify prognosis for patients with HNC. Advanced age and comorbidity are associated with decreased survival.[114–116] Tobacco use before, during, and after treatment for HNC has been associated with decreased overall survival and progression-free survival, worse response to treatment, and increased risk of second primary malignancy.[117–121] Finally, race and SES are associated with prognosis.[122] In the United States, blacks with HNC have double the mortality of whites.[28,122,123] Although this is in part explained by the higher incidence of

HPV-HNC among whites than blacks,[28,122] initial studies suggest that even when limiting to HPV-positive oropharyngeal cancer, there may still be better survival among whites compared with blacks.[124] Poverty also has been associated with an increased risk of death that is not entirely explained by demographics or comorbidities.[123]

Disease Recurrence and Second Primary Malignancies

There is a high rate of second primary, recurrent, and synchronous tumors of the upper aerodigestive tract (head and neck region and lungs) in patients with HNC, which may be related to the molecular mechanisms of tobacco-induced and alcohol-induced carcinogenesis. Tobacco use results in what is known as "field cancerization," with widespread genetic alterations throughout the upper aerodigestive mucosa despite the absence of gross malignancy. Even after excision of a primary cancer, surrounding tissue may harbor malignant or premalignant clones with similar tobacco-induced molecular alterations, leading to increased risk of recurrent or second primary cancers.[125] Approximately 50% of patients with locally advanced HNC will develop a recurrence, often within two years after treatment.[126] Synchronous tumors of the head and neck are found in 2% to 10% of patients with HNC.[127–129] The 20-year cumulative risk of a second primary malignancy after HNC is as high as 36%,[130] and smokers have a fourfold increase in risk of a second aerodigestive cancer compared with non-smokers and former smokers.[131]

Of note, the risk of disease recurrence is lower for HPV-positive compared with HPV-negative oropharyngeal cancer (local-regional recurrence 13.6% compared with 35.1% at 3 years, $P<.001$), as is the risk of second primary malignancy (5.9% compared with 14.6% at 3 years, $P = .02$).[9] These patterns may be secondary to a lack of analogous "field cancerization" in HPV-HNC.[132] Even when HPV-HNC disease progression does occur, HPV-positive tumor status still confers improved prognosis compared with HPV-negative disease (overall survival 54.6% compared with 27.6% at 2 years, $P<.001$).[133]

SUMMARY

HNC is a heterogeneous disease that is caused primarily by tobacco use and HPV. Although the incidence of tobacco-related HNC is decreasing in the United States, following a decline in tobacco-smoking prevalence, the incidence of HPV-HNC is rising rapidly. HPV-HNC is mostly observed in middle-aged white men, which may be explained by patterns of oral sexual behavior in this demographic and age cohort. HNC incidence trends vary considerably by country and by patterns of tobacco use. Although some developed countries are observing decreasing tobacco-related HNC and increasing HPV-HNC incidence, like in the United States, many other countries are experiencing increasing or stable tobacco-related HNC rates without evidence of an HPV-HNC epidemic. HNC prognosis is determined by anatomic site and stage, with HPV-positive tumor status conferring significantly improved survival.

REFERENCES

1. Ferlay J, Shin HR, Bray F, et al. Estimates of worldwide burden of cancer in 2008: GLOBOCAN 2008. Int J Cancer 2010;127(12):2893–917.
2. Howlander N, Noone AM, Krapcho M, et al. SEER cancer statistics review (CSR) 1975-2011. Bethesda (MD): National Cancer Institute; 2014.
3. Licitra L, Locati LD, Bossi P, et al. Head and neck tumors other than squamous cell carcinoma. Curr Opin Oncol 2004;16(3):236–41.

4. Gillison ML, D'Souza G, Westra W, et al. Distinct risk factor profiles for human papillomavirus type 16-positive and human papillomavirus type 16-negative head and neck cancers. J Natl Cancer Inst 2008;100(6):407–20.

5. Agrawal N, Frederick MJ, Pickering CR, et al. Exome sequencing of head and neck squamous cell carcinoma reveals inactivating mutations in NOTCH1. Science 2011;333(6046):1154–7.

6. Stransky N, Egloff AM, Tward AD, et al. The mutational landscape of head and neck squamous cell carcinoma. Science 2011;333(6046):1157–60.

7. D'Souza G, Kreimer AR, Viscidi R, et al. Case-control study of human papillomavirus and oropharyngeal cancer. N Engl J Med 2007;356:1944–56.

8. Fakhry C, Westra WH, Li S, et al. Improved survival of patients with human papillomavirus-positive head and neck squamous cell carcinoma in a prospective clinical trial. J Natl Cancer Inst 2008;100(4):261–9.

9. Ang KK, Harris J, Wheeler R, et al. Human papillomavirus and survival of patients with oropharyngeal cancer. N Engl J Med 2010;363(1):24–35.

10. Chaturvedi AK, Engels EA, Anderson WF, et al. Incidence trends for human papillomavirus-related and -unrelated oral squamous cell carcinomas in the United States. J Clin Oncol 2008;26(4):612–9.

11. Chaturvedi AK, Engels EA, Pfeiffer RM, et al. Human papillomavirus and rising oropharyngeal cancer incidence in the United States. J Clin Oncol 2011;29(32): 4294–301.

12. Simard EP, Torre LA, Jemal A. International trends in head and neck cancer incidence rates: differences by country, sex and anatomic site. Oral Oncol 2014; 50(5):387–403.

13. Blot WJ, McLaughlin JK, Winn DM, et al. Smoking and drinking in relation to oral and pharyngeal cancer. Cancer Res 1988;48(11):3282–7.

14. Hashibe M, Brennan P, Benhamou S, et al. Alcohol drinking in never users of tobacco, cigarette smoking in never drinkers, and the risk of head and neck cancer: pooled analysis in the International Head and Neck Cancer Epidemiology Consortium. J Natl Cancer Inst 2007;99(10):777–89.

15. Vineis P, Alavanja M, Buffler P, et al. Tobacco and cancer: recent epidemiological evidence. J Natl Cancer Inst 2004;96(2):99–106.

16. Franceschi S, Talamini R, Barra S, et al. Smoking and drinking in relation to cancers of the oral cavity, pharynx, larynx, and esophagus in northern Italy. Cancer Res 1990;50(20):6502–7.

17. Schlecht NF, Franco EL, Pintos J, et al. Effect of smoking cessation and tobacco type on the risk of cancers of the upper aero-digestive tract in Brazil. Epidemiology 1999;10(4):412–8.

18. Secretan B, Straif K, Baan R, et al. A review of human carcinogens–Part E: tobacco, areca nut, alcohol, coal smoke, and salted fish. Lancet Oncol 2009; 10(11):1033–4.

19. Boffetta P, Hecht S, Gray N, et al. Smokeless tobacco and cancer. Lancet Oncol 2008;9(7):667–75.

20. Zhou J, Michaud DS, Langevin SM, et al. Smokeless tobacco and risk of head and neck cancer: evidence from a case-control study in New England. Int J Cancer 2013;132:1911–7.

21. Anantharaman D, Marron M, Lagiou P, et al. Population attributable risk of tobacco and alcohol for upper aerodigestive tract cancer. Oral Oncol 2011;47(8):725–31.

22. Hashibe M, Boffetta P, Zaridze D, et al. Contribution of tobacco and alcohol to the high rates of squamous cell carcinoma of the supraglottis and glottis in Central Europe. Am J Epidemiol 2007;165(7):814–20.

23. Brugere J, Guenel P, Leclerc A, et al. Differential effects of tobacco and alcohol in cancer of the larynx, pharynx, and mouth. Cancer 1986;57(2):391–5.

24. Menvielle G, Luce D, Goldberg P, et al. Smoking, alcohol drinking and cancer risk for various sites of the larynx and hypopharynx. A case-control study in France. Eur J Cancer Prev 2004;13(3):165–72.

25. Hashibe M, Brennan P, Chuang SC, et al. Interaction between tobacco and alcohol use and the risk of head and neck cancer: pooled analysis in the International Head and Neck Cancer Epidemiology Consortium. Cancer Epidemiol Biomarkers Prev 2009;18(2):541–50.

26. Howlader N, Noone AM, Krapcho M, et al. SEER cancer statistics review, 1975-2011. 2014; based on November 2013 SEER data submission, posted to the SEER web site, April 2014. Available at: http://seer.cancer.gov/csr/1975_2011/. Accessed October 15, 2014.

27. Thun M, Peto R, Boreham J, et al. Stages of the cigarette epidemic on entering its second century. Tob Control 2012;21(2):96–101.

28. Settle K, Posner MR, Schumaker LM, et al. Racial survival disparity in head and neck cancer results from low prevalence of human papillomavirus infection in black oropharyngeal cancer patients. Canc Prev Res 2009;2(9):776–81.

29. Boing AF, Antunes JL, de Carvalho MB, et al. How much do smoking and alcohol consumption explain socioeconomic inequalities in head and neck cancer risk? J Epidemiol Community Health 2011;65(8):709–14.

30. Menvielle G, Luce D, Goldberg P, et al. Smoking, alcohol drinking, occupational exposures and social inequalities in hypopharyngeal and laryngeal cancer. Int J Epidemiol 2004;33(4):799–806.

31. Hwang E, Johnson-Obaseki S, McDonald JT, et al. Incidence of head and neck cancer and socioeconomic status in Canada from 1992 to 2007. Oral Oncol 2013;49(11):1072–6.

32. Conway DI, Brenner DR, McMahon AD, et al. Estimating and explaining the effect of education and income on head and neck cancer risk: INHANCE consortium pooled analysis of 31 case-control studies from 27 countries. Int J Cancer 2014;36:1125–39.

33. Cavelaars AE, Kunst AE, Geurts JJ, et al. Educational differences in smoking: international comparison. BMJ 2000;320(7242):1102–7.

34. Agaku I, King B, Dube SR, Office on Smoking and Health, National Center for Chronic Disease Prevention and Health Promotion, CDC. Current cigarette smoking among adults - United States, 2011. MMWR Morb Mortal Wkly Rep 2012;61(44):889–94.

35. Grulich AE, van Leeuwen MT, Falster MO, et al. Incidence of cancers in people with HIV/AIDS compared with immunosuppressed transplant recipients: a meta-analysis. Lancet 2007;370(9581):59–67.

36. Adami J, Gabel H, Lindelof B, et al. Cancer risk following organ transplantation: a nationwide cohort study in Sweden. Br J Canc 2003;89(7):1221–7.

37. Jensen P, Hansen S, Moller B, et al. Skin cancer in kidney and heart transplant recipients and different long-term immunosuppressive therapy regimens. J Am Acad Dermatol 1999;40(2 Pt 1):177–86.

38. Piselli P, Serraino D, Segoloni GP, et al. Risk of de novo cancers after transplantation: results from a cohort of 7217 kidney transplant recipients, Italy 1997-2009. Eur J Canc 2013;49(2):336–44.

39. Long JL, Engels EA, Moore RD, et al. Incidence and outcomes of malignancy in the HAART era in an urban cohort of HIV-infected individuals. AIDS 2008;22(4):489–96.

40. Begum S, Cao D, Gillison M, et al. Tissue distribution of human papillomavirus 16 DNA integration in patients with tonsillar carcinoma. Clin Cancer Res 2005; 11(16):5694–9.
41. Gillison ML, Koch WM, Capone RB, et al. Evidence for a causal association between human papillomavirus and a subset of head and neck cancers. J Natl Cancer Inst 2000;92(9):709–20.
42. Lin BM, Wang H, D'Souza G, et al. Long-term prognosis and risk factors among patients with HPV-associated oropharyngeal squamous cell carcinoma. Cancer 2013;119:3462–71.
43. Weinberger PM, Yu Z, Haffty BG, et al. Molecular classification identifies a subset of human papillomavirus–associated oropharyngeal cancers with favorable prognosis. J Clin Oncol 2006;24(5):736–47.
44. Lewis JS Jr, Thorstad WL, Chernock RD, et al. p16 positive oropharyngeal squamous cell carcinoma: an entity with a favorable prognosis regardless of tumor HPV status. Am J Surg Pathol 2010;34(8):1088–96.
45. Mehanna H, Beech T, Nicholson T, et al. Prevalence of human papillomavirus in oropharyngeal and nonoropharyngeal head and neck cancer—systematic review and meta-analysis of trends by time and region. Head Neck 2012;35:747–55.
46. Park K, Cho KJ, Lee M, et al. p16 immunohistochemistry alone is a better prognosticator in tonsil cancer than human papillomavirus in situ hybridization with or without p16 immunohistochemistry. Acta Otolaryngol 2013;133(3):297–304.
47. Lingen MW, Xiao W, Schmitt A, et al. Low etiologic fraction for high-risk human papillomavirus in oral cavity squamous cell carcinomas. Oral Oncol 2013;49(1): 1–8.
48. Tota JE, Chevarie-Davis M, Richardson LA, et al. Epidemiology and burden of HPV infection and related diseases: implications for prevention strategies. Prev Med 2011;53(Suppl 1):S12–21.
49. Herrero R, Castellsague X, Pawlita M, et al. Human papillomavirus and oral cancer: the International Agency for Research on Cancer multicenter study. J Natl Cancer Inst 2003;95(23):1772–83.
50. Gillison ML, Alemany L, Snijders PJ, et al. Human papillomavirus and diseases of the upper airway: head and neck cancer and respiratory papillomatosis. Vaccine 2012;30(Suppl 5):F34–54.
51. Gillison ML, Broutian T, Pickard RK, et al. Prevalence of oral HPV infection in the United States, 2009-2010. JAMA 2012;307(7):693–703.
52. Mork J, Lie AK, Glattre E, et al. Human papillomavirus infection as a risk factor for squamous-cell carcinoma of the head and neck. N Engl J Med 2001;344(15): 1125–31.
53. Kreimer AR, Johansson M, Waterboer T, et al. Evaluation of human papillomavirus antibodies and risk of subsequent head and neck cancer. J Clin Oncol 2013;31(21):2708–15.
54. Schwartz SM, Daling JR, Doody DR, et al. Oral cancer risk in relation to sexual history and evidence of human papillomavirus infection. J Natl Cancer Inst 1998;90(21):1626–36.
55. Bajos N, Bozon M, Beltzer N, et al. Changes in sexual behaviours: from secular trends to public health policies. AIDS 2010;24(8):1185–91.
56. D'Souza G, Cullen K, Bowie J, et al. Differences in oral sexual behaviors by gender, age, and race explain observed differences in prevalence of oral human papillomavirus infection. PLoS One 2014;9:e86023.
57. Turner CF, Danella RD, Rogers SM. Sexual behavior in the United States 1930-1990: trends and methodological problems. Sex Transm Dis 1995;22(3):173–90.

58. Schmidt G, Sigusch V. Changes in sexual behavior among young males and females between 1960-1970. Arch Sex Behav 1972;2(1):27–45.
59. Pickard RK, Xiao W, Broutian TR, et al. The prevalence and incidence of oral human papillomavirus infection among young men and women, aged 18-30 years. Sex Transm Dis 2012;39(7):559–66.
60. Beachler DC, Weber KM, Margolick JB, et al. Risk factors for oral HPV infection among a high prevalence population of HIV-positive and at-risk HIV-negative adults. Cancer Epidemiol Biomarkers Prev 2012;21(1):122–33.
61. Read TR, Hocking JS, Vodstrcil LA, et al. Oral human papillomavirus in men having sex with men: risk-factors and sampling. PLoS One 2012;7:e49324.
62. D'Souza G, Agrawal Y, Halpern J, et al. Oral sexual behaviors associated with prevalent oral human papillomavirus infection. J Infect Dis 2009;199(9): 1263–9.
63. Lang Kuhs KA, Gonzalez P, Struijk L, et al. Prevalence of and risk factors for oral human papillomavirus among young women in Costa Rica. J Infect Dis 2013; 208(10):1643–52.
64. Kreimer AR, Alberg AJ, Daniel R, et al. Oral human papillomavirus infection in adults is associated with sexual behavior and HIV serostatus. J Infect Dis 2004;189(4):686–98.
65. Videla S, Darwich L, Canadas MP, et al. Natural history of human papillomavirus infections involving anal, penile, and oral sites among HIV-positive men. Sex Transm Dis 2013;40(1):3–10.
66. Hafkamp HC, Manni JJ, Haesevoets A, et al. Marked differences in survival rate between smokers and nonsmokers with HPV 16-associated tonsillar carcinomas. Int J Cancer 2008;122(12):2656–64.
67. D'Souza G, Gross ND, Pai SI, et al. Oral human papillomavirus (HPV) infection in HPV-positive patients with oropharyngeal cancer and their partners. J Clin Oncol 2014;32:2408–15.
68. Fakhry C, Gillison ML, D'Souza G. Tobacco use and oral HPV-16 infection. JAMA 2014;312(14):1465–7.
69. Rischin D, Young RJ, Fisher R, et al. Prognostic significance of p16INK4A and human papillomavirus in patients with oropharyngeal cancer treated on TROG 02.02 phase III trial. J Clin Oncol 2010;28(27):4142–8.
70. Schwartz SR, Yueh B, McDougall JK, et al. Human papillomavirus infection and survival in oral squamous cell cancer: a population-based study. Otolaryngol Head Neck Surg 2001;125(1):1–9.
71. Sethi S, Ali-Fehmi R, Franceschi S, et al. Characteristics and survival of head and neck cancer by HPV status: a cancer registry-based study. Int J Cancer 2012;131(5):1179–86.
72. Mellin H, Friesland S, Lewensohn R, et al. Human papillomavirus (HPV) DNA in tonsillar cancer: clinical correlates, risk of relapse, and survival. Int J Cancer 2000;89(3):300–4.
73. De Petrini M, Ritta M, Schena M, et al. Head and neck squamous cell carcinoma: role of the human papillomavirus in tumour progression. New Microbiol 2006;29(1):25–33.
74. Kumar B, Cordell KG, Lee JS, et al. EGFR, p16, HPV Titer, Bcl-xL and p53, sex, and smoking as indicators of response to therapy and survival in oropharyngeal cancer. J Clin Oncol 2008;26(19):3128–37.
75. Worden FP, Kumar B, Lee JS, et al. Chemoselection as a strategy for organ preservation in advanced oropharynx cancer: response and survival positively associated with HPV16 copy number. J Clin Oncol 2008;26(19):3138–46.

76. Heath S, Willis V, Allan K, et al. Clinically significant human papilloma virus in squamous cell carcinoma of the head and neck in UK practice. Clin Oncol 2012;24(1):e18–23.
77. Gayar OH, Ruterbusch JJ, Elshaikh M, et al. Oropharyngeal carcinoma in young adults: an alarming national trend. Otolaryngol Head Neck Surg 2014;150(4): 594–601.
78. D'Souza G, Kluz N, Wentz A, et al. Oral human papillomavirus (HPV) infection among unvaccinated high-risk young adults. Cancers 2014;6(3):1691–704.
79. Leichliter JS, Chandra A, Liddon N, et al. Prevalence and correlates of heterosexual anal and oral sex in adolescents and adults in the United States. J Infect Dis 2007;196:1852–9.
80. Sturgis EM, Cinciripini PM. Trends in head and neck cancer incidence in relation to smoking prevalence: an emerging epidemic of human papillomavirus-associated cancers? Cancer 2007;110(7):1429–35.
81. U.S. Department of Health and Human Services. The Health Consequences of Smoking: 50 Years of Progress. A Report of the Surgeon General. Atlanta (GA): U.S. Department of Health and Human Services, Centers for Disease Control and Prevention, National Center for Chronic Disease Prevention and Health Promotion, Office on Smoking and Health; 2014.
82. Jemal A, Simard EP, Dorell C, et al. Annual Report to the Nation on the Status of Cancer, 1975-2009, featuring the burden and trends in human papillomavirus(HPV)-associated cancers and HPV vaccination coverage levels. J Natl Cancer Inst 2013;105(3):175–201.
83. Forte T, Niu J, Lockwood GA, et al. Incidence trends in head and neck cancers and human papillomavirus (HPV)-associated oropharyngeal cancer in Canada, 1992-2009. Cancer Causes Control 2012;23(8):1343–8.
84. Mayor S. Tobacco atlas illustrates shift to low income countries. BMJ 2009;338: b981.
85. Eriksen MP, Mackay J, Ross H, et al. The tobacco atlas. 4th ed. Completely revised and updated. ed. Atlanta (GA): American Cancer Society; 2012.
86. Dobrossy L. Epidemiology of head and neck cancer: magnitude of the problem. Cancer Metastasis Rev 2005;24(1):9–17.
87. Warnakulasuriya S. Global epidemiology of oral and oropharyngeal cancer. Oral Oncol 2009;45(4–5):309–16.
88. Samet JM. Tobacco smoking: the leading cause of preventable disease worldwide. Thorac Surg Clin 2013;23(2):103–12.
89. Chaturvedi AK, Anderson WF, Lortet-Tieulent J, et al. Worldwide trends in incidence rates for oral cavity and oropharyngeal cancers. J Clin Oncol 2013; 31(36):4550–9.
90. McCormack VA, Boffetta P. Today's lifestyles, tomorrow's cancers: trends in lifestyle risk factors for cancer in low- and middle-income countries. Ann Oncol 2011;22(11):2349–57.
91. Danaei G, Vander Hoorn S, Lopez AD, et al. Causes of cancer in the world: comparative risk assessment of nine behavioural and environmental risk factors. Lancet 2005;366(9499):1784–93.
92. Conway DI, Stockton DL, Warnakulasuriya KA, et al. Incidence of oral and oropharyngeal cancer in United Kingdom (1990-1999)–recent trends and regional variation. Oral Oncol 2006;42(6):586–92.
93. Patel SC, Carpenter WR, Tyree S, et al. Increasing incidence of oral tongue squamous cell carcinoma in young white women, age 18 to 44 years. J Clin Oncol 2011;29(11):1488–94.

94. Koch WM, Lango M, Sewell D, et al. Head and neck cancer in nonsmokers: a distinct clinical and molecular entity. Laryngoscope 1999;109(10):1544–51.
95. Li R, Faden DL, Fakhry C, et al. Clinical, genomic, and metagenomic characterization of oral tongue squamous cell carcinoma in patients who do not smoke. Head Neck 2014. [Epub ahead of print].
96. Hammarstedt L, Lindquist D, Dahlstrand H, et al. Human papillomavirus as a risk factor for the increase in incidence of tonsillar cancer. Int J Cancer 2006; 119(11):2620–3.
97. Edge SB, American Joint Committee on Cancer. AJCC cancer staging manual. 7th edition. New York: Springer; 2010.
98. Pfister DG, Ang K, Brockstein B, et al. NCCN practice guidelines for head and neck cancers. Oncology 2000;14(11A):163–94.
99. Pulte D, Brenner H. Changes in survival in head and neck cancers in the late 20th and early 21st century: a period analysis. Oncologist 2010;15(9):994–1001.
100. Straetmans JM, Olthof N, Mooren JJ, et al. Human papillomavirus reduces the prognostic value of nodal involvement in tonsillar squamous cell carcinomas. Laryngoscope 2009;119(10):1951–7.
101. Fischer CA, Kampmann M, Zlobec I, et al. p16 expression in oropharyngeal cancer: its impact on staging and prognosis compared with the conventional clinical staging parameters. Ann Oncol 2010;21(10):1961–6.
102. O'Rorke MA, Ellison MV, Murray LJ, et al. Human papillomavirus related head and neck cancer survival: a systematic review and meta-analysis. Oral Oncol 2012;48(12):1191–201.
103. Posner MR, Lorch JH, Goloubeva O, et al. Survival and human papillomavirus in oropharynx cancer in TAX 324: a subset analysis from an international phase III trial. Ann Oncol 2011;22(5):1071–7.
104. Masterson L, Moualed D, Liu ZW, et al. De-escalation treatment protocols for human papillomavirus-associated oropharyngeal squamous cell carcinoma: a systematic review and meta-analysis of current clinical trials. Eur J Canc 2014; 50(15):2636–48.
105. Isayeva T, Li Y, Maswahu D, et al. Human papillomavirus in non-oropharyngeal head and neck cancers: a systematic literature review. Head Neck Pathol 2012; 6(Suppl 1):S104–20.
106. Johnson JT, Myers EN, Bedetti CD, et al. Cervical lymph node metastases. Incidence and implications of extracapsular carcinoma. Arch Otolaryngol 1985; 111(8):534–7.
107. Bernier J, Cooper JS, Pajak TF, et al. Defining risk levels in locally advanced head and neck cancers: a comparative analysis of concurrent postoperative radiation plus chemotherapy trials of the EORTC (#22931) and RTOG (# 9501). Head Neck 2005;27(10):843–50.
108. Soo KC, Carter RL, O'Brien CJ, et al. Prognostic implications of perineural spread in squamous carcinomas of the head and neck. Laryngoscope 1986; 96(10):1145–8.
109. Ravasz LA, Slootweg PJ, Hordijk GJ, et al. The status of the resection margin as a prognostic factor in the treatment of head and neck carcinoma. J Craniomaxillofac Surg 1991;19(7):314–8.
110. Spiro RH, Guillamondegui O Jr, Paulino AF, et al. Pattern of invasion and margin assessment in patients with oral tongue cancer. Head Neck 1999;21(5):408–13.
111. Skinner HD, Sandulache VC, Ow TJ, et al. TP53 disruptive mutations lead to head and neck cancer treatment failure through inhibition of radiation-induced senescence. Clin Cancer Res 2012;18(1):290–300.

112. Koch WM, Brennan JA, Zahurak M, et al. p53 mutation and locoregional treatment failure in head and neck squamous cell carcinoma. J Natl Cancer Inst 1996;88(21):1580–6.

113. Ang KK, Berkey BA, Tu X, et al. Impact of epidermal growth factor receptor expression on survival and pattern of relapse in patients with advanced head and neck carcinoma. Cancer Res 2002;62(24):7350–6.

114. Bourhis J, Overgaard J, Audry H, et al. Hyperfractionated or accelerated radiotherapy in head and neck cancer: a meta-analysis. Lancet 2006;368(9538): 843–54.

115. Pignon JP, le Maitre A, Maillard E, et al. Meta-analysis of chemotherapy in head and neck cancer (MACH-NC): an update on 93 randomised trials and 17,346 patients. Radiother Oncol 2009;92(1):4–14.

116. Paleri V, Wight RG, Silver CE, et al. Comorbidity in head and neck cancer: a critical appraisal and recommendations for practice. Oral Oncol 2010;46(10): 712–9.

117. Gillison ML, Zhang Q, Jordan R, et al. Tobacco smoking and increased risk of death and progression for patients with p16-positive and p16-negative oropharyngeal cancer. J Clin Oncol 2012;30:2102–11.

118. Browman GP, Mohide EA, Willan A, et al. Association between smoking during radiotherapy and prognosis in head and neck cancer: a follow-up study. Head Neck 2002;24(12):1031–7.

119. Browman GP, Wong G, Hodson I, et al. Influence of cigarette smoking on the efficacy of radiation therapy in head and neck cancer. N Engl J Med 1993;328(3): 159–63.

120. Chen AM, Chen LM, Vaughan A, et al. Head and neck cancer among lifelong never-smokers and ever-smokers: matched-pair analysis of outcomes after radiation therapy. Am J Clin Oncol 2011;34(3):270–5.

121. Do KA, Johnson MM, Doherty DA, et al. Second primary tumors in patients with upper aerodigestive tract cancers: joint effects of smoking and alcohol (United States). Cancer Causes Control 2003;14(2):131–8.

122. Schrank TP, Han Y, Weiss H, et al. Case-matching analysis of head and neck squamous cell carcinoma in racial and ethnic minorities in the United States–possible role for human papillomavirus in survival disparities. Head Neck 2011;33(1):45–53.

123. Molina MA, Cheung MC, Perez EA, et al. African American and poor patients have a dramatically worse prognosis for head and neck cancer: an examination of 20,915 patients. Cancer 2008;113(10):2797–806.

124. Isayeva T, Xu J, Dai Q, et al. African Americans with oropharyngeal carcinoma have significantly poorer outcomes despite similar rates of human papillomavirus-mediated carcinogenesis. Hum Pathol 2014;45(2):310–9.

125. Ha PK, Califano JA. The molecular biology of mucosal field cancerization of the head and neck. Crit Rev Oral Biol Med 2003;14(5):363–9.

126. Argiris A, Karamouzis MV, Raben D, et al. Head and neck cancer. Lancet 2008; 371(9625):1695–709.

127. Hordijk GJ, de Jong JM. Synchronous and metachronous tumours in patients with head and neck cancer. J Laryngol Otol 1983;97(7):619–21.

128. Erkal HS, Mendenhall WM, Amdur RJ, et al. Synchronous and metachronous squamous cell carcinomas of the head and neck mucosal sites. J Clin Oncol 2001;19(5):1358–62.

129. Schwartz LH, Ozsahin M, Zhang GN, et al. Synchronous and metachronous head and neck carcinomas. Cancer 1994;74:1933–8.

130. Chuang SC, Scelo G, Tonita JM, et al. Risk of second primary cancer among patients with head and neck cancers: a pooled analysis of 13 cancer registries. Int J Cancer 2008;123(10):2390–6.
131. Day GL, Blot WJ, Shore RE, et al. Second cancers following oral and pharyngeal cancer: patients' characteristics and survival patterns. Eur J Canc B Oral Oncol 1994;30B(6):381–6.
132. Koch WM. Clinical features of HPV-related head and neck squamous cell carcinoma: presentation and work-up. Otolaryngol Clin North Am 2012;45(4):779–93.
133. Fakhry C, Zhang Q, Nguyen-Tan PF, et al. Human papillomavirus and overall survival after progression of oropharyngeal squamous cell carcinoma. J Clin Oncol 2014;32(30):3365–73.

Molecular Biology and Immunology of Head and Neck Cancer

Theresa Guo, MD*, Joseph A. Califano, MD

KEYWORDS

- Molecular biology • Targeted therapy • Immunology • Head and neck cancer

KEY POINTS

- Most head and neck squamous cell carcinomas are associated with smoking and alcohol, but an emerging subset of tumors is associated with human papillomavirus. These patients have improved clinical outcomes and a distinct genetic profile.
- Genetic sequencing of head and neck cancer revealed mutations in key cancer pathways, including p53, epidermal growth factor receptor (EGFR)/Ras/phosphatidylinositol 3-kinase (PI3K), Notch and apopototic pathways.
- Therapies targeted toward these pathways are limited but under investigation.
- Head and neck cancers may progress by immune evasion, which is another potential targetable mechanism under investigation.

In recent years, our knowledge and understanding of head and neck squamous cell carcinoma (HNSCC) has expanded dramatically. New high-throughput sequencing technologies have accelerated these discoveries since the first reports of whole-exome sequencing of HNSCC tumors in 2011.[1,2] In addition, the discovery of human papillomavirus (HPV) in relationship with oropharyngeal squamous cell carcinoma (SCC) has shifted our molecular understanding of the disease.[3] New investigation into the role of immune evasion in HNSCC has also led to potential novel therapies based on immune-specific systemic therapies.

DISTINCT ETIOLOGIC SUBSETS OF HEAD AND NECK SQUAMOUS CELL CARCINOMA

HNSCC forms after accumulation of genetic events, which are accelerated by genomic instability related to carcinogen exposures, particularly tobacco and alcohol. These tumors may occur throughout the upper aerodigestive tract (oral cavity, oropharynx, larynx) and are found in older patients, usually with history of smoking

Department of Otolaryngology, Head and Neck Surgery, Johns Hopkins Medical Institutions, 1550 Orleans St, Baltimore, MD 21231, USA
* Corresponding author. Cancer Research Building CRB II, 5M, 1550 Orleans Street, Baltimore, MD 21231.
E-mail address: tguo5@jhmi.edu

Surg Oncol Clin N Am 24 (2015) 397–407
http://dx.doi.org/10.1016/j.soc.2015.03.002
1055-3207/15/$ – see front matter © 2015 Elsevier Inc. All rights reserved.

or alcohol use. They are also associated with p53 mutations and poor clinical outcomes, with 5-year survival of 33.8% to 66.8%, depending on subsite.[4,5]

Recently, HPV has been associated with a subset of HNSCC, chiefly in the oropharynx and primarily in younger, white, nonsmokers.[3,6] HPV is a double-stranded DNA virus that infects the squamous epithelium. High-risk subtypes, particularly HPV-16 and HPV-18, are associated with development of malignancy in both HNSCC and cervical cancer. The mechanism of oncogenesis is attributed to viral proteins E6 (which binds and degrades p53) and E7 (which inhibits retinoblastoma protein, a tumor suppressor gene that inhibits cell cycle progression).[7,8] Patients with HPV-related HNSCC have improved prognosis with longer overall survival, decreased rate of recurrence, and improved response to chemoradiation.[3,9]

GENETIC ALTERATIONS

In 2011, the first whole-exome sequencing of HNSCC was published.[1,2] Recently, the Cancer Genome Atlas (TCGA) Research Network performed integrated genomic analysis, including genome sequencing, copy number and loss of heterozygosity arrays, whole-genome methylation, and RNA sequencing on 279 head and neck cancers, constituting the largest cohort of sequenced tumors studied.[10]

Gene mutations were segregated by HPV tumor status. HPV-positive tumors harbored fewer mutations compared with HPV-negative tumors.[1,10,11] TP53 mutations were found almost exclusively in HPV-negative tumors,[1,10] whereas activating mutations and amplifications of PIK3CA (phosphatidylinositol 3-kinase, catalytic subunit alpha) were commonly seen in HPV-positive tumors (**Fig. 1**).[10] This finding is consistent with prior data showing the same distinct genetic alterations.[12]

Beyond sequencing, gene promoter methylation of several genes, including CDKN2A (cyclin-dependent kinase inhibitor 2A), CDH1 (cadherin 1 type 1, E-cadherin), MGMT (O-6-methylguanine-DNA methyltransferase), and DAPK1 (death-associated protein kinase 1), has been established in oral SCC.[13] CDKN2A, a tumor suppressor gene, is one of the first genes in HNSCC to be associated with promoter methylation as a mechanism of downregulation.[14]

MAJOR PATHWAYS
TP53 and CDKN2A

The TP53 (tumor protein p53) gene encodes for the p53 protein, "guardian of the genome."[15] TP53 is one of the most frequently mutated genes in HNSCC[1,2,10,15] tumors and even premalignant lesions.[16] The p53 protein acts as a tumor suppressor that accumulates in response to stress, including DNA damage.[17] Accumulation of p53 induces cell cycle arrest to allow the cell to perform DNA repair. If damage is beyond repair, p53 induces apoptosis.[15] The expression of p53 is regulated by MDM2 (MDM2 proto-oncogene, E3 ubiquitin protein ligase), which inactivates and degrades p53.[18] The CDKN2A locus at 9p21 codes for 2 alternatively spliced proteins p14ARF and p16INK4A, which both regulate p53 function (**Fig. 2**).[19]

Most p53 mutations in HNSCC (50%–63%) are missense mutations.[1,2] Missense mutations in p53 can result in a stable protein with loss of key binding function or even act in a dominant negative fashion inactivating any remaining wild-type p53.[15] Tobacco exposure is associated with increased rates of TP53 mutations.[4,20] Mutations in TP53 have been associated with decreased overall survival,[21] increased locoregional recurrence rates,[22] and decreased response to therapy.[23,24]

In recent sequencing data, it was found that CDKN2A was mutated in 9% to 12% of tumors.[1,2] Loss of heterozygosity is frequently seen at the CDKN2A locus in HNSCC,

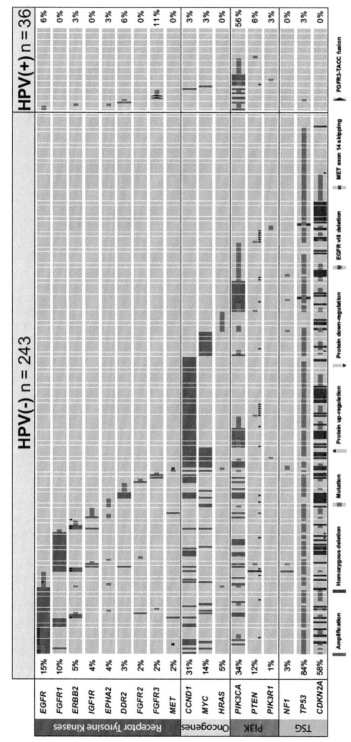

Fig. 1. Genetic alterations in key oncogenic pathways from TCGA. TSG, tumor supressor genes. (*From* The Cancer Genome Atlas Network. Comprehensive genomic characterization of head and neck squamous cell carcinomas. Nature 2015;517(7536):579; with permission.)

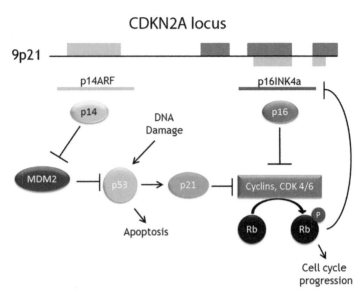

Fig. 2. CDKN2A gene products and p53 regulation. CDKN2A codes for alternatively spliced p14ARF and p16INK4a genes. The p14 protein inhibits MDM2, which ubiquitinates p53. Both p21, induced by p53, and p16 inhibit cyclins that promote cell cycle progression through phosphorylation of retinoblastoma protein (Rb). Rb feeds back to inhibit p16 production. CDK, cyclin-dependent kinase; MDM2, MDM2 proto-oncogene E3 ubiquitin protein ligase; P, phosphorylation.

including premalignant lesions.[25] Additionally, p16 protein overexpression is consistently seen in HPV-related oropharyngeal cancers.[26] The mechanism is related to the inactivation of retinoblastoma protein by the E7 viral protein, resulting in unregulated overexpression of p16.[27]

Epidermal Growth Factor Receptor, Ras, and PI3K (Phosphatidylinositol 3-Kinase Pathways)

Epidermal growth factor receptor (EGFR) is part of the ErbB family of receptor tyrosine kinases. After ligand binding (ligands include epidermal growth factor or transforming growth factor-α), activated EGFR forms a dimer and activates downstream pathways. These pathways include phosphoinositide 3-kinase (PI3K), Akt and Ras pathways that promote cell growth, proliferation, and inhibit apoptosis (**Fig. 3**). Activation of PI3K results in conversion of phosphatidylinositol biphosphate (PIP2) to phosphatidylinositol triphosphate (PIP3). PIP3 can then bind and phosphorylate Akt, triggering inhibition of apoptosis, mammalian target of rapamycin (mTOR) pathway activation, and activation of MDM2.[28] PTEN (phosphatase and tensin homolog) negatively regulates this signaling by dephosphorylating PIP3 to PIP2, thus, preventing downstream signaling.

In HNSCC, overexpression of the EGFR gene is seen in about 90% of tumors.[29] Increased EGFR expression correlates with increased local recurrence[30] and worse overall survival.[30,31] EGFR overexpression plays a clear role in HNSCC; interestingly, few mutations have been observed in EGFR (see **Fig. 1**).[11,29] HRAS (Harvey rat sarcoma viral oncogene homolog), a target downstream of EGFR, is mutated in 4% to 5% of tumors.[1,2,10]

In HNSCC, PI3KCA (catalytic subunit of PI3 kinase) is mutated in 6% to 21% of tumors.[1,2,32] Advanced stage HNSCC harbor increased mutations along the PI3K

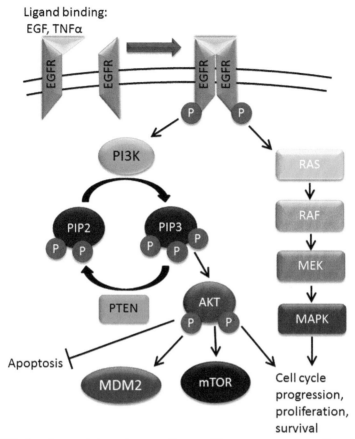

Fig. 3. EGFR signaling and downstream pathways. When an extracellular ligand binds to EGFR, dimerization occurs, promoting cross-phosphorylation. This cross-phosphorylation activates Ras signaling and activates PI3K to produce phosphatidylinositol triphosphate (PIP3). PIP3 phosphorylates Akt, which promotes mamalian target of rapamycin (mTOR) signaling, promotes MDM2 (inhibits p53), and inhibits apoptosis. EGF, epidermal growth factor; MAPK, mitogen-activated protein kinase; MDM2, MDM2 proto-onocogene E3 ubiquitin protein ligase; MEK, MAPK/ERK (extracellular signal regulated kinase) kinase; mTOR, mammalian target of rapamycin; P, phosphorylation; PIP2, phosphatidylinositol biphosphate; PTEN, phosphatase and tensin homolog; TNFα, tumor necrosis factor α.

pathway.[33] PI3K pathway genes are the main genes mutated in HPV-related tumors (see **Fig. 1**).[10,33]

Notch Signaling

Notch is a cell surface receptor that binds to ligands on an adjacent cell surface, such as Jagged or Delta.[28] Next, proteolytic cleavage releases an intracellular fragment that travels to the nucleus, affecting gene transcription. Downstream targets include HES1 [hes family basic helix-loop-helix (bHLH) transcription factor 1] and HEY1 (hes-related family bHLH transcription factor with YRPW motif 1), which promote cell cycle progression and survival.[34]

Inactivating mutations of NOTCH1 were found in 10% to 19% of head and neck tumors.[1,2,10] This finding suggests that NOTCH1 acts as a tumor suppressor in

HNSCC. In oral SCC cell lines, reactivation of the wild-type NOTCH1 gene blocked cell proliferation.[35] However, NOTCH1 also acts as an oncogene in hematologic malignancies.[36] Within sequencing data of HNSCC, some mutations in NOTCH1 were not inactivating, suggesting that its role in HNSCC may be mixed.[32,37] Accordingly, recent data have shown that a subset of HNSCC tumors actually show downstream activation of NOTCH.[37]

Apoptotic Pathways

Apoptotic pathways are regulated by intrinsic signals (such as p53) or extrinsic signals through cell surface receptors. Multiple signals, such as p53 response to DNA damage, UV radiation, or influx of calcium ions, can trigger apoptotic signaling. When the balance tips toward apoptosis, cytochrome c is released from the mitochondria, and the caspase cascade executes programmed cell death. Cell surface receptors, such as Fas and death receptors, may also trigger apoptosis through activation of caspase 8 (CASP8) and other downstream caspases.[28]

With head and neck cancer, mutations in CASP8 have been observed in 8% to 9% of tumors[2] (TCGA data) with most occurring in oral cavity SCC.[10] TRAF3 (TNF receptor-associated factor 3), BIRC2 (baculoviral inhibitor of apoptosis protein repeat containing 2), and FADD (Fas-associated via death domain) interact with the cell surface death receptors and were found to harbor mutations in head and neck cancer.[10] TRAF3 mutations were noted primarily in HPV-positive tumors.

Implications for Targeted Therapy

Current chemotherapy treatments for head and neck cancer are not targeted but instead primarily platinum based treatments (primarily cisplatin and carboplatin) with concurrent radiation are the mainstay of treatment.[38]

Therapies Targeting Epidermal Growth Factor Receptor

The main targeted therapy currently available for HNSCC is cetuximab, an anti-EGFR immunoglobulin G1 (IgG1) antibody. Cetuximab was approved for the treatment of HNSCC after a study showed significantly improved progression-free and overall survival when concurrent cetuximab with radiation was compared with radiation alone.[39] Recent data have not shown improved outcomes when combining cetuximab with concurrent cisplatin in primary chemoradiation.[40] Questions still remain regarding the mechanism of cetuximab activity. Despite frequent EGFR overexpression, response rates to cetuximab as a single agent are around 10% to 15% in recurrent HNSCC[41]; efficacy has not been found to correlate with EGFR expression (**Fig. 4**).[40,42]

Other anti-EGFR antibodies (panitumumab, zalutumumab, nimotuzumab) have shown promising results in preclinical studies.[43] In phase II clinical trials, panitumumab did not show improvement in overall survival[44]; the efficacy of the other antibodies has yet to be determined (clinical trials: NCT01054625, NCT00401401, NCT01425736).

Food and Drug Administration (FDA)–approved small molecule tyrosine kinase inhibitors (TKI) of EGFR in other cancers include gefitinib, erlotinib, lapatinib, and afatinib.[43] In preclinical studies, these TKI treatments have been shown to increase cell death in response to radiation therapy, especially when combined with vascular endothelial growth factor (VEGF) inhibitors.[45,46] In clinical trials, they have not been shown to improve outcomes[47,48]; but lapatinib may improve progression-free survival in HPV-negative patients.[49]

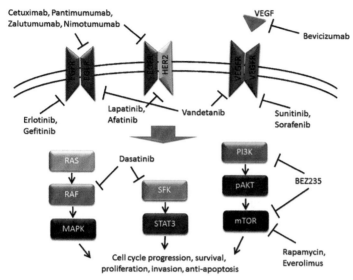

Fig. 4. Potential targets for therapy in head and neck cancer. HER2, human epidermal growth factor receptor 2; MAPK, mitogen-activated protein kinase; mTOR, mammalian target of rapamycin; pAKT, phosphorylated Akt; PI3K, phosphatidylinositol 3-kinase; SFK, Src family kinases; STAT3, signal transducer and activator of transcription 3; VEGF, vascular endothelial growth factor; VEGFR, vascular endothelial growth factor receptor. (*Adapted from* Du Y, Peyser ND, Grandis JR. Integration of molecular targeted therapy with radiation in head and neck cancer. Pharmacol Therapeut 2014;142(1):89; with permission.)

Vascular Endothelial Growth Factor and Other Tyrosine Kinase Inhibitors

Inhibition of VEGF may sensitize HNSCC to radiation treatment.[50] However, treatment with bevacizumab, an anti-VEGF antibody, has not shown improved outcomes. Importantly in clinical trials, it was associated with locoregional progression[51] as well as an increased incidence of osteoradionecrosis.[52]

Small molecule TKIs with multiple kinase targets approved for other cancers include vandetanib, sunitinib, sorafenib, and dasatinib.[43] Preclinical studies of these TKIs in HNSCC have shown promise, particularly in increasing radiation-induced cytotoxicity.[53–55] Ongoing trials have not yet shown significant clinical results.[56,57]

PI3K and mTOR Inhibitors

The PI3K/mTOR pathway is another potential target in HNSCC, highlighted in recent genomic data (see **Fig. 1**, TCGA). Preclinical studies of BEZ235, a small molecule inhibitor of PI3K and mTOR, have shown efficacy in head and neck cells harboring PIK3CA mutations[33]; it may be more effective for HPV-related tumors.[58] Rapamycin and everolimus, mTOR inhibitors that have been used for transplant immunosuppression, are currently under clinical trial investigation in patients with HNSCC (NCT00935961, NCT01283334, NCT01195922).

Immunology

Recent studies have explored the role of immune system evasion in the progression of HNSCC.[59] One major pathway of interest is the cosignaling of the programmed cell death protein 1 (PD-1) and its ligand (PD-L1). PD-L1 is normally expressed by antigen-presenting cells and is overexpressed in solid tumor cells.[60] The interaction between PD-1 and PD-L1 dampens the immune response.[60] Currently, antibodies directed toward PD-1 and PD-L1 are in clinical trials for patients with other solid tumors. Recently, nivolumab, an IgG4 monoclonal anti-PD-1, has shown dramatic results in advanced melanoma and was approved by the (this is a recent change since our submission) FDA.[61] HNSCC, especially HPV-positive tumors, show increased expression of PD-L1.[62] However, PD-L1 expression in head and neck tumors has not been clearly associated with clinical prognosis.[59] Clinical trials are beginning to investigate pembrolizumab (anti–PD-1) in head and neck cancer (NCT02255097, NCT02252042).

Another potential method of immune system modulation currently under investigation is with the use of phosphodiesterase-5 (PDE5) inhibitors, such as tadalafil. PDE5 inhibitors act by increasing cGMP to inhibit myeloid-derived suppressor cells (MDSC), which may dampen the immune response to tumors.[63] Preclinical studies showed that treatment with tadalafil reduced tumor growth.[63] In patients with head and neck cancer, tadalafil has been shown to significantly decrease T-regulatory and MDSC in patient serum[64]; phase II trials are currently accruing to assess treatment efficacy (NCT01697800).

REFERENCES

1. Agrawal N, Frederick MJ, Pickering CR, et al. Exome sequencing of head and neck squamous cell carcinoma reveals inactivating mutations in NOTCH1. Science 2011;333(6046):1154–7.
2. Stransky N, Egloff AM, Tward AD, et al. The mutational landscape of head and neck squamous cell carcinoma. Science 2011;333(6046):1157–60.
3. Ang KK, Harris J, Wheeler R, et al. Human papillomavirus and survival of patients with oropharyngeal cancer. N Engl J Med 2010;363(1):24–35.
4. Brennan JA, Boyle JO, Koch WM, et al. Association between cigarette smoking and mutation of the p53 gene in squamous-cell carcinoma of the head and neck. N Engl J Med 1995;332(11):712–7.
5. Pulte D, Brenner H. Changes in survival in head and neck cancers in the late 20th and early 21st century: a period analysis. Oncologist 2010;15(9):994–1001.
6. D'Souza G, Kreimer AR, Viscidi R, et al. Case-control study of human papillomavirus and oropharyngeal cancer. N Engl J Med 2007;356:1944–56.
7. Scheffner M, Huibregtse JM, Vierstra RD, et al. The HPV-16 E6 and E6-AP complex functions as a ubiquitin-protein ligase in the ubiquitination of p53. Cell 1993; 75(3):495–505.
8. Pagano M, Durst M, Joswig S, et al. Binding of the human E2F transcription factor to the retinoblastoma protein but not to cyclin A is abolished in HPV-16-immortalized cells. Oncogene 1992;7(9):1681–6.
9. Fakhry C, Westra WH, Li S, et al. Improved survival of patients with human papillomavirus-positive head and neck squamous cell carcinoma in a prospective clinical trial. J Natl Cancer Inst 2008;100(4):261–9.
10. The Cancer Genome Atlas Network. Comprehensive genomic characterization of head and neck squamous cell carcinomas. Nature 2015;517(7536):576–82.
11. Sun W, Califano J. Sequencing the head and neck cancer genome- Impact on therapy. Ann N Y Acad Sci 2014;1333:33–42.
12. Lechner M, Frampton GM, Fenton T, et al. Targeted next-generation sequencing of head and neck squamous cell carcinoma identifies novel genetic alterations in HPV+ and HPV- tumors. Genome Med 2013;5(5):49.

13. Ha PK, Califano JA. Promoter methylation and inactivation of tumour-suppressor genes in oral squamous-cell carcinoma. Lancet Oncol 2006;7(1):77–82.
14. Reed AL, Califano J, Cairns P, et al. High frequency of p16 (CDKN2/MTS-1/INK4A) inactivation in head and neck squamous cell carcinoma. Cancer Res 1996;56(16):3630–3.
15. Lane DP. Cancer. p53, guardian of the genome. Nature 1992;358(6381):15–6.
16. Califano J, van der Riet P, Westra W, et al. Genetic progression model for head and neck cancer: implications for field cancerization. Cancer Res 1996;56(11):2488–92.
17. Carr AM. Cell cycle. Piecing together the p53 puzzle. Science 2000;287(5459):1765–6.
18. Haupt Y, Maya R, Kazaz A, et al. Mdm2 promotes the rapid degradation of p53. Nature 1997;387(6630):296–9.
19. Roussel MF. The INK4 family of cell cycle inhibitors in cancer. Oncogene 1999;18(38):5311–7.
20. Ronchetti D, Neglia CB, Cesana BM, et al. Association between p53 gene mutations and tobacco and alcohol exposure in laryngeal squamous cell carcinoma. Arch Otolaryngol Head Neck Surg 2004;130(3):303–6.
21. Poeta ML, Manola J, Goldwasser MA, et al. TP53 mutations and survival in squamous-cell carcinoma of the head and neck. N Engl J Med 2007;357(25):2552–61.
22. Skinner HD, Sandulache VC, Ow TJ, et al. TP53 disruptive mutations lead to head and neck cancer treatment failure through inhibition of radiation-induced senescence. Clin Cancer Res 2012;18(1):290–300.
23. Ganly I, Soutar DS, Brown R, et al. p53 alterations in recurrent squamous cell cancer of the head and neck refractory to radiotherapy. Br J Cancer 2000;82(2):392–8.
24. Perrone F, Bossi P, Cortelazzi B, et al. TP53 mutations and pathologic complete response to neoadjuvant cisplatin and fluorouracil chemotherapy in resected oral cavity squamous cell carcinoma. J Clin Oncol 2010;28(5):761–6.
25. Ha PK, Chang SS, Glazer CA, et al. Molecular techniques and genetic alterations in head and neck cancer. Oral Oncol 2009;45(4–5):335–9.
26. Begum S, Gillison ML, Ansari-Lari MA, et al. Detection of human papillomavirus in cervical lymph nodes: a highly effective strategy for localizing site of tumor origin. Clin Cancer Res 2003;9(17):6469–75.
27. Li Y, Nichols MA, Shay JW, et al. Transcriptional repression of the D-type cyclin-dependent kinase inhibitor p16 by the retinoblastoma susceptibility gene product pRb. Cancer Res 1994;54(23):6078–82.
28. Weinberg RA. The biology of cancer. New York: Garland Science; 2007.
29. Kalyankrishna S, Grandis JR. Epidermal growth factor receptor biology in head and neck cancer. J Clin Oncol 2006;24(17):2666–72.
30. Psyrri A, Yu Z, Weinberger PM, et al. Quantitative determination of nuclear and cytoplasmic epidermal growth factor receptor expression in oropharyngeal squamous cell cancer by using automated quantitative analysis. Clin Cancer Res 2005;11(16):5856–62.
31. Chung CH, Ely K, McGavran L, et al. Increased epidermal growth factor receptor gene copy number is associated with poor prognosis in head and neck squamous cell carcinomas. J Clin Oncol 2006;24(25):4170–6.
32. Sun W, Gaykalova DA, Ochs MF, et al. Activation of the NOTCH pathway in head and neck cancer. Cancer Res 2014;74(4):1091–104.
33. Lui VW, Hedberg ML, Li H, et al. Frequent mutation of the PI3K pathway in head and neck cancer defines predictive biomarkers. Cancer Discov 2013;3(7):761–9.

34. Ntziachristos P, Lim JS, Sage J, et al. From fly wings to targeted cancer therapies: a centennial for notch signaling. Canc cell 2014;25(3):318–34.

35. Pickering CR, Zhang J, Yoo SY, et al. Integrative genomic characterization of oral squamous cell carcinoma identifies frequent somatic drivers. Cancer Discov 2013;3(7):770–81.

36. Weng AP, Ferrando AA, Lee W, et al. Activating mutations of NOTCH1 in human T cell acute lymphoblastic leukemia. Science 2004;306(5694):269–71.

37. Song X, Xia R, Li J, et al. Common and complex Notch1 mutations in Chinese oral squamous cell carcinoma. Clin Cancer Res 2014;20(3):701–10.

38. Head and neck cancers. NCCN clinical practice guidelines in oncology (NCCN guidelines). 2014. Available at: http://www.nccn.org/professionals/physician_gls/pdf/head-and-neck.pdf. Accessed October 24, 2014.

39. Bonner JA, Harari PM, Giralt J, et al. Radiotherapy plus cetuximab for squamous-cell carcinoma of the head and neck. N Engl J Med 2006;354(6):567–78.

40. Ang KK, Zhang Q, Rosenthal DI, et al. Randomized phase III trial of concurrent accelerated radiation plus cisplatin with or without cetuximab for stage III to IV head and neck carcinoma: RTOG 0522. J Clin Oncol 2014;32:2940–50.

41. Vermorken JB, Herbst RS, Leon X, et al. Overview of the efficacy of cetuximab in recurrent and/or metastatic squamous cell carcinoma of the head and neck in patients who previously failed platinum-based therapies. Cancer 2008;112(12):2710–9.

42. Licitra L, Mesia R, Rivera F, et al. Evaluation of EGFR gene copy number as a predictive biomarker for the efficacy of cetuximab in combination with chemotherapy in the first-line treatment of recurrent and/or metastatic squamous cell carcinoma of the head and neck: EXTREME study. Ann Oncol 2011;22(5):1078–87.

43. Du Y, Peyser ND, Grandis JR. Integration of molecular targeted therapy with radiation in head and neck cancer. Pharmacol Therapeut 2014;142(1):88–98.

44. Vermorken JB, Stohlmacher-Williams J, Davidenko I, et al. Cisplatin and fluorouracil with or without panitumumab in patients with recurrent or metastatic squamous-cell carcinoma of the head and neck (SPECTRUM): an open-label phase 3 randomised trial. Lancet Oncol 2013;14(8):697–710.

45. Huang SM, Li J, Armstrong EA, et al. Modulation of radiation response and tumor-induced angiogenesis after epidermal growth factor receptor inhibition by ZD1839 (Iressa). Cancer Res 2002;62(15):4300–6.

46. Chinnaiyan P, Huang S, Vallabhaneni G, et al. Mechanisms of enhanced radiation response following epidermal growth factor receptor signaling inhibition by erlotinib (Tarceva). Cancer Res 2005;65(8):3328–35.

47. Caponigro F, Romano C, Milano A, et al. A phase I/II trial of gefitinib and radiotherapy in patients with locally advanced inoperable squamous cell carcinoma of the head and neck. AntiCanc Drugs 2008;19(7):739–44.

48. Rodriguez CP, Adelstein DJ, Rybicki LA, et al. Single-arm phase II study of multiagent concurrent chemoradiotherapy and gefitinib in locoregionally advanced squamous cell carcinoma of the head and neck. Head Neck 2012;34(11):1517–23.

49. Harrington K, Berrier A, Robinson M, et al. Randomised phase II study of oral lapatinib combined with chemoradiotherapy in patients with advanced squamous cell carcinoma of the head and neck: rationale for future randomised trials in human papilloma virus-negative disease. Eur J Cancer 2013;49(7):1609–18.

50. Hoang T, Huang S, Armstrong E, et al. Enhancement of radiation response with bevacizumab. J Exp Clin Cancer Res 2012;31:37.

51. Salama JK, Haraf DJ, Stenson KM, et al. A randomized phase II study of 5-fluorouracil, hydroxyurea, and twice-daily radiotherapy compared with bevacizumab

plus 5-fluorouracil, hydroxyurea, and twice-daily radiotherapy for intermediate-stage and T4N0-1 head and neck cancers. Ann Oncol 2011;22(10):2304–9.

52. Yoo DS, Kirkpatrick JP, Craciunescu O, et al. Prospective trial of synchronous bevacizumab, erlotinib, and concurrent chemoradiation in locally advanced head and neck cancer. Clin Cancer Res 2012;18(5):1404–14.

53. Sano D, Matsumoto F, Valdecanas DR, et al. Vandetanib restores head and neck squamous cell carcinoma cells' sensitivity to cisplatin and radiation in vivo and in vitro. Clin Cancer Res 2011;17:1815–27.

54. Schueneman AJ, Himmelfarb E, Geng L, et al. SU11248 maintenance therapy prevents tumor regrowth after fractionated irradiation of murine tumor models. Cancer Res 2003;63(14):4009–16.

55. Yadav A, Kumar B, Teknos TN, et al. Sorafenib enhances the antitumor effects of chemoradiation treatment by downregulating ERCC-1 and XRCC-1 DNA repair proteins. Mol Cancer Ther 2011;10(7):1241–51.

56. Limaye S, Riley S, Zhao S, et al. A randomized phase II study of docetaxel with or without vandetanib in recurrent or metastatic squamous cell carcinoma of head and neck (SCCHN). Oral Oncol 2013;49(8):835–41.

57. Brooks HD, Glisson BS, Bekele BN, et al. Phase 2 study of dasatinib in the treatment of head and neck squamous cell carcinoma. Cancer 2011;117:2112–9.

58. Sewell A, Brown B, Biktasova A, et al. Reverse-phase protein array profiling of oropharyngeal cancer and significance of PIK3CA mutations in HPV-associated head and neck cancer. Clin Cancer Res 2014;20(9):2300–11.

59. Bauman JE, Ferris RL. Integrating novel therapeutic monoclonal antibodies into the management of head and neck cancer. Cancer 2014;120(5):624–32.

60. Zandberg DP, Strome SE. The role of the PD-L1: PD-1 pathway in squamous cell carcinoma of the head and neck. Oral Oncol 2014;50(7):627–32.

61. Topalian SL, Sznol M, McDermott DF, et al. Survival, durable tumor remission, and long-term safety in patients with advanced melanoma receiving nivolumab. J Clin Oncol 2014;32(10):1020–30.

62. Ukpo OC, Thorstad WL, Lewis JS Jr. B7-H1 expression model for immune evasion in human papillomavirus-related oropharyngeal squamous cell carcinoma. Head Neck Pathol 2013;7(2):113–21.

63. Serafini P, Meckel K, Kelso M, et al. Phosphodiesterase-5 inhibition augments endogenous antitumor immunity by reducing myeloid-derived suppressor cell function. J Trace Elem Exp Med 2006;203(12):2691–702.

64. Weed DT, Vella JL, Reis I, et al. Tadalafil reduces myeloid derived suppressor cells and regulatory T cells and promotes tumor immunity in patients with head and neck squamous cell carcinoma. Clin Cancer Res 2014;21:39–48.

Examination of the Patient with Head and Neck Cancer

Rachel Georgopoulos, MD[a], Jeffrey C. Liu, MD[a,b],*

KEYWORDS

- Oral cavity • Larynx • Nasopharynx • Oropharynx • Neck • Salivary • Malignancies

KEY POINTS

- The head and neck is a complex region, with many anatomic sites.
- A thorough detailed head and neck examination can adequately evaluate and stage patients with head and neck cancer.
- Endoscopic evaluation is an important complement to the head and neck examination.

Head and neck cancer typically refers to epithelial malignancies of the upper aerodigestive tract, which include the oral cavity, the oropharynx, larynx/hypopharynx, nasopharynx, nasal cavity, and paranasal sinuses. In addition, the term may also include neoplasms of the thyroid, salivary glands, and soft tissue, bone sarcomas, and skin cancers.[1,2] Head and neck cancer accounts for an estimated 3% to 5% of all cancer in the United States.[3] Two-thirds of patients present with advanced disease involving regional lymph nodes at the time of diagnosis.[4] In view of the broad range of disease and discrete anatomic relationships, a thorough history and detailed examination of the patient with head and neck cancer are often required to define the clinical problem. This careful examination is integral to oncologic staging and treatment planning.

This article begins with an overview of the head and neck examination (with special attention to detailed findings with clinical implications), followed by a discussion of the major head and neck subsites, and clinical pearls surrounding the examination.

HISTORY TAKING IN THE HEAD AND NECK

Evaluation of the patient with head and neck cancer begins with the patient's history. This history should be solicited, with attention to time course of symptom onset and progression. Symptoms such as shortness of breath, hoarseness, dysphagia, odynophagia, otalgia, globus sensation, hearing loss, aural fullness, epiphora, or trismus may be elicited

The authors have nothing to disclose.
[a] Department of Otolaryngology, Temple University School of Medicine, 3440 North Broad Street, Kresge West 3rd Floor, Philadelphia, PA 19140, USA; [b] Head and Neck Section, Fox Chase Cancer Center, 333 Cottman Avenue, Philadelphia, PA 19111, USA
* Corresponding author.
E-mail address: jeffrey.liu@temple.edu

Surg Oncol Clin N Am 24 (2015) 409–421
http://dx.doi.org/10.1016/j.soc.2015.03.003
1055-3207/15/$ – see front matter © 2015 Elsevier Inc. All rights reserved.

surgonc.theclinics.com

while obtaining the history and often direct the examiner to the primary malignancy. A mass in the neck, or of the face, scalp, mouth, or nose, may be the presenting complaint.

A detailed history of previous malignancies and previous treatments should be obtained. Patients with a previous head and neck malignancy harbor substantial risk for developing a second primary lesion. The annual risk of patients with head and neck cancer developing a metachronous second primary malignancy is estimated between 1.5% and 5.1%.[5,6] In addition, a variety of tumors can metastasize to the head and neck, with melanoma, breast, lung, kidney, and gynecologic malignancies having been reported in the literature.[7,8]

In addition to the patient's comorbid conditions, a family history should be obtained. Birthplace and ethnicity may play a role in head and neck cancer because of ethnic and regional predilections of some diseases. For example, nasopharyngeal carcinoma (NPC) is an uncommon malignancy in most countries of the world, with an average annual incidence of less than 1 per 100,000 per year. However, in the central region of Guangdong province of southern China, the incidence is more than 24 cases per 100,000 per year.[9,10] Increased incidence of NPC is observed in patients from North Africa, the Middle East, and the Arctic.[9,10] Although the risk of NPC among Chinese individuals who immigrate to North America remains high, American-born Chinese have significantly lower rates of NPC, approaching the geographic average.[11]

Substance Abuse and Occupational Risk Factors

A focused social and occupational history should be secured. Tobacco use and alcohol consumption account for an estimated 74% of squamous cell carcinoma (SCC) of the head and neck (SCCHN).[12–14] In individuals who smoke 2 or more packs of cigarettes a day and drink 4 or more alcoholic beverages, there is a 35-fold increased risk in the development of oropharyngeal cancer.[12] Similarly, smokeless tobacco products, such as chewing tobacco and snuff, are well-established risk factors in the development of oral and oropharyngeal cancer.[13,15] Betel quid, with and without tobacco, which is commonly used by South Asians, is a risk factor in the development of oral cavity as well as larynx, esophageal, liver, and pancreatic cancer.[16] Occupational exposures to asbestos, cement dust, and arsenic are also known risk factors for head and neck cancer.[17,18] Nickel refining and exposure to wood and leather dust are established risk factors for the development of sinonasal cancers.[19]

OVERALL FUNCTION

It is important to assess the patient's baseline functional status and recent changes in their ability to perform activities of daily living (ADLs). The Eastern Cooperative Oncology Group performance status scale is a commonly used clinical tool for patient assessment.[20] Because head and neck malignancies affect eating, drinking, breathing, swallowing, and talking, progressive disease often has a dramatic impact on performance status, as a result of trouble eating, weakness, and inability to perform ADLs. A patient's performance status influences treatment planning. Low performance status suggests a poor surgical candidate, problems completing radiation, or an inability to tolerate high-dose cisplatin chemotherapy. Such information informs the patient's treatment plan.

It is important to assess the patient's nutritional status, inquiring about weight loss and dysphagia. Dysphagia is an independent predictor of poor survival outcomes.[21] A variety of validated questionnaires, such as EAT-10 (eating assessment tool-10) and SWAL-QOL (swallowing quality of life) , can be used in the office to assess baseline dysphagia.[22–24] Patients with severe dysphagia and weight loss may need nutritional support, which may include tube feeding.

An assessment of shortness of breath or difficulty breathing should always be performed. Patients with some head and neck cancer (such as larynx cancer) may present with progressive airway obstruction. These patients must be urgently identified and treated. Indirect laryngoscopy to evaluate the airway is probably the best approach to rapid evaluation.

PHYSICAL EXAMINATION

A complete head and neck examination should be performed for all patients with suspected head and neck cancer, even if the location of the primary malignancy is already known. Of patients with head and neck cancer, 3% to 4% present with a synchronous second primary lesion in the head and neck.[25,26]

Evaluation begins with an assessment of the patient's general appearance. Difficulty breathing or stridor, nutritional status, affect, and mood are readily assessed by observation alone. Smell of smoke and tar-stained teeth may be signs of heavy tobacco use.

Stridor presents as a high-pitched respiratory sound resulting from turbulent airflow through a partially obstructed airway. Inspiratory stridor is commonly associated with obstructive supraglottic masses, whereas biphasic stridor usually accompanies fixed obstruction either of the trachea or at the level of the glottis (such as in bilateral vocal cord paralysis). Individuals with significant dysphagia and difficulty tolerating secretions may drool. Drooling should be considered a worrisome sign. All such patients should undergo timely evaluation including airway inspection by indirect laryngoscopy.

Stertor is an inspiratory sound comparable with snoring and occurs when there is an airway obstruction above the level of the larynx. Stertor often occurs with benign presentations such as obstructive sleep apnea, or in patients with Pickwickian syndrome. It can also be a presenting sign of malignancy. For example, new onset stertor may be reported with a cancer of the uvula, tonsil, or nasopharynx.

Appreciate the quality and power of the patient's voice. A breathy voice suggests a unilateral vocal cord paralysis and may be seen in lung cancer, thyroid cancer, larynx cancer, or with other lesions along the vagus nerve tract (eg, vagal paraganglioma). Hoarseness may be a sign of laryngeal disease. A hot potato voice or inability to articulate words clearly suggests posterior oral cavity or oropharyngeal disease. Hyponasality may be a sign of a mass involving the nasopharynx.

Inspect the face for symmetry. Masses of the parotid gland may be appreciated. Tumors causing incomplete facial nerve paralysis may present with asymmetric facial wrinkling, asymmetric eye blink, blunting of the nasolabial fold, or ptosis of the oral commissure.

Skin and Scalp

Evaluation of the skin should be performed systematically, with particular attention to sun-exposed areas such as the ears, scalp, and posterior neck. Note any chronic burns, scars, and ulcers. Inspect all masses and lesions for color variegation and asymmetry. Note the size of all lesions and whether there is ulceration or bleeding.

Intralymphatic regional metastases in the form of satellite or in-transit metastases may be appreciated surrounding a primary melanoma.[1] Satellite metastases occur within 2 cm of the primary lesion, whereas in-transit metastases occur more than 2 cm from the primary lesion.

Neurologic

A complete cranial nerve examination provides considerable information surrounding the affected patient. The cranial nerves course throughout the head and neck, and therefore, cranial neuropathies may indicate the location of a primary malignancy and the extent of tumor invasion.

Although the olfactory nerve is not routinely tested in the office, patients may present with subjective changes in their sense of smell, or its complete loss. Tumors of the olfactory epithelium such as esthesioneuroblastomas, primary sinonasal tumors, and other nasal tumors may present with hyposmia/anosmia.

With tumors involving the nasopharynx, sinuses, orbital cavity, or suprasellar masses such as craniopharyngiomas, visual acuity and extraocular movements should be assessed. The oculomotor, trochlear, and abducens nerves are assessed through evaluation of eye mobility. Tumors of the sphenoid or other paranasal sinuses may extend into the orbit and result in palsy. In the case of a suprasellar mass, bitemporal hemianopsia may be the presenting symptom.

The trigeminal system should be tested. Numbness or paresthesias can greatly inform the clinical scenario. A forehead SCC with V_1 numbness suggests perineural invasion. Loss of V_2 sensation in conjunction with a maxillary sinus mass may suggest invasion into the nerve. Some oral cavity cancers present with a loss of sensation to the chin during shaving, caused by cancer involving the mandibular canal and disruption of mental nerve. Paresthesias of the trigeminal system are not to be taken lightly; anatomic imaging should be used to evaluate the course of these nerves with any dysfunction.

Facial nerve deficits may occur from disruption anywhere along its course and could reflect tumors of the parotid, an acoustic neuroma, or perineural invasion from cutaneous malignancies.

Masses along the course of the main trunk of the vagus nerve such as vagal paragangliomas can result in asymmetric palatal elevation or vocal cord paralysis. Loss of laryngeal sensation may result in symptoms of aspiration or choking. Evaluation of vocal cord movement is discussed separately.

The spinal accessory nerve innervates the sternocleidomastoid and trapezius muscles and is therefore important in rotation of the head, shoulder elevation, and adduction of the arm. Cervical metastasis may also invade the spinal accessory nerve. It is best assessed through shoulder adduction.

The hypoglossal nerve innervates the tongue and is responsible for movement. Invasion of the hypoglossal nerve may result in the inability to protrude the involved side of the tongue. Unilateral weakness results in deviation of the tongue to the ipsilateral side. Loss of function of the hypoglossal nerve may accompany deep tongue invasion into the extrinsic muscles of the tongue within the oral cavity, involvement of the nerve near the external carotid artery caused by metastatic lymphadenopathy, or direct invasion at the skull base by tumor. These possibilities should all be considered on examination.

Ear Examination

Inspect the outer ear for any masses, lesions, or signs of deformity. The ears are particularly prone to solar damage and are a common site of cutaneous malignancies.[27,28] Inspect the tympanic membrane. Malignancies of the nasopharynx may result in eustachian tube dysfunction and unilateral serous effusions. Hearing loss may be a presenting symptom. Pneumatic otoscopy allows for assessment of the mobility of the tympanic membrane. Normally, the middle ear space is filled with air, and the tympanic membrane is highly mobile. An effusion dampens the mobility of the tympanic membrane.

Nasal Examination

Anterior rhinoscopy should be performed with a nasal speculum. The anterior septum, inferior and middle turbinate, and middle meatus should be readily seen. The nasal cavity should be examined for masses, ulcers, polyps, or evidence of bleeding.

Oral Cavity

The oral cavity begins at the white line or the junction between the skin and the vermilion border of the lip. The oral cavity is subdivided into the lips, tongue (to the level of the circumvallate papillae), hard palate, floor of mouth, retromolar trigone (RMT), and buccal membranes. The RMT is a triangular region with its base of the last mandibular molar and apex at the maxillary tuberosity. It is composed of the ascending ramus of the mandible with its overlying mucosa. Each of these subsites within the oral cavity should be examined for masses, lesions, ulcers, or asymmetry.

Oral cavity examination begins with inspection of the lips and competence of the oral commissure. Next, the dentition, gums, floor of mouth, tongue, alveolar ridge, RMT, and palate should be inspected. Dentures should be removed.

Assess for trismus by instructing the patient to open their mouth as much as they can. Trismus has many causes. It may be caused by pain, for example as a result of a cancer of the buccal mucosa. It may also be a sign of invasion of pterygoid musculature, as seen with advanced oropharynx cancers. When patients present with an oral cancer, resectability of oral cavity lesions should be evaluated.

A gloved finger should be used to palpate for any submucosal masses. The Wharton ducts should be appreciated as they open on either side of the lingual frenulum in the floor of the mouth. The papilla of the Stenson ducts may be seen exiting the buccal mucosa adjacent to the second maxillary molar tooth. A bimanual examination is performed using a gloved finger to palpate the floor of the mouth while providing external neck manipulation.

Evaluate tongue protrusion and mobility. As noted earlier, tumors of the tongue or floor of mouth may limit tongue mobility.

Oropharynx

The oropharynx is subdivided into the tonsil/tonsillar pillars, soft palate/uvula, posterior pharyngeal wall, and tongue base. The oropharynx should be inspected for symmetry. A gloved finger should be used to palpate the tonsillar fossae and tongue base. A mirror may be used to inspect the vallecula.

Neck, Parotid, and Submandibular Gland

The trachea and larynx are palpable in the midline neck. The hyoid bone, thyroid cartilage, and cricoid should be appreciated. Visible and palpable pulsations in the suprasternal notch may herald a high-riding innominate artery and should be noted. The thyroid may be palpated below the level of the cricoid and any masses noted. Fixation of thyroid nodules to the musculature or overlying skin is a worrisome sign of potentially aggressive thyroid disease.

The neck is divided into 7 levels (**Fig. 1**). Laterality, size, mobility, and firmness of all lymph nodes should be noted. Submandibular lymphadenopathy should be differentiated from prominent submandibular glands.

The parotid gland should be palpated. Tumors may arise from the parenchyma of the parotid gland. In addition, lymph nodes reside in the parotid tail, and the gland may be a site of metastatic disease either from the head and neck or elsewhere. The parotid is one of the most common sites for nodal metastases from cutaneous SCCHN.[29] Enlarged intraparotid nodes may reflect lymphoma.

Indirect Laryngoscopy

Indirect laryngoscopy by mirror examination is a quick means of examining the vallecula, base of tongue, hypopharynx, and vocal cords in the office. A handheld

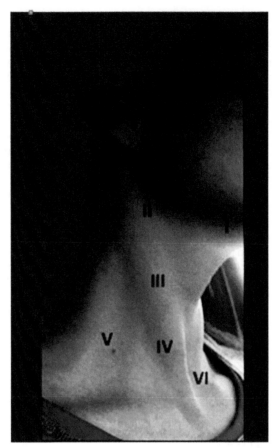

Fig. 1. Levels of the neck.

mirror and headlight are used. Use of the mirror is a learned skill and, although worthwhile, not easily mastered. The patient's legs should not be crossed, and patients should be positioned so that that they are leaning forward with their chin extended. Before inserting the mirror into the oral cavity, it should be warmed to prevent fogging. The mirror may be warmed using a glass bead mirror warmer or the back of the examiner's hand or warming the mirror on the patient's buccal mucosa. The patient should extrude their tongue, and the examiner should stabilize it with a piece of gauze, using the nondominant hand. The patient is instructed to breathe through the mouth. The mirror is inserted with the glass pointing downwards into the oropharynx, and with careful motion the oropharynx, hypopharynx, and larynx can be examined.

Fiber-Optic Laryngoscopy

Flexible fiberoptic laryngoscopy (FFL) may be used to augment the mirror examination.[30] It allows for inspection of the nasal cavity, septum/turbinates, nasopharynx, base of tongue, hypopharynx, and larynx. Both anatomic and functional deficits of the larynx can be defined. Before performing the examination, a combination decongestant and topical anesthetic is often sprayed in the nasal cavity. Neosynephrine and 2% lidocaine 50/50 mixture is commonly used. However, it is almost invariably possible to examine the patient without topical anesthesia, which may lead to misleading pooling of secretions (which suggest underlying tumor).

Flexible laryngoscopy should begin with a bilateral nasal endoscopy. The anterior nasal cavity is inspected on each side, noting nasal structures, including the septum, turbinates, and their respective meatus. The nasal cavity is inspected for masses or polyps. The inferior turbinate and middle turbinate are examined, as well as the middle meatus. As the scope is advanced superiorly, the sphenoethmoidal recess may be appreciated. The scope is then advanced into the nasopharynx. The torus tubarius should be seen bilaterally, and the nasopharynx should be inspected for any masses. Nasopharynx cancers often arise in the fossa of Rosenmuller, which is posterior and superior to the torus tubarius (**Fig. 2**). Lymphomas of the nasopharynx and other tumors may arise from the posterior wall in the nasopharynx. Instructing the patient to speak plosive sounds (eg, "coca cola") allows for evaluation of velopharyngeal function and closure.

As the scope is advanced, the vallecula, base of tongue, and hypopharynx come into view. Examination of the tongue base can be improved by having the patient extrude their tongue. The epiglottis should have a sharp edge. Irregularities in the mucosa raise suspicion for carcinoma. The aryepiglottic folds, arytenoids, false, and true cords should be individually inspected. Having the patient say "ee" adducts the vocal cords, allowing assessment of vocal cord mobility. Short inspiration (sniffing) causes vocal cord adduction. Puffing the cheeks with air causes distention of the piriform sinuses. Pooling of secretions in the piriform is abnormal and may be seen in instances of decreased laryngeal sensation and vocal fold immobility. The piriform sinuses are not completely seen during FFL.

SPECIAL CONSIDERATIONS BY ANATOMIC SITE
Neck Levels and Patterns of Metastasis

Assessment of regional lymph node status is essential in the evaluation of all patients with head and neck cancer. The status of regional lymph nodes is prognostically important and often dictates treatment. The neck is divided into 7 levels; nomenclature and boundaries are listed in **Table 1**.

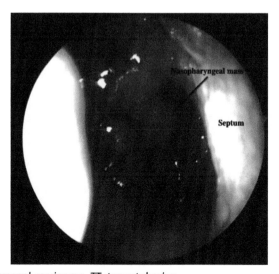

Fig. 2. Nasopharyngeal carcinoma. TT, torus tubarius.

Table 1
Levels of the neck

Level	Anatomic Location
I	1A: submental triangle Bound by the anterior digastric and mylohyoid muscle 1B: submandibular triangle Bound by the anterior and posterior digastrics and mandible
II	Upper jugulodigastric lymph nodes Extent: skull base to hyoid bone IIA: anterior to spinal accessory nerve IIB: posterior to spinal accessory nerve
III	Midjugulodigastric Extent: hyoid bone to inferior border of cricoid Bound by the lateral border of the sternohyoid muscle and the posterior border of the SCM
IV	Lower jugulodigastric Extent: inferior border of the cricoid cartilage to clavicle
V	Posterior triangle Boundaries: SCM trapezius superiorly, clavicle inferiorly, posterior boarder of SCM anteriorly, and the trapezius posteriorly VA: above the inferior border of the cricoid VB: below the inferior border of the cricoid
VI	Anterior compartment Boundaries: hyoid superiorly, suprasternal notch inferiorly, carotid arteries laterally
VII	Superior mediastinal nodes Boundaries: manubrium superiorly, carotid arteries laterally

Abbreviation: SCM, sternocleidomastoid.

In 2 landmarks studies, Lindberg[31] and then Shah[32] described predictable patterns of cervical lymph node drainage based on the subsite of the primary head and neck malignancy. First echelon drainage of oral cavity cancers is into levels I, II, and III. In cancers that are lateralized, such as buccal mucosa, lateral tongue, or floor of mouth, the ipsilateral level I/II/III are at highest risk. However, lesions that approach or cross the midline (eg, in the midline tongue or floor of mouth) may have bilateral drainage, and right and left I/II/III level lymph nodes should be considered at risk.

Cancers of the oropharynx, hypopharynx, and larynx primarily drain into lymph nodes in levels II, III, and IV.[2,31–33] Although cancers of the tonsil usually have only ipsilateral lymph nodes at risk, base of tongue and supraglottic cancers have rich lymphatics, and bilateral level II/III/IV lymph nodes are at risk for metastatic spread. Cancers confined to the glottis rarely metastasize and regional lymph nodes are seldom a consideration.

Malignancies of the nasopharynx and posterior skin lesions have a predilection for the posterior cervical lymph nodes of level V.[31]

Neck masses are one of the most common reasons for referral to a head and neck surgeon/otolaryngologist. A detailed history, with attention to context, time course, progression, and associated symptoms inform the index of suspension for malignancy. Reactive cervical lymphadenopathy is not uncommon in the presence of a viral upper respiratory infection. These lymph nodes should regress in size over the ensuing weeks. Persistent or enlarging lymphadenopathy, particularly in adults with a history of tobacco or alcohol abuse, regardless of antecedent infection, should be considered worrisome for a possible malignancy. Although the location of the cervical lymph node metastasis can confer information about the primary site, unknown primary carcinoma with neck metastasis accounts for approximately 3% to 7% of all head and neck cancers.[34]

Cervical lymph nodes should be evaluated systematically. Lymph nodes should be assessed for their tethering to surrounding structures including musculature and skin, because these are concerning for ease of resectability. In addition, size and number of lymph nodes should be noted. Matted lymph nodes are associated with worse outcomes in some oropharynx cancers.[35] Despite a thorough evaluation, the sensitivity for identifying cervical lymphadenopathy by physical examination alone is significantly less than that provided by imaging.[36] Radiologic imaging is recommended in the staging of most patients with head and neck cancer.

Oral Cavity

Individuals with cancers of the oral cavity may present with symptoms of pain, newly loose teeth, odynophagia, nonhealing ulcers, cervical lymphadenopathy, and problems with articulation, trismus, and dysphagia. Oral cavity bleeding with minimal provocation is not uncommon.

Lesions of the oral cavity are often characterized by color, referring to erythroplakia (red) and leukoplakia (white). Leukoplakia is a white premalignant lesion commonly seen in the oral cavity, with a potential for malignant transformation ranging from 0.13% to 17.5%.[37] Some studies suggest that there is a higher potential of malignant transformation of leukoplakia involving the tongue and floor of the mouth than the gums and buccal mucosa.[38,39] Erythroplakia is a red lesion, which has a significantly higher rate of malignant transformation than leukoplakia, with carcinoma being found in nearly 50% of these lesions.[40,41]

Lip

The location of the lesion on the upper versus lower lip is important, because the lymph node basins at risk differ. The lower lip tends to drain to the submental and submandibular lymph nodes, whereas the upper lip and commissure drain to the ipsilateral submandibular, submental, preauricular, and infraparotid lymph nodes. Bilateral lymph node involvement is more common in centrally located lesions.[42] Size or involvement of the vermilion border and oral commissure are important in the resectability of lip lesions. There should be a heightened concern for lymphatic spread through the mental foramen, perineural invasion, and direct extension through the mandible in individuals with paresthesias or hypesthesia in the distribution of the mandibular division of the trigeminal (V_3) nerve.

Floor of Mouth

Tumors of the floor of mouth may extend into the ventral tongue, resulting in tethering and decreased tongue mobility. These tumors can cause dysphagia or difficulty with articulation. The size of the lesion and the projected size of the defect are important when considering reconstructive options.

Tongue

When considering cancer of the oral tongue, it is important to take note of the proximity of the lesion to the midline. Involvement of the midline results in a significantly increased rate of contralateral lymph node metastasis.[43] A gloved finger should be used to palpate the mass. Depth of invasion has a significant impact on local regional control.[44–46] Tumors more than 4 mm thick are associated with increased regional recurrence and worse overall survival. Thickness may be difficult to determine on physical examination alone.[44–46]

Buccal Mucosa

Laterally, the oral cavity is bound by the buccal mucosa. Posteriorly, the buccal mucosa extends from the RMT to the pterygomandibular raphae, reaching the oral commissure anteriorly and the alveolar ridge inferiorly. The buccal mucosa lacks any significant barriers to tumor extension. Lesions may be deeper and larger than they seem, so reconstructive options should be considered when evaluating these patients.

Alveolar Ridge

The tooth-bearing bone of the mandible and maxilla with their overlying mucosa and gingiva comprise the alveolar ridges. In the edentulous patient, the tooth sockets serve as routes for tumor invasion and should be noted. Assess tumor fixation to the underlying bone. Extent of bony invasion dictates whether a portion of the bone or an entire segment of mandible must be resected. One-third of clinically mobile cancers show bony invasion on histopathology.[47] In light of this finding, radiologic imaging is often recommended for treatment planning.

In the case of malignancies of the upper alveolar ridge or hard palate, tumor may extend to the incisive foramen or pterygopalatine fossa via the palatine foramina.[48] The incisive foramen allows for extension of tumor into the anterior nose, and for this reason, nasal endoscopy should be performed.

Larynx

The larynx serves 3 main functions: it assists in respiration, phonation, and deglutition.[49] The timing and way in which a larynx cancer affects these functions largely depends on its location within the larynx.

Supraglottic tumors tend to present with symptoms of sore throat, dysphagia, and referred otalgia. On the other hand, glottic tumors tend to present with hoarseness.[50] For this reason, hoarseness that fails to resolve within several weeks of onset raises the suspicion for possible malignancy, and therefore, the larynx should be examined.[51] Flexible laryngoscopy significantly improves the ability to diagnose laryngeal malignancies in the office and should be performed in instances in which there is a high clinical suspicion.[52] In many cases, the presenting sign of a supraglottic laryngeal malignancy is a neck mass. Larynx cancer has a propensity for spread to levels II, III, and IV, and therefore, laryngeal malignancy should be considered as part of the differential diagnosis in patients with cervical metastasis in these levels.[2,32,33] Conversely, subglottic tumors often present in an advanced stage with signs of airway obstruction.[49]

Examination of a patient with suspected laryngeal cancer begins by listening to the quality of the patient's breathing. The larynx should be examined in a systematic manner by mirror or flexible FFL. The appearance and size of any masses should be noted, as well as the number of subsites within the larynx that they involve. Some laryngeal masses are submucosal, and therefore, physical findings are subtle. Vocal fold mobility is important in staging, because it suggests extension into the cricoarytenoid joint or paraglottic space.[49] The subglottis is often difficult to see during office examination. It is not advisable to pass the scope through the vocal cords because of possible laryngospasm. Any suspicious lesions should prompt operative direct laryngoscopy with biopsy.[53]

Of utmost importance in evaluating patients with laryngeal cancer is assessing the patency and stability of their airway. Hemorrhage or an obstructing mass may require tracheotomy.

SUMMARY

Examination of the patient with head and neck cancer should be performed systematically. A thorough and accurate examination can confer considerable information surrounding the nature and extent of tumor involvement. This strategy improves staging, appropriate treatment planning, and patient outcomes.

REFERENCES

1. Greene FL, editor. AJCC cancer staging atlas. Chicago (IL): Springer; 2006. p. 13–66.
2. Shah JP, Medina JE, Shaha AR, et al. Cervical lymph node metastasis. Curr Probl Surg 1993;30(3):1–335.
3. Siegel R, Ma J, Zou Z, et al. Cancer statistics. CA Cancer J Clin 2014;64:9–29.
4. Howlader N, Noone A, Krapcho M, et al. SEER cancer statistics review, 1975–2008. Bethesda (MD): National Cancer Institute; 2010.
5. Argiris A, Brockstein BE, Haraf DJ, et al. Competing causes of death and second primary tumors in patients with locoregionally advanced head and neck cancer treated with chemoradiotherapy. Clin Cancer Res 2004;10(6):1956–62.
6. Leon X, Ferlito A, Myer CM 3rd, et al. Second primary tumors in head and neck cancer patients. Acta Otolaryngol 2002;122(7):765–78.
7. Giridharan W, Hughes J, Fenton JE, et al. Lymph node metastases in the lower neck. Clin Otolaryngol Allied Sci 2003;28:221–6.
8. Irani S. Metastasis to head and neck area: a 16-year retrospective study. Am J Otolaryngol 2011;32:24–7.
9. Chang ET, Adami HO. The enigmatic epidemiology of nasopharyngeal carcinoma. Cancer Epidemiol Biomarkers Prev 2006;15(10):1765–77.
10. Yu MC, Yuan JM. Epidemiology of nasopharyngeal carcinoma. Semin Cancer Biol 2002;12(6):421–9.
11. Dickson RI, Flores AD. Nasopharyngeal carcinoma: an evaluation of 134 patients treated between 1971–1980. Laryngoscope 1985;95(3):276–83.
12. Blot WJ, McLaughlin JK, Winn DM, et al. Smoking and drinking in relation to oral and pharyngeal cancer. Cancer Res 1988;48(11):3282–7.
13. Lee PN, Hamling J. Systematic review of the relation between smokeless tobacco and cancer in Europe and North America. BMC Med 2009;7:36.
14. Vineis P, Alavanja M, Buffler P, et al. Tobacco and cancer: recent epidemiological evidence. J Natl Cancer Inst 2004;96(2):99–106.
15. Bhattacharyya N. Trends in the use of smokeless tobacco in United States, 2000–2010. Laryngoscope 2012;122(10):2175–8.
16. Wen CP, Tsai MK, Chung WS, et al. Cancer risks from betel quid chewing beyond oral cancer: a multiple-site carcinogen when acting with smoking. Cancer Causes Control 2010;21(9):1427–35.
17. Purdue MP, Järvholm B, Bergdahl IA, et al. Occupational exposures and head and neck cancers among Swedish construction workers. Scand J Work Environ Health 2006;32(4):270–5.
18. Yu HS, Liao WT, Chai CY. Arsenic carcinogenesis in the skin. J Biomed Sci 2006; 13(5):657–66.

19. Straif K, Benbrahim-Tallaa L, Baan R, et al. A review of human carcinogens–part C: metals, arsenic, dusts, and fibres. Lancet Oncol 2009;10(5):453–4.
20. Correa GT, Bandeira GA, Cavalcanti BG, et al. Analysis of ECOG performance status in head and neck squamous cell carcinoma patients: association with sociodemographical and clinical factors, and overall survival. Support Care Cancer 2012;20(11):2679–85.
21. Lango MN, Egleston B, Fang C, et al. Baseline health perceptions, dysphagia, and survival in patients with head and neck cancer. Cancer 2014;120(6):840–7.
22. Belafsky PC, Mouadeb DA, Rees CJ, et al. Validity and reliability of the Eating Assessment Tool (EAT-10). Ann Otol Rhinol Laryngol 2008;117(12):919–24.
23. McHorney CA, Bricker DE, Robbins J, et al. The SWAL-QOL outcomes tool for oropharyngeal dysphagia in adults: II. Item reduction and preliminary scaling. Dysphagia 2000;15(3):122–33.
24. McHorney CA, Martin-Harris B, Robbins J, et al. Clinical validity of the SWAL-QOL and SWAL-CARE outcome tools with respect to bolus flow measures. Dysphagia 2006;21(3):141–8.
25. Chinn SB, Schwartz SM, Prince ME, et al. Synchronous and metachronous tumors in head and neck cancer: analysis of the SEER database. Otolaryngol Head Neck Surg 2013;149(5):198.
26. Hujala K, Sipila J, Grenman R. Panendoscopy and synchronous second primary tumors in head and neck cancer patients. Eur Arch Otorhinolaryngol 2005;262(1):17–20.
27. Armstrong BK, Kricker A. The epidemiology of UV induced skin cancer. J Photochem Photobiol B 2001;63(1–3):8–18.
28. Atillasoy ES, Elenitsas R, Sauter ER, et al. UVB induction of epithelial tumors in human skin using a RAG-1 mouse xenograft model. J Invest Dermatol 1997;109(6):704–9.
29. D'Souza J, Clark J. Management of the neck in metastatic cutaneous squamous cell carcinoma of the head and neck. Curr Opin Otolaryngol Head Neck Surg 2011;19(2):99–105.
30. Sham JS, Wei WI, Zong YS, et al. Detection of subclinical nasopharyngeal carcinoma by fibreoptic endoscopy and multiple biopsy. Lancet 1990;335(8686):371–4.
31. Lindberg R. Distribution of cervical lymph node metastases from squamous cell carcinoma of the upper respiratory and digestive tracts. Cancer 1972;29(6):1446–9.
32. Shah JP. Patterns of cervical lymph node metastasis from squamous carcinomas of the upper aerodigestive tract. Am J Surg 1990;160(4):405–9.
33. Jia S, Wang Y, He H, et al. Incidence of level IIB lymph node metastasis in supraglottic laryngeal squamous cell carcinoma with clinically negative neck–a prospective study. Head Neck 2013;35(7):987–91.
34. Miller FR, Hussey D, Beeram M, et al. Positron emission tomography in the management of unknown primary head and neck carcinoma. Arch Otolaryngol Head Neck Surg 2005;131(7):626–9.
35. Spector ME, Gallagher KK, Light E, et al. Matted nodes: poor prognostic marker in oropharyngeal squamous cell carcinoma independent of HPV and EGFR status. Head Neck 2012;34(12):1727–33.
36. Merritt RM, Williams MF, James TH, et al. Detection of cervical metastasis. A meta-analysis comparing computed tomography with physical examination. Arch Otolaryngol Head Neck Surg 1997;123(2):149–52.

37. Amagasa T, Yamashiro M, Uzawa N. Oral premalignant lesions: from a clinical perspective. Int J Clin Oncol 2011;16(1):5–14.

38. Amagasa T, Yamashiro M, Ishikawa H. Oral leukoplakia related to malignant transformation. Oral Sci Int 2006;3:45–55.

39. Pogrel MA. Sublingual keratosis and malignant transformation. J Oral Pathol 1979;8(3):176–8.

40. Reichart PA, Philipsen HP. Oral erythroplakia–a review. Oral Oncol 2005;41(6): 551–61.

41. Villa A, Villa C, Abati S. Oral cancer and oral erythroplakia: an update and implication for clinicians. Aust Dent J 2011;56(3):253–6.

42. Wurman LH, Adams GL, Meyerhoff WL. Carcinoma of the lip. Am J Surg 1975; 130(4):470–4.

43. Lloyd S, Yu JB, Wilson LD, et al. The prognostic importance of midline involvement in oral tongue cancer. Am J Clin Oncol 2012;35(5):468–73.

44. Asakage T, Yokose T, Mukai K, et al. Tumor thickness predicts cervical metastasis in patients with stage I/II carcinoma of the tongue. Cancer 1998;82(8):1443–8.

45. Fukano H, Matsuura H, Hasegawa Y, et al. Depth of invasion as a predictive factor for cervical lymph node metastasis in tongue carcinoma. Head Neck 1997; 19(3):205–10.

46. Kurokawa H, Yamashita Y, Takeda S, et al. Risk factors for late cervical lymph node metastases in patients with stage I or II carcinoma of the tongue. Head Neck 2002;24(8):731–6.

47. Tsue TT, McCulloch TM, Girod DA, et al. Predictors of carcinomatous invasion of the mandible. Head Neck 1994;16(2):116–26.

48. Ginsberg LE, DeMonte F. Imaging of perineural tumor spread from palatal carcinoma. AJNR Am J Neuroradiol 1998;19(8):1417–22.

49. Chu EA, Kim YJ. Laryngeal cancer: diagnosis and preoperative work-up. Otolaryngol Clin North Am 2008;41(4):673–95, v.

50. Thekdi AA, Ferris RL. Diagnostic assessment of laryngeal cancer. Otolaryngol Clin North Am 2002;35(5):953–69, v.

51. Schwartz SR, Cohen SM, Dailey SH, et al. Clinical practice guideline: hoarseness (dysphonia). Otolaryngol Head Neck Surg 2009;141(3 Suppl 2):S1–31.

52. Paul BC, Chen S, Sridharan S, et al. Diagnostic accuracy of history, laryngoscopy, and stroboscopy. Laryngoscope 2013;123(1):215–9.

53. Djukic V, Milovanovic J, Jotic AD, et al. Stroboscopy in detection of laryngeal dysplasia effectiveness and limitations. J Voice 2014;28(2):262.e13–21.

Radiation Treatment of Head and Neck Cancer

Sue S. Yom, MD, PhD

KEYWORDS

- Radiation • Treatment • Head and neck • Cancer

KEY POINTS

- Intensity-modulated radiation therapy is now the dominant mode of head and neck radiotherapeutic treatment but is challenging because of its technical complexity.
- For definitive treatment of most advanced-stage head and neck cancers which are not treated with primary surgery, concurrent chemoradiation produces the greatest efficacy, at a cost of significantly increased toxicity over radiation therapy alone.
- For human papillomavirus–associated oropharyngeal cancers, active investigation into deintensification strategies is likely to reshape the landscape of treatment options over the next several years.
- The worst prognostic factors in the postoperative setting are positive margins of resection or nodal extracapsular extension, and even with adjuvant chemoradiation, rates of locoregional recurrence are high in these patients.
- Future developments in radiation therapy technology will require substantial capital investments, with the understanding that most of these technical improvements are likely to decrease toxicities rather than improve oncologic outcomes.

INTRODUCTION

Radiation therapy plays a central and continuously evolving role in the treatment of head and neck cancer. In part, the uses of radiation are varied because of the diversity of histology and natural history within subsites of the head and neck. Although the basic principles of radiation therapy have not changed over the past decades, a greater understanding of clinically applicable aspects of radiation biology and the wide availability of technologically based advances have contributed to the increasing sophistication of radiation-based treatment, with quantifiable benefits in improved tumor control and quality of life. In addition, ongoing discovery in surgical and systemic therapy are informing multimodality approaches involving radiation therapy.

In this review, some basic principles of radiation oncology are explained and common clinical scenarios are addressed in which radiation therapy forms part of the

Dr Yom receives clinical trial support from Genentech, Inc.
Department of Radiation Oncology, Helen Diller Family Comprehensive Cancer Center, University of California, San Francisco, Box 1708, 1600 Divisadero Street, MZ Building R H1031, San Francisco, CA 94143-1708, USA
E-mail address: Sue.Yom@ucsf.edu

treatment course, with a focus on issues most pertinent to the interaction of radiation oncology with surgical treatment. These issues include refinement of the indications guiding the choice of adjuvant radiation therapy or chemoradiotherapy, sequencing and timing of therapies before or after definitive surgical management, and scientific and technical advances with the potential to reduce radiation-related toxicity.

TECHNICAL PRINCIPLES OF MODERN HEAD AND NECK RADIATION THERAPY

Ionizing radiation as known to most practitioners is a far remove from that delivered by the machines used in the 1950s and 1960s. Modern linear accelerators are capable of producing deeply penetrating photon beams that are shaped by high-attenuating tungsten collimation in space and over time, creating intricate three-dimensional (3D) distributions of the radiation dose. They may be imagined as dose clouds in concentric arrangements falling off to lesser and lesser dose levels.[1]

Intensity-modulated radiation therapy (IMRT) is a photon-based ionizing radiation treatment. IMRT was developed to improve the conformality of the dose cloud to the shape of the tumor, sparing (avoiding) the normal tissues in proximity. The underlying concept is to modify the intensity of the radiation beam as it is delivered across and around the site of the cancer. This complex planning process requires computer assistance, and hence, IMRT is almost always inverse planned, meaning that instead of designing the apertures and then calculating the resulting doses (forward planning), the desired shapes of the dose clouds (called contours) are drawn by the radiation oncologist using a 3D computed tomography (CT) scan, and the computer defines the radiation beam angles to optimize the intensity modulation so that the resultant dose cloud mimics the contours to the highest degree possible.[2]

IMRT found some of its earliest uses in prostate and head and neck cancer although its subsequent adoption in general radiation oncology practice was rapid.[3] It is estimated that IMRT is used for greater than 85% of head and neck cancer treatments across the United States, and the prevalence is similar in other developed nations. IMRT is used more frequently in head and neck cancer cases than for any other major class of cancer.[4]

This situation presents ongoing challenges, because of the complexity of IMRT. To specify the areas where the dose cloud should be delivered, the contours delineating the anatomic boundaries of the tumor mass and normal anatomic structures must be precisely drawn on the CT scan using for planning. The Hounsfield units of that CT scan are used to determine the density of the tissues (and thus to calculate the delivered dose to each small volume of the body). The radiation dose is specified in units of Gray (Gy), corresponding to 1 J of energy deposited per kilogram of material.[5] Because of the anatomic expertise needed to delineate normal and abnormal structures on the CT scan, typically incorporating margins of error of a few to several millimeters, IMRT is an order of magnitude more demanding to prescribe, at least at the tumor delineation step, than less conformal techniques. IMRT-related quality assurance of the delivered treatments and the required machine maintenance is also more demanding.[6]

However, IMRT is not the only form of radiotherapy suitable for head and neck cancers. For skin cancers or other superficially located tumors, low-penetrating photons (in the kilovoltage rather than megavoltage energy range) or electron therapy can be useful, and for well-circumscribed, physically accessible tumors, some large centers maintain an active practice of brachytherapy, or "short therapy," in which radioactive wires or seeds are introduced directly into the intended treatment volume. **Fig. 1** depicts these forms of radiation delivery.

As another alternative to IMRT, traditional conformal techniques using less conformal two-dimensional (2D) radiograph-based forward planning (eg, anterior

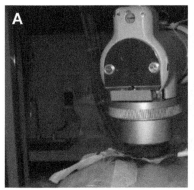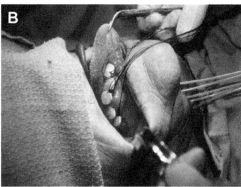

Fig. 1. (*A*) Superficial orthovoltage radiograph treatment for skin cancer. These highly effective treatments are set up based on clinical inspection and directly applied to the skin. Only thin lead shielding is required to cover the areas not intended for treatment. (*B*) High-dose-rate brachytherapy treatment of the oral tongue after an initial surgical resection. Because of minor perineural invasion and absence of other negative features, it was decided to treat the primary lateral tongue area only. The hollow catheters are inserted through the intended treatment site. A small radioactive source is fed from the computer-controlled brachytherapy unit through these catheters into the patient.

and posterior beams or opposed lateral beams) or 3D CT-based forward planning (using more beam angles to encircle the central target and achieve greater conformality) are highly effective if the normal tissues close to the treatment volume are able to tolerate high levels of radiation. Concomitant with their relative technical simplicity, these less conformal 2D or 3D techniques carry the burden of a heavier side effect profile, because more normal tissue is typically irradiated.[7,8]

Fig. 2 shows the initial delineations that are considered basic requirements in designing an IMRT treatment. According to International Commission on Radiation Units and Measurements Report 50, the gross tumor volume (GTV) encompasses all disease that can be appreciated on physical examination or radiologic imaging.[9] The clinical target volume (CTV) is the area considered to be at high risk for microscopic disease spread. The planning target volume (PTV) is an additional envelope around the CTV (to account for a few millimeters of daily patient setup and machine variance). The PTVs are fed into the computational algorithm that generates the beam angles and intensity-modulated segments that are delivered from the head of the linear accelerator machine (**Fig. 3**).

The prescribed standard dose to volumes encompassing the GTV is typically 7000 cGy over 6 to 7 weeks. For example, the recently concluded RTOG 1016 (Radiation Therapy Oncology Group 1016) protocol (a phase 3 randomized study of human papillomavirus [HPV]-associated oropharyngeal cancer) assigned, randomized patients to receive radiation therapy with either concurrent cisplatin or with concurrent cetuximab. The protocol prescription was 7000 cGy over 6 weeks, with a dose of 5600 cGy delivered to the areas of likely microscopic disease involvement and 5000 to 5250 cGy delivered to areas at very low risk for presence of tumor.

CLINICAL EVIDENCE IN SUPPORT OF HIGHLY CONFORMAL THERAPY

For the most part, radiation oncologists have considerable faith in radiation physics; a rationally derived preferred dose distribution is considered acceptable evidence of clinical superiority. Despite this tendency to embrace technological superiority in

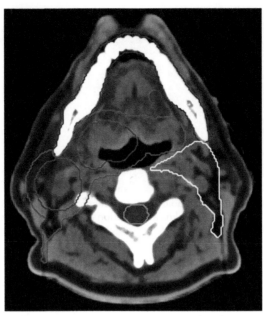

Fig. 2. Clinical target volumes (CTVs) drawn in preparation for planning an IMRT treatment. The red CTV is the highest dose area (typically prescribed to a dose in the range of 6600–7400 cGy), followed by the blue subclinical volume (typical range of 5600–6300 cGy) and the yellow elective or low-risk volume (typical range of 5000–5600 cGy). PTVs are created with a few millimeters of margin around the CTVs to account for tiny machine and setup errors; these PTVs are fed into the computer to generate the optimized algorithm of beam angles and intensity modulation to achieve the desired dose clouds.

the absence of clinically proven superiority, distinct lines of evidence support the improvements believed to result from the use of IMRT. A randomized study of patients with nasopharyngeal carcinoma[10] showed a reduction from 82% to 39% in the rates of observer-rated severe xerostomia at 1 year in the patients who received IMRT with concurrent chemotherapy, compared with those treated similarly but with 2D radiation therapy (based on grading by clinicians according to the RTOG/European Organization for Research and Treatment of Cancer [EORTC] scale). Another trial in patients with early-stage nasopharyngeal carcinoma[11] showed improvements in stimulated saliva flow rates as well as EORTC-scored quality of life at 1 year in patients treated with IMRT rather than 3D conformal radiation therapy.

It might be considered a problem that in the United States, expensive and technically demanding IMRT was adopted quickly and widely, without testing for which applications it would be best suited or when its advantages would be most profound over 3D radiation therapy. A multicenter randomized study of parotid-sparing IMRT (PARSPORT) was conducted in the United Kingdom, at a time when the implementation of IMRT was not yet universal. Thus, the PARSPORT trial was able to test these issues in a relatively technique-neutral environment. The study reported that at 12 and 24 months, IMRT produced statistically significant benefits in recovery of salivary secretion and in dry-mouth-specific and global quality of life scores.[12]

The very long-term results of IMRT have yet to be fully appreciated in realms outside xerostomia, but generally, the side effect profile seems to be positive.[13] A few institutional reports[14,15] have reported lower risks of major radiation-related complications

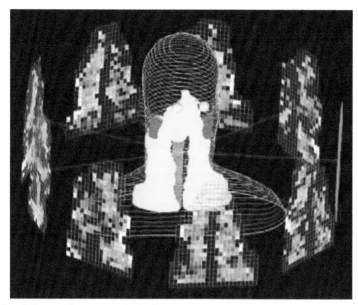

Fig. 3. The delivery of IMRT. Multiple beam angles are used, with intensity modulation carried out over each segment by opening and closing of the multileaf collimator leaves for varying amounts of time. (*From* Intensity Modulated Radiation Therapy Collaborative Working Group. Intensity-modulated radiotherapy: current status and issues of interest. Int J Radiat Oncol Biol Phys 2001;51(4):882; with permission.)

using IMRT, focusing most notably on a reduction in the rates of osteoradionecrosis. Other investigators[16,17] have proposed deployment of IMRT to reduce dose to the swallowing structures, especially the pharyngeal constrictors, in an attempt to mitigate the long-term swallowing dysfunction associated with long-term radiation-induced fibrosis of these areas. When tumor anatomy is in close apposition to the mandible or pharyngeal constrictors, it is not possible to avoid those structures even with IMRT. Furthermore, the physics of IMRT require that when dose is shifted away from a designated high-priority critical structure, there may be a price to pay elsewhere. On the other hand, a few reports now associate IMRT with novel toxicities resulting from the beam path.[18] These toxicities include nausea related to brainstem irradiation, alopecia of the posterior scalp, and oral cavity mucositis from beams passing through the mouth. Investigational efforts are under way to identify and ameliorate these IMRT-associated toxicities, potentially adding to the complexity of planning these treatments.

RESULTS OF INDUCTION AND CONCURRENT CHEMORADIATION

Induction chemotherapy before radiation therapy was developed as a successful strategy for treating moderately advanced-stage laryngeal cancer in the 1980s, most convincingly affirmed as a reasonable alternative to laryngectomy for select advanced-stage tumors in the standard-setting Veterans Administration trial.[19] Subsequently, RTOG 9111[20] compared the use of cisplatin-based chemotherapy as an induction regimen or as a concurrent radiosensitizer in combination with radiation therapy versus radiation therapy alone. Long-term follow-up confirmed the superiority of the laryngeal preservation rate obtained with concurrent chemoradiation over the other 2 approaches.

Induction chemotherapy was also used in a phase 3 randomized trial of patients with cancers of the piriform sinus, comparing initial surgery followed by adjuvant therapy with induction cisplatin and 5-fluorouracil chemotherapy followed by radiation for responders, with the result of higher overall survival in the chemotherapy arm.[21] Induction chemotherapy thus remains an acceptable initial treatment strategy for hypopharyngeal and laryngeal cancers, more so than in oropharyngeal cancers, in which induction chemotherapy has not produced clear advantages over concurrent chemoradiation, or in nasopharyngeal cancers, in which induction chemotherapy does not seem to improve outcomes, at least in the absence of more sophisticated biological assessment indices such as high levels of the Epstein-Barr viral DNA in plasma assays.[22–24] Other, more intensified induction regimens may have higher efficacy than cisplatin with 5-fluorouracil, but these have not been tested so rigorously in a randomized comparison with concurrent chemoradiation alone, and the comparative long-term toxicities are not yet known.[25]

Concurrent chemoradiotherapy is the usual recommended treatment plan for advanced-stage head and neck cancers that are not initially treated with surgery. Two early randomized studies in advanced-stage head and neck cancer reported the clear benefits of concomitant chemoradiotherapy over radiation therapy alone, and several subsequent studies specific to nasopharyngeal cancer have also shown statistically significant benefits from concurrent chemoradiation.[26–29] An influential set of meta-analyses[30] has reinforced the more impressive survival benefits derived from the use of concomitant chemoradiation regimens, with little proven benefit from induction chemotherapy schedules. However, the toxicity and morbidity of concurrent chemoradiation therapy are not trivial; systematically derived estimates based on prospective data are that the acute toxicity may be increased by 2-fold or 3-fold when concurrent systemic chemotherapy is added to a radiation-based treatment plan.[31]

UNIQUELY EVOLVING ISSUES IN OROPHARYNGEAL CARCINOMA

There is some dispute over whether the advantage of concurrent chemoradiation seen in these studies applies equally to HPV-associated oropharyngeal cancers. Large retrospective experiences at major institutions have reported excellent locoregional control (LRC) and overall survival for oropharyngeal cancers treated with radiation therapy alone.[32] In RTOG 0129[33] (a study of concurrent chemotherapy given with 2 different schedules of radiation therapy), certain classes of oropharyngeal tumors were found in a recursive partitioning analysis to confer low risk for death using HPV-positive (HPV[+]) status and a smoking history of equal to or less than 10 pack-years. These low-risk classes of tumors were similarly identified by investigators at Princess Margaret Hospital in a review of their experience with HPV(+) oropharyngeal cancers, many of which were treated with radiation alone.[34]

Particularly in view of the younger, healthier patients in this population, many believe that an excessive toxicity burden should be avoided if possible, in the interests of maximizing quality of life as well as longevity. Deintensification proposals attempting to address the issue of whether concurrent chemotherapy is required to achieve high cure rates include reduction or elimination of chemotherapy in these patients, reduction of the radiation dose, use of induction chemotherapy in combination with deintensified concurrent programs, and surgical resection followed by reduced-intensity adjuvant radiation or chemoradiation. Deintensification should be considered investigational, and applied only in the setting of a research protocol.[35]

POSTTREATMENT SURVEILLANCE

Posttreatment surveillance can be challenging in patients treated with radiation. The current National Comprehensive Cancer Network guidelines, presumably applicable to all patients with head and neck cancer, advise a single cross-sectional imaging study, then continued physical examination in the absence of symptoms.[36] This is probably a practical policy because most patients in the United States treated with either initial radiation or chemoradiation have cancers of oropharyngeal or laryngeal origin, with either low failure rates or robust surgical salvage options. Among those who have undergone resection before adjuvant therapy, the success of additional surgical or radiotherapeutic interventions is highly dependent on the conditions of the recurrence, and the requirements for imaging should be tailored accordingly.[37,38] Surveillance strategies have not been clearly established in a widely acceptable fashion for the variety of cancer types found in the head and neck. General guidelines often cannot account for the contributions of different imaging modalities and clinical setting, with resultant substantial variance in practice.[39,40]

Practically all strategies of posttreatment surveillance share the common characteristic of a high negative predictive value in the population with oropharyngeal cancer because so few patients recur.[41] On the other hand, there are clearly patients who are a higher risk for locoregional failure (such as higher T stage and N stage cancers or those with a heavy smoking history); after chemoradiation, it can be difficult to examine these patients, especially in the neck, where the examination is frustrated by edema and late-evolving fibrosis. A complex post surgical reconstruction may likewise make evaluation of the primary site highly challenging. In these patients harboring a higher risk for recurrence, continued imaging surveillance may be helpful, although present guidelines do not differentiate between these classes of risk or specify the appropriate imaging modality.[42] No trials have been able to demonstrate a quantifiable benefit from surveillance imaging in the absence of clinical signs or symptoms of recurrence.

POSTRADIATION RESECTION

The practice of consolidative or salvage neck dissection, even with findings of residual positive disease, may be beneficial to overall survival, and recent data show that patients with oropharyngeal HPV(+) cancers can achieve lengthy survival after surgery undertaken for recurrence.[43] Although the question has not been entirely answered, a purely consolidative preplanned neck dissection is believed by many to be necessary only for larger-volume residual disease that is only slowly (or not) responding after treatment ends.[44] Formerly, planned consolidative neck dissections were conducted for all patients presenting with N2-N3 disease based on the expectation that these patients remained at high risk for locoregional relapse.[45] At least in the case of oropharyngeal cancers, in most patients a residual nodal mass in the neck of a centimeter or less resolves. Additional favorable features include disease that is no longer palpable or avid on PET/CT or that shows clear response on serial physical examinations.[46,47] The rates of consolidative neck dissections have declined, although certain subclasses of patients with truly bulky initial presentation likely remain at higher risk for regional recurrence. These factors have not been clearly delineated with respect to useful practice guidelines.[48,49]

SEQUENCING OF OTHER THERAPIES AROUND SURGERY

The delivery of radiation in the postoperative setting is challenging because of patient, tumor, and treatment factors. After operation, patients typically experience impairment of nutritional status and reduced performance status. The tumor itself may show accelerated postsurgical repopulation, which imposes some degree of urgency on initiation of postoperative therapy.[50,51] The postoperative radiation planning process can be complex because of altered anatomy, which does not match the original imaging studies, as well as the delicacy of recently operated tissues, requiring additional supportive care.

Several factors are considered indications for the delivery of postoperative radiation therapy. However, it is uncertain whether combinations of minor adverse factors merit consideration for chemoradiation. An early trial at University of Texas – M.D. Anderson Cancer Center (MDACC) classified patients as lower or higher risk based on several clinicopathologic features, including T and N stage, margin status, perineural invasion, number of nodes, number of nodal groups, size of node, extracapsular extension (ECE), and direct invasion of adjacent tissues. The study did not show local-regional control (LRC) benefit for mild levels of radiation dose escalation, except for patients with ECE, who did benefit from a higher dose. However, the heterogeneity of the many assessed clinicopathologic features may have obscured any benefit of increasing dosage. The LRC at 2 to 5 years in patients declined with clusters of 2 or more risk factors, and with 4 or more minor risk factors, the LRC became similar to that obtained in patients with ECE, who experienced high rates of recurrence even with higher radiation dose.[52] To address these questions, investigators are accruing to RTOG 0920, a randomized trial of postoperative radiation therapy versus radiation therapy with concurrent cetuximab. RTOG 0920 includes patients with multiple intermediate- risk factors but excludes those with positive margins or ECE.

Another common issue in postoperative therapy is the timing of adjuvant treatment relative to resection. Timing questions were most carefully explored in another early trial.[53] This trial examined the effect of total treatment package time, starting from the initial operation date until the conclusion of postoperative radiation therapy. In the group considered at highest risk for recurrence, a total treatment package time of 11 weeks or less produced statistically significant survival advantages compared with patients who experienced a more prolonged package time. Thus, for high-risk patients to achieve a treatment package time of 11 weeks or less, including 6 weeks of radiation therapy, the patient can initiate the treatment with radiation therapy no later than the fifth week after the operation.

The factors warranting chemoradiation were established by 2 large trials simultaneously published in 2004. These 2 protocols, EORTC 22931 and RTOG 9501,[54,55] both were relatively large phase 3 randomized trials of postoperative radiation versus chemoradiation. The 2 studies reported similar improvements in LRC and overall survival, but only the European trial reported a significant difference in overall survival between the arms. This incongruence may have arisen because of the different populations enrolled in the 2 studies. When a combined analysis was performed (including data from the total population in these 2 trials), the advantage of chemoradiation was established only in patients who had positive margins or ECE.[56] As a result, patients with those strong postoperative indications are now typically treated with chemoradiation. The RTOG 1216 protocol is intended for these high-risk patients; all receive postoperative radiation and are randomized to receive a concurrent systemic regimen of cisplatin, docetaxel, or docetaxel and cetuximab.

RTOG 0024[57] studied the feasibility and safety of delivery of chemotherapy as soon as 2 weeks after surgery, based on the theory that surgical resection might itself stimulate proliferative factors in the tumor bed, leading to accelerated repopulation of the cancer cells. This regimen was reasonably well tolerated and did produce encouraging results in LRC and disease-free survival. However, this strategy was not pursued, in part because of concerns surrounding intensification in view of the potentially fragile state of the patients in the first several weeks after resection.

The delivery of preoperative radiation is seldom practiced in the United States, based on the results of RTOG 7303,[58] which showed improved LRC from the delivery of postoperative rather than preoperative radiation therapy. However, isolated centers continue to practice preoperative therapy, particularly for oral cavity cancers, and the retrospective results reported from these centers are acceptable.[59–62] There is no substantial advantage to the delivery of preoperative therapy in most settings, although it is claimed that this approach benefits from better patient tolerance to the radiation course given before surgery, immediate initiation of a therapy during the waiting time before the scheduled operation, and a theoretic advantage in reducing tumor bulk by the time of surgery. These general indications have not been established as clearly advantageous in any modern head-to-head comparisons against the current standard of postoperative radiation therapy.

Recently, a few studies have evaluated administration of chemotherapy before surgery.[63,64] None has shown survival improvements, although there seems to be a beneficial effect in obtaining negative margins. In the research setting, several so-called window trials have been initiated, using the time between consultation and the surgical procedure to deliver a short course of targeted or molecular therapy. These studies are experimental and typically are designed to explore a biological end point rather than a clinical one.

FUTURE ADVANCES IN RADIATION THERAPY

Technical advances may affect how radiation therapy is administered to patients with head and neck cancer over the next decade. Image-guided radiation therapy (IGRT) is already offered by most commercial practices. This is a generic term, which indicates that some form of real-time imaging takes place shortly before (or while) the patient is receiving an individual radiation dose, the better to ensure the exact positioning of the patient without setup errors. IGRT solutions are increasingly technically appealing and will continue to improve, although the impact on clinical outcomes will probably be limited. However, a related technology, deformable image registration (DIR) may, in combination with IGRT, result in more substantive evolution. DIR can be used to deform imaging studies to overlay them on one another or to sum a series over time. If the sites included in the imaging study are associated with anticipated or delivered radiation doses, the dose clouds can be deformed in concert with the imaging studies. It will be possible to sum associated dose clouds over a series of imaging studies that differ anatomically and thus predict excessive levels of dose delivery to critical structures in response to positional or anatomic changes (such as when the patient loses weight during the radiation therapy course). Ideally, the radiation plan would be altered, perhaps on a daily basis, in response to these undesired effects. Furthermore, magnetic resonance imaging-based solutions now in development may offer promise in their greater DIR precision. Because these technologies remain in early development, it is not yet clear what the impact on clinical outcomes will be, although the most promising improvements may be found in reducing doses to normal structures.

Several different particle therapies now have clinical commercialization. The available forms of particle therapy in clinical use include fast neutrons, protons, and carbon ions. Fast neutrons interact with atomic nuclei, producing a dense ionizing track of heavy charged particles passing through nearby tissue. The linear energy transfer of neutron therapy is dramatically higher than that of standard photon-based therapy, such as used in IMRT, and thus the destructive capability is higher. Neutron therapy was investigated successfully in cooperative group trials focused on salivary gland cancer,[65] with improvements in LRC but lingering concerns about secondary effects. Its limited indications have curtailed its widespread adoption.

Proton therapy has a biological effect that may be similar to standard photon-based therapy but offers greater conformality to the targeted areas. Proton dose plans deliver a sudden, steep gradient once they reach a specified depth within tissue (known as the Bragg peak), such that the dose that travels through the body beyond the target to the other side is dramatically less than that seen with photon therapy. Clinical experiences with proton therapy are increasing in head and neck cancer, although the most substantial experiences involve rare tumors of the skull base, such as chordoma. Further technical development is to be expected in the near future. Currently, most proton therapy centers support 3D conformal planning, although intensity-modulated proton therapy (IMPT) is being actively implemented in select clinics, and the commercial enthusiasm to develop this feature is robust. It remains to be seen to what degree 3D conformal proton therapy, or IMPT, will supplant standard IMRT.[66] The most likely advantage may be in the reduction of secondary effects attributable to the reduction of fall-off dose delivered beyond the target. However, the cost of proton therapy is high, limiting its widespread use. Special applications may be justified in cases of reirradiation or other classes of patients in whom limitation of toxicity is of paramount importance.

Although proton therapy incurs a substantial capital investment cost, carbon ion therapy is even more costly. Carbon ions share with proton therapy the properties of low fall-off dose beyond the target and high conformality, but they produce a greater biological effect estimated at 3 to 4 times that of photon-based or proton-based particle therapies. Carbon ion therapy is offered in Europe and Asia at select centers, with reported excellent outcomes. Single-institution experiences have documented impressive results in LRC of typically resistant tumors, such as adenoid cystic carcinoma.[67] Despite its desirability from a technical perspective, carbon ion therapy has not yet been widely used in the United States because of its cost and unwillingness of insurance carriers to reimburse facilities for its administration.

SUMMARY

Radiation therapy is an essential component of the multidisciplinary treatment of head and neck cancer. Improvements in surgical and radiotherapeutic techniques, refinements in the specific indications to administer radiation in combination with systemic therapies, and technological developments leading to reductions in radiation-induced secondary effects will actuate increasingly nuanced and complex deployments of radiation therapy in the future.

REFERENCES

1. Thwaites DI, Tuohy JB. Back to the future: the history and development of the clinical linear accelerator. Phys Med Biol 2006;51:R343–62.
2. Intensity Modulated Radiation Therapy Collaborative Working Group. Intensity-modulated radiotherapy: current status and issues of interest. Int J Radiat Oncol Biol Phys 2001;51:880–914.
3. Bucci MK, Bevan A, Roach M 3rd. Advances in radiation therapy: conventional to 3D, to IMRT, to 4D, and beyond. CA Cancer J Clin 2005;55:117–34.
4. Mell LK, Mehrotra AK, Mundt AJ. Intensity-modulated radiation therapy use in the US, 2004. Cancer 2005;104:1296–303.

5. Wyckoff HO, Allisy A, Liden K. The new special names of SI units in the field of ionizing radiation. Acta Radiol Ther Phys Biol 1975;14:590–1.

6. Kubicek GJ, Machtay M. New advances in high-technology radiotherapy for head and neck cancer. Hematol Oncol Clin North Am 2008;22:1165–80, viii.

7. Rusthoven KE, Raben D, Ballonoff A, et al. Effect of radiation techniques in treatment of oropharynx cancer. Laryngoscope 2008;118:635–9.

8. Lohia S, Rajapurkar M, Nguyen SA, et al. A comparison of outcomes using intensity-modulated radiation therapy and 3-dimensional conformal radiation therapy in treatment of oropharyngeal cancer. JAMA Otolaryngol Head Neck Surg 2014;140:331–7.

9. Prescribing, recording, and reporting photon-beam intensity-modulated radiation therapy (IMRT): contents. J ICRU 2010;10:NP.

10. Kam MK, Leung SF, Zee B, et al. Prospective randomized study of intensity-modulated radiotherapy on salivary gland function in early-stage nasopharyngeal carcinoma patients. J Clin Oncol 2007;25:4873–9.

11. Pow EH, Kwong DL, McMillan AS, et al. Xerostomia and quality of life after intensity-modulated radiotherapy vs conventional radiotherapy for early-stage nasopharyngeal carcinoma: initial report on a randomized controlled clinical trial. Int J Radiat Oncol Biol Phys 2006;66:981–91.

12. Nutting CM, Morden JP, Harrington KJ, et al. Parotid-sparing intensity modulated versus conventional radiotherapy in head and neck cancer (PARSPORT): a phase 3 multicentre randomised controlled trial. Lancet Oncol 2011;12:127–36.

13. Studer G, Linsenmeier C, Riesterer O, et al. Late term tolerance in head neck cancer patients irradiated in the IMRT era. Radiat Oncol 2013;8:259.

14. Ben-David MA, Diamante M, Radawski JD, et al. Lack of osteoradionecrosis of the mandible after intensity-modulated radiotherapy for head and neck cancer: likely contributions of both dental care and improved dose distributions. Int J Radiat Oncol Biol Phys 2007;68:396–402.

15. Studer G, Studer SP, Zwahlen RA, et al. Osteoradionecrosis of the mandible: minimized risk profile following intensity-modulated radiation therapy (IMRT). Strahlenther Onkol 2006;182:283–8.

16. Eisbruch A, Schwartz M, Rasch C, et al. Dysphagia and aspiration after chemoradiotherapy for head-and-neck cancer: which anatomic structures are affected and can they be spared by IMRT? Int J Radiat Oncol Biol Phys 2004;60:1425–39.

17. Roe JW, Carding PN, Dwivedi RC, et al. Swallowing outcomes following intensity modulated radiation therapy (IMRT) for head & neck cancer–a systematic review. Oral Oncol 2010;46:727–33.

18. Rosenthal DI, Chambers MS, Fuller CD, et al. Beam path toxicities to non-target structures during intensity-modulated radiation therapy for head and neck cancer. Int J Radiat Oncol Biol Phys 2008;72:747–55.

19. Induction chemotherapy plus radiation compared with surgery plus radiation in patients with advanced laryngeal cancer. The Department of Veterans Affairs Laryngeal Cancer Study Group. N Engl J Med 1991;324:1685–90.

20. Forastiere AA, Zhang Q, Weber RS, et al. Long-term results of RTOG 91–11: a comparison of three nonsurgical treatment strategies to preserve the larynx in patients with locally advanced larynx cancer. J Clin Oncol 2013;31:845–52.

21. Lefebvre JL, Chevalier D, Luboinski B, et al. Larynx preservation in pyriform sinus cancer: preliminary results of a European Organization for Research and Treatment of Cancer phase III trial. EORTC Head and Neck Cancer Cooperative Group. J Natl Cancer Inst 1996;88:890–9.

22. Chua M, Sze OW, Wee J, et al. Plasma EBV DNA as a predictive biomarker in patients with endemic nasopharyngeal carcinoma treated with induction chemotherapy and concurrent chemoradiation therapy. Int J Radiat Oncol Biol Phys 2014;90:S120–1.

23. Cohen EE, Karrison TG, Kocherginsky M, et al. Phase III randomized trial of induction chemotherapy in patients with N2 or N3 locally advanced head and neck cancer. J Clin Oncol 2014;32:2735–43.

24. Haddad R, O'Neill A, Rabinowits G, et al. Induction chemotherapy followed by concurrent chemoradiotherapy (sequential chemoradiotherapy) versus concurrent chemoradiotherapy alone in locally advanced head and neck cancer (PARADIGM): a randomised phase 3 trial. Lancet Oncol 2013;14:257–64.

25. Posner MR, Hershock DM, Blajman CR, et al. Cisplatin and fluorouracil alone or with docetaxel in head and neck cancer. N Engl J Med 2007;357:1705–15.

26. Adelstein DJ, Li Y, Adams GL, et al. An intergroup phase III comparison of standard radiation therapy and two schedules of concurrent chemoradiotherapy in patients with unresectable squamous cell head and neck cancer. J Clin Oncol 2003;21:92–8.

27. Denis F, Garaud P, Bardet E, et al. Final results of the 94-01 French Head and Neck Oncology and Radiotherapy Group randomized trial comparing radiotherapy alone with concomitant radiochemotherapy in advanced-stage oropharynx carcinoma. J Clin Oncol 2004;22:69–76.

28. Al-Sarraf M, LeBlanc M, Giri PG, et al. Chemoradiotherapy versus radiotherapy in patients with advanced nasopharyngeal cancer: phase III randomized Intergroup study 0099. J Clin Oncol 1998;16:1310–7.

29. Wee J, Tan EH, Tai BC, et al. Randomized trial of radiotherapy versus concurrent chemoradiotherapy followed by adjuvant chemotherapy in patients with American Joint Committee on Cancer/International Union against cancer stage III and IV nasopharyngeal cancer of the endemic variety. J Clin Oncol 2005;23:6730–8.

30. Pignon JP, le Maitre A, Maillard E, et al. Meta-analysis of chemotherapy in head and neck cancer (MACH-NC): an update on 93 randomised trials and 17,346 patients. Radiother Oncol 2009;92:4–14.

31. Trotti A, Pajak TF, Gwede CK, et al. TAME: development of a new method for summarising adverse events of cancer treatment by the Radiation Therapy Oncology Group. Lancet Oncol 2007;8:613–24.

32. Garden AS, Kies MS, Morrison WH, et al. Outcomes and patterns of care of patients with locally advanced oropharyngeal carcinoma treated in the early 21st century. Radiat Oncol 2013;8:21.

33. Ang KK, Harris J, Wheeler R, et al. Human papillomavirus and survival of patients with oropharyngeal cancer. N Engl J Med 2010;363:24–35.

34. O'Sullivan B, Huang SH, Siu LL, et al. Deintensification candidate subgroups in human papillomavirus-related oropharyngeal cancer according to minimal risk of distant metastasis. J Clin Oncol 2013;31:543–50.

35. Kimple RJ, Harari PM. Is radiation dose reduction the right answer for HPV-positive head and neck cancer? Oral Oncol 2014;50:560–4.

36. Pfister DG, Ang KK, Brizel DM, et al. Head and neck cancers, version 2.2013. Featured updates to the NCCN guidelines. J Natl Compr Canc Netw 2013;11:917–23.

37. Ridge JA. Squamous cancer of the head and neck: surgical treatment of local and regional recurrence. Semin Oncol 1993;20:419–29.

38. Goodwin WJ Jr. Salvage surgery for patients with recurrent squamous cell carcinoma of the upper aerodigestive tract: when do the ends justify the means? Laryngoscope 2000;110:1–18.

39. Manikantan K, Khode S, Dwivedi RC, et al. Making sense of post-treatment surveillance in head and neck cancer: when and what of follow-up. Cancer Treat Rev 2009;35:744–53.

40. Paniello RC, Virgo KS, Johnson MH, et al. Practice patterns and clinical guidelines for posttreatment follow-up of head and neck cancers: a comparison of 2 professional societies. Arch Otolaryngol Head Neck Surg 1999;125:309–13.

41. Ryan WR, Fee WE Jr, Le QT, et al. Positron-emission tomography for surveillance of head and neck cancer. Laryngoscope 2005;115:645–50.

42. Mancuso AA. The "third-best" strategy for treating head and neck cancer. AJNR Am J Neuroradiol 1999;20:1191–2.

43. Fakhry C, Zhang Q, Nguyen-Tan PF, et al. Human papillomavirus and overall survival after progression of oropharyngeal squamous cell carcinoma. J Clin Oncol 2014;32:3365–73.

44. Yao M, Hoffman HT, Chang K, et al. Is planned neck dissection necessary for head and neck cancer after intensity-modulated radiotherapy? Int J Radiat Oncol Biol Phys 2007;68:707–13.

45. McHam SA, Adelstein DJ, Rybicki LA, et al. Who merits a neck dissection after definitive chemoradiotherapy for N2-N3 squamous cell head and neck cancer? Head Neck 2003;25:791–8.

46. Soltys SG, Choi CY, Fee WE, et al. A planned neck dissection is not necessary in all patients with N2-3 head-and-neck cancer after sequential chemoradiotherapy. Int J Radiat Oncol Biol Phys 2012;83:994–9.

47. Nayak JV, Walvekar RR, Andrade RS, et al. Deferring planned neck dissection following chemoradiation for stage IV head and neck cancer: the utility of PET-CT. Laryngoscope 2007;117:2129–34.

48. Igidbashian L, Fortin B, Guertin L, et al. Outcome with neck dissection after chemoradiation for N3 head-and-neck squamous cell carcinoma. Int J Radiat Oncol Biol Phys 2010;77:414–20.

49. Brizel DM, Prosnitz RG, Hunter S, et al. Necessity for adjuvant neck dissection in setting of concurrent chemoradiation for advanced head-and-neck cancer. Int J Radiat Oncol Biol Phys 2004;58:1418–23.

50. Hofer SO, Shrayer D, Reichner JS, et al. Wound-induced tumor progression: a probable role in recurrence after tumor resection. Arch Surg 1998;133:383–9.

51. Sieweke MH, Bissell MJ. The tumor-promoting effect of wounding: a possible role for TGF-beta-induced stromal alterations. Crit Rev Oncog 1994;5:297–311.

52. Peters LJ, Goepfert H, Ang KK, et al. Evaluation of the dose for postoperative radiation therapy of head and neck cancer: first report of a prospective randomized trial. Int J Radiat Oncol Biol Phys 1993;26:3–11.

53. Ang KK, Trotti A, Brown BW, et al. Randomized trial addressing risk features and time factors of surgery plus radiotherapy in advanced head-and-neck cancer. Int J Radiat Oncol Biol Phys 2001;51:571–8.

54. Bernier J, Domenge C, Ozsahin M, et al. Postoperative irradiation with or without concomitant chemotherapy for locally advanced head and neck cancer. N Engl J Med 2004;350:1945–52.

55. Cooper JS, Pajak TF, Forastiere AA, et al. Postoperative concurrent radiotherapy and chemotherapy for high-risk squamous-cell carcinoma of the head and neck. N Engl J Med 2004;350:1937–44.

56. Bernier J, Cooper JS, Pajak TF, et al. Defining risk levels in locally advanced head and neck cancers: a comparative analysis of concurrent postoperative radiation plus chemotherapy trials of the EORTC (#22931) and RTOG (# 9501). Head Neck 2005;27:843–50.

57. Rosenthal DI, Harris J, Forastiere AA, et al. Early postoperative paclitaxel followed by concurrent paclitaxel and cisplatin with radiation therapy for patients with resected high-risk head and neck squamous cell carcinoma: report of the phase II trial RTOG 0024. J Clin Oncol 2009;27:4727–32.

58. Tupchong L, Scott CB, Blitzer PH, et al. Randomized study of preoperative versus postoperative radiation therapy in advanced head and neck carcinoma: long-term follow-up of RTOG study 73-03. Int J Radiat Oncol Biol Phys 1991; 20:21–8.

59. Puc MM, Chrzanowski FA Jr, Tran HS, et al. Preoperative chemotherapy-sensitized radiation therapy for cervical metastases in head and neck cancer. Arch Otolaryngol Head Neck Surg 2000;126:337–42.

60. Wanebo HJ, Glicksman AS, Landman C, et al. Preoperative cisplatin and accelerated hyperfractionated radiation induces high tumor response and control rates in patients with advanced head and neck cancer. Am J Surg 1995;170:512–6.

61. Klug C, Berzaczy D, Voracek M, et al. Preoperative chemoradiotherapy in the management of oral cancer: a review. J Craniomaxillofac Surg 2008;36:75–88.

62. Onizawa K, Yoshida H, Ohara K, et al. Predictive factors for the histologic response to preoperative radiotherapy in advanced oral cancer. J Oral Maxillofac Surg 2006;64:81–6.

63. Licitra L, Grandi C, Guzzo M, et al. Primary chemotherapy in resectable oral cavity squamous cell cancer: a randomized controlled trial. J Clin Oncol 2003;21: 327–33.

64. Grau JJ, Domingo J, Blanch JL, et al. Multidisciplinary approach in advanced cancer of the oral cavity: outcome with neoadjuvant chemotherapy according to intention-to-treat local therapy. A phase II study. Oncology 2002;63:338–45.

65. Laramore GE. Role of particle radiotherapy in the management of head and neck cancer. Curr Opin Oncol 2009;21:224–31.

66. Ahn PH, Lukens JN, Teo BK, et al. The use of proton therapy in the treatment of head and neck cancers. Cancer J 2014;20:421–6.

67. Kamada T, Tsujii H, Blakely EA, et al. Carbon ion radiotherapy in Japan: an assessment of 20 years of clinical experience. Lancet Oncol 2015;16:e93–100.

Systemic Therapy for Squamous Cell Carcinoma of the Head and Neck

 CrossMark

Philip Pancari, MD, Ranee Mehra, MD*

KEYWORDS

- Squamous cell head and neck cancer • Platinum chemotherapy
- Epidermal growth factor receptor • Chemoradiation

KEY POINTS

- The use of systemic therapy for squamous cell cancer of the head and neck (SCCHN) has evolved, and cytotoxic therapy is now an integral component of the combined-modality treatment of locally advanced disease.
- An increasing understanding of the molecular basis of SCCHN has led to the development of agents targeting epidermal growth factor receptor, such as cetuximab and afatinib.
- Further advances are required for the treatment human papillomavirus–negative disease, which often is associated with a poor prognosis.

SYSTEMIC THERAPY FOR LOCALIZED DISEASE
Definitive Chemotherapy with Radiation

Meta-analyses evaluating the efficacy of multimodality approaches to the treatment of squamous cell cancer of the head and neck (SCCHN) have consistently supported concurrent chemoradiation (CCRT), reporting an improved overall survival (OS) of 8% to 11% in both surgically resectable and unresectable patients.[1] However, higher locoregional dose density delivered with CCRT results, predictably, in a higher degree of regional toxicity, including severe mucositis with associated pain and diminished nutritional intake.[2,3] Despite the demonstrated regional control and survival benefits, analysis of failure patterns has not demonstrated consistent decline in distant metastasis with CCRT in comparison with radiotherapy alone.[4] Similarly, studies of induction chemotherapy, followed by chemoradiation, have failed to improve survival or decrease the risk of distant metastases.[5,6]

Employee of GSK. Consulting Novartis, Bayer, Genentech.
Department of Medical Oncology, Fox Chase Cancer Center, 333 Cottman Avenue, Philadelphia, PA 19111, USA
* Corresponding author.
E-mail address: Ranee.Mehra@fccc.edu

Thus, for locally advanced cancers of the head and neck, definitive CCRT is the current treatment standard.

Long-term results of a trial evaluating the contribution of platinum-based chemotherapy added to radiotherapy demonstrated a significant improvement in locoregional control (LRC) and larynx preservation compared with either induction chemotherapy or radiation therapy alone.[7,8] Locoregional failure has traditionally been the predominant manner of recurrence; nearly 90% of patients who present with distant metastasis also harbor concurrent locoregional cancer.[9] CCRT has become an essential component of the treatment paradigm in patients with potentially curable disease. Disease-free survival (DFS) was demonstrated in the Radiation Therapy Oncology Group (RTOG) 91-11 study[8] to be significantly prolonged in patients who received CCRT compared with radiotherapy alone (5-year OS and DFS were 22% and 27% vs 16% and 15%, respectively). There were disconcerting late deaths after CCRT that were not readily explained by tumor or treatment toxicity.

Single-Agent Platinum-Based Therapy

For patients in whom the primary site of malignancy is truly unresectable, OS after standard single-modality local radiotherapy was measured at less than 25%.[10,11] A phase III randomized trial conducted by the Head and Neck Intergroup from 1982 to 1987 compared radiotherapy alone to CCRT with weekly cisplatin at 20 mg/m^2.[12] The median survival of 13 months did not differ significantly between the two treatment arms, and the CCRT regimen was not adopted. This study was followed in 1987 by an RTOG phase II trial evaluating the efficacy of concurrent radiation and high-dose cisplatin, using a dose of 100 mg/m^2 given every 21 days. This schedule yielded a complete response (CR) in 71% of patients, with a 4-year survival of 34%.[13] The results suggested dose dependency of the observed improvement in response and survival, and the study was followed in 1992 by a second-generation trial by the Head and Neck Intergroup.[14]

This phase III Intergroup trial compared radiotherapy alone with 2 different schedules of chemoradiotherapy in patients with locally unresectable disease. The first regimen used concurrent high-dose cisplatin and radiation (the RTOG regimen, 100 mg/m^2 on days 1, 22, and 43), and the second involved a split course of single-daily fractionated radiation and 3 cycles of concurrent infusional 5-fluorouracil (5-FU) plus bolus cisplatin (cisplatin at 75 mg/m^2 given every 4 weeks). With a median follow-up of 41 months, the 3-year projected OS for patients receiving high-dose cisplatin-based chemoradiation was 37% compared with 23% for those in the arm receiving radiotherapy alone ($P = .014$). The addition of concurrent single-agent cisplatin at 100 mg/m^2 significantly improved survival over radiotherapy alone. Toxicities of grade 3 or greater occurred in 89% of patients receiving high-dose cisplatin, predominantly mucositis with dysphagia (43 of 95 patients), leukopenia (40 of 95 patients), and to a lesser extent nausea with vomiting.

Patients receiving high-dose cisplatin are at risk of auditory toxicity, for which they may be monitored with serial comprehensive hearing tests during the course of therapy. This approach is warranted for such symptoms as diminished auditory acuity or tinnitus. Patients receiving CCRT with cisplatin also require regular assessment and repletion of volume status, particularly during high-dose therapy, to minimize renal complications from potential insults, including direct cisplatin-induced nephrotoxicity and prerenal insufficiency secondary to diminished oral fluid and nutritional intake. Patients typically receive liberal amounts of intravenous fluid immediately surrounding each cisplatin administration (approximately 2.5 L), and frequently require additional intravenous hydration during the course of each 21-day cycle. Many continue to benefit from intravenous hydration for several weeks after formal completion of the course of therapy.

For patients unable to tolerate high-dose cisplatin at baseline, or for those who require a dose alteration during the course of definitive CCRT, an acceptable consideration is transition to a weekly cisplatin dosing schedule using either 30 mg/m^2 or 40 mg/m^2 (category 2B as per National Comprehensive Cancer Network guidelines).[15] This regimen has been shown to achieve a high rate of LRC and survival (demonstrated 2-year OS of 67% with a median relapse-free survival time of 31 months).[16] However, no randomized phase III trials compare high dosing with weekly dosing in the definitive locally advanced setting.

Agents Targeting Epidermal Growth Factor Receptor Combined with Radiation

The epidermal growth factor receptor (EGFR) is expressed at very high levels in most SCCHN.[17] EGFR is activated by several ligands including the epidermal growth factor (EGF), or transforming growth factor α, resulting in a signal transduction cascade leading to tumorigenic activity such as resistance to apoptosis and transcription of proangiogenic proteins. The RTOG 90-03 trial demonstrated that high EGFR expression measured by immunohistochemistry was associated with a higher risk of both locoregional recurrence and death in comparison with tumors with EGFR expression below the median.[18] Preclinical data show synergy between EGFR inhibition and radiation, prompting further study of this class of agents.[19,20]

Cetuximab

Cetuximab is an immunoglobulin G1 (IgG1) EGFR-targeting monoclonal antibody which, like cisplatin, has been demonstrated to improve both LRC and survival when added to definitive radiation therapy in the treatment of patients with locally advanced head and neck cancer.[21] When cetuximab was initially investigated, CCRT had not yet been established as the standard of care, so EGFR-targeted therapy was initially compared with radiotherapy alone rather than with cisplatin-based CCRT. A phase III randomized clinical trial conducted by Bonner and colleagues[21,22] randomized patients to either radiotherapy alone or radiotherapy plus cetuximab (400 mg/m^2 loading dose followed by 7 weekly doses at 250 mg/m^2). The primary end point was local tumor control, and OS was included within the secondary end points. The updated median OS at long-term follow-up in 2009 was reported as 49.0 months (95% confidence interval [CI] 32.8–69.5) in the combined-modality arm, compared with 29.3 months (95% CI 20.6–41.4) for those receiving radiotherapy alone. This result appears to represent a significant improvement over historical data. Development of the common cetuximab-associated acneiform rash of grade 2 or greater severity was associated with a significant improvement in OS compared with those who developed either no rash or a grade 1 rash (hazard ratio [HR] 0.49, 95% CI 0.34–0.72; P = 002), suggesting that this toxicity may serve as an early indicator of outcome. However, in the absence of level 1 evidence from a phase III noninferiority trial demonstrating equivalence, cisplatin remains the agent of choice for fit patients receiving chemoradiation for locally advanced SCCHN.

Cetuximab constitutes a form of targeted therapy using a mechanism markedly different from that of traditional cytotoxic therapy, so it was hypothesized that its combination with platinum-based CCRT might act synergistically to improve survival in the locally advanced setting. This question was addressed in RTOG-0522, a phase III clinical trial that compared results of cisplatin-based CCRT with or without cetuximab.[23] Published in 2014, results failed to meet either the primary end point of improved progression-free survival (PFS) or the secondary end points of prolonged OS, improved LRC, and decreased incidence of distant metastasis. Furthermore, patients receiving the added cetuximab had a greater number of high-grade toxicities, primarily an increase in grade 3 to 4 acneiform rash and radiation dermatitis. Thus there would seem to be no benefit from cetuximab and platinum-based therapy with radiation in the curative setting.

Panitumumab

Additional EGFR inhibitors investigated in the locally advanced setting include panitumumab, which differs from cetuximab in that it is fully humanized and is based on an IgG2 isotype (potentially affecting its mechanism of action). A phase II randomized trial of CCRT with or without panitumumab in patients with stage III, IVA, or IVB disease (CONCERT-1) reported disappointing results in 2012.[24] The 2-year LRC rate (95% CI) was found to be 61% (50%–71%) for CCRT plus panitumumab, versus 68% (54%–78%) for CCRT alone. PFS events occurred in 40% of the panitumumab group and 35% of the standard CCRT arm, whereas death occurred in 36% of the patients in the experimental arm compared with 24% in the control arm. Like RTOG-0522, this was considered a negative study. The addition of panitumumab demonstrated no increase in efficacy compared with standard platinum-based CCRT alone. Toxicities worsened along with the addition of this EGFR-inhibitor in a manner similar to those noted with the addition of cetuximab: grade 3 or higher adverse events (AEs) occurred in 85% of patients in the experimental arm versus 68% in the control arm, primarily mucosal inflammation (55% vs 24%), radiation skin toxicity (28% vs 13%), dysphagia (40% vs 27%), and acneiform rash (11% vs 0%).

As already noted, no formal completed phase III study compares cisplatin-based CCRT with radiotherapy plus EGFR-inhibitor therapy for locally advanced disease. RTOG 10-16 has pursued this question with cetuximab, and a phase II randomized trial (CONCERT-II) has recently been conducted comparing panitumumab plus radiotherapy with standard high-dose platinum-based CCRT.[25] LRC was the primary end point, with results revealing a 2-year LRC rate of 61% among patients assigned to standard CCRT compared with 51% among patients assigned to panitumumab plus radiotherapy. Secondary end points included OS, which also favored the CCRT group (HR 1.59, 95% CI 0.91–2.79). AEs of grade 3 or higher were again notable for greater skin toxicity in the experimental arm, with such AEs affecting 85% of the panitumumab arm versus a slightly lower 81% of the standard CCRT arm. The patients receiving cisplatin-based therapy experienced more neutropenia and febrile neutropenia, whereas grade 3 or higher neutropenia was absent in the panitumumab arm. The study revealed a significant worsening of outcome for those patients receiving panitumumab in lieu of standard platinum-based CCRT.

Lapatinib

Lapatinib is an oral agent that targets multiple transmembrane receptors within the EGFR family, and has been investigated as a potential agent in the treatment of head and neck cancers. It is a selective and potent inhibitor of the tyrosine kinase domains of HER2 and EGFR, with preclinical data demonstrating the potential inhibition of HER2 in SCCHN cell lines and within xenograft mouse models.[26] In addition, breast cancer cell lines treated with lapatinib have decreased levels of phosphorylated Akt and ERK1/2, with termination of proliferative signals, consequent growth arrest, and apoptosis.[27]

Two phase II studies demonstrated modest clinical activity of single-agent lapatinib, one in the recurrent/metastatic setting[28] and the other as induction therapy before definitive chemoradiation.[29] A phase II study of definitive chemoradiotherapy with or without oral lapatinib (1500 mg daily) in patients with stage III to IVB squamous cell carcinoma of the head and neck, followed by maintenance lapatinib or placebo, suggested a statistically significant investigator-assessed improvement in complete response rate (CRR) in the lapatinib arm compared with placebo (50% vs 24%, $P = .009$).[30] With independent assessment, however, the improvement in CRR did not achieve statistical significance (53% vs 36%, $P = .093$). Other reported outcomes included improved PFS with addition of lapatinib to 35.3 months (compared with 12.1 months in the control arm; HR 0.74, $P = .184$) and an HR for OS of 0.9 ($P = .382$). Although the latter measures did not meet statistical significance, the HPV-negative population experienced an improved PFS in favor of the addition of lapatinib (median PFS = not reached vs 10.3 months). Recent and currently ongoing trials include a phase II study (RTOG 3501: TRYHARD trial) combining lapatinib with platinum-based CCRT in patients with human papillomavirus (HPV)-negative (HPV(−)) disease,[31] and a phase II study combining lapatinib with carboplatin and paclitaxel in the induction setting before surgery followed by risk-guided adjuvant therapy.[32]

Combination Cytotoxic Therapy

Multiagent systemic regimens as a component of definitive CCRT in the locally advanced and unresectable setting have been studied, reporting excellent outcomes. Although cisplatin remains the current standard of care, phase III trials in favor of the concurrent chemoradiotherapy approach have been conducted with multiagent regimens.[33–36] The phase III Intergroup trial compared standard radiotherapy and 2 different schedules of CCRT in patients with unresectable disease.[14] The results of this study favored the single-agent cisplatin arm (versus cisplatin and infusion of 5-FU), although the radiation therapy schedule deviated significantly from the standard at that time.

An additional phase III randomized trial of 2 cisplatin-based CCRT regimens for locally advanced disease (cisplatin vs cisplatin plus 5-FU) concluded that the outcomes were similar (primary end point of recurrence-free survival at 2 years was 94% in the cisplatin arm versus 88% in the in the cisplatin/5-FU arm; $P = .86$).[37] The toxicity profile differed considerably between the two arms, suggesting that the choice of regimen may hinge on this difference.

Carboplatin/5-fluorouracil

Citing the overall poor results of radiotherapy alone for locally advanced oropharyngeal carcinomas, the French Head and Neck Oncology and Radiotherapy Group (GORTEC) initiated in 1994 a phase III randomized clinical trial evaluating the benefit of CCRT with a combination of carboplatin and 5-FU compared with radiotherapy alone. The 5-year results were reported in 2004.[36] OS was 22% in the multiagent CCRT arm compared with 16% in the radiotherapy arm ($P = .05$). DFS was also improved in the CCRT arm (27% vs 15%; $P = .01$), as was the rate of LRC (48% vs 25%; $P = .002$). Late grade III or IV toxicities were not increased in the CCRT arm when compared with the arm receiving radiotherapy alone (56% vs 30%; P not significant), although there was a trend toward increased toxicity.

Hemoglobin (Hgb) level in patients before treatment was found to be one of the most important factors for shortened survival, with an Hgb level of less than 12.5 g/dL associated with a 92% rate of death within 2 years (OR 10.36, 95% CI 3.07–34.97; $P<.0001$). This factor was found to be more prognostic than either the presence of stage IV disease (vs stage III) or randomization to the radiotherapy arm. Based on the hypothesis that correction of anemia would decrease tumor hypoxia and thus enhance response to therapy, a review of 5 randomized controlled trials (1397 patients) was undertaken, which concluded that the addition of erythropoietin to CCRT actually results in an adverse effect on outcomes.[38]

Platinum plus paclitaxel

To further explore the role of multiagent CCRT in the locally advanced setting, the RTOG conducted a 3-arm randomized phase II trial (RTOG 97-03) comparing outcomes with 3 doublet regimens in combination with radiotherapy.[39] Eligible patients had stage III or IV squamous cell carcinoma (SCC) of the oral cavity, oropharynx, or hypopharynx, and received either weekly cisplatin (20 mg/m^2) plus paclitaxel (30 mg/m^2), cisplatin (10 mg/m^2) plus fluorouracil (400 mg/m^2 continuous infusion for the final 10 days of treatment), or hydroxyurea (1 g every 12 hours) plus fluorouracil (800 mg/m^2/d infusion with each fraction of radiation).

The investigators reported an estimated 2-year DFS of 51.3% and OS of 66.6% for the arm receiving CCRT with weekly cisplatin plus paclitaxel. The number of patients in this arm who completed the scheduled radiotherapy was 83%, and 66% received both drugs for the entire prescribed course. The CR rate in the platinum-taxane arm was 82%, with only 27.5% (95% CI 17.4–37.6) of patients experiencing locoregional failure at 2 years (compared with 41.1% and 40.8% in the other 2 arms, respectively). Analysis of first-failure patterns revealed a lower percentage of patients with persistent local disease in the platinum-taxane arm, and a decreased number of patients with regional nodal relapse. The incidence of grade 3 or greater toxicity in this arm was measured at 87%, which proved very similar to the 89% reported by the Head and Neck Intergroup with high-dose single-agent cisplatin-based CCRT.[14] Overall, all 3 approaches with multiagent CCRT were feasible.

5-Fluorouracil plus hydroxyurea

As one of the regimens used in RTOG 97-03, patients received a single 5-FU dose of 800 mg/m^2 with each fraction of radiotherapy rather than a prolonged infusion. In contrast to standard continuous daily treatment, this was an every-other-week regimen. Hydroxyurea was administered at 1 g twice per day throughout the course of treatment. The 2-year OS for this group was estimated at 69% (range 59.0%–79.8%), which was slightly higher than that for the platinum-taxane arm, and 2-year DFS was estimated at 49%, which was comparatively slightly lower. Although these outcomes were similar (including estimated survival), the rate of estimated locoregional failure was reported to be 41% (95% CI 29.6–51.9), which compared unfavorably with the 28% reported in the platinum-taxane group. Hematologic toxicity of grade 3 or higher in the 5-FU plus hydroxyurea group was reported in 44% of patients. In view of the similar rates of OS and DFS when compared with platinum-based therapy, this is an acceptable and recommended CCRT regimen along with cisplatin-paclitaxel and carboplatin–5-FU for the definitive treatment of locally advanced SCCHN. Additional trials have investigated the backbone of 5-FU, hydroxyurea, and hyperfractionated radiation with taxanes, cetuximab, and bevacizumab.[40–42] These combinations are active, but at the expense of elevated acute toxicity.

Considerations for the Definitive Treatment of Locally Advanced Human Papillomavirus–Positive Disease

Patients with human papillomavirus–positive (HPV(+))-associated SCCHN have different patterns of disease progression, and a better prognosis. Investigators from the Eastern Cooperative Oncology Group (ECOG) conducted a planned analysis of a prospective trial of induction chemotherapy followed by chemoradiation to determine the impact of HPV status on prognosis.[43] This study was one of the first to establish the superior prognosis of HPV(+) patients, with a 2-year survival of 95% ($P = .005$). An additional retrospective analysis published in 2010 explored the association between tumor HPV status and survival among stage III or IV patients with oropharyngeal cancer treated with cisplatin-based CCRT, and found tumor HPV status to be a strong and independent prognostic factor for survival.[44] After adjustment for age, tumor and nodal stage, race, tobacco exposure, and treatment randomization, there was a 58% reduction in the risk of death over a 3-year period (HR 0.42, 95% CI 0.27–0.66).

HPV(+) patients typically present with oropharyngeal malignancy at a younger age than those who are HPV(−), making the long-term toxicities of definitive therapy for those with potentially cured disease of even greater importance than for patients whose cancer is caused by substance abuse. As HPV(+) disease now represents at least 60% of new diagnoses of squamous cell oropharyngeal cancers, amelioration of toxicity has received considerable attention.

One area of recent investigation has aimed to determine whether the standard dose of radiotherapy during CCRT may be safely lowered in HPV-associated disease without adverse outcomes. ECOG 1308 was a phase II trial evaluating reduced-dose intensity-modulated radiation therapy (IMRT) in HPV-associated resectable oropharyngeal SCCs among patients who derived a clinical complete response (cCR) to platinum-based induction chemotherapy.[45] The investigators hypothesized that reduced-dose IMRT given at 54 Gy (representing a 23% reduction to the standard dose) with ongoing weekly cetuximab could maintain a high rate of LRC and a 2-year PFS of at least 85% in patients with stage III, IVa, or IVb HPV(+) disease who had achieved a cCR to induction chemotherapy with paclitaxel (90 mg/m^2 on days 1, 15, 18), cisplatin (75 mg/m^2 on day 1), and cetuximab. At a median follow-up of 23 months, lower-dose radiotherapy had achieved a PFS of 84% and a 2-year survival rate of 95%. In patients with a less than 10-year smoking history and T1-3 N0-2b disease, the PFS was 96%. Patients with lower PFS and OS included those with greater than 10-pack-year smoking history, T4 stage, and advanced N2c nodal stage. Late toxicities with this approach were reported as minimal. These results demonstrated that reduced-dose IMRT in patients with chemoresponsive disease can produce very high tumor control rates, although this does not represent a current standard of care. Phase III comparative studies are warranted.

Although EGFR expression is not predictive of sensitivity to EGFR inhibition, the lower EGFR expression noted in p16-positive tumors has raised questions regarding the activity of cetuximab in HPV(+) disease.[46,47] RTOG 1016, a phase III trial of radiotherapy plus cetuximab versus cisplatin and radiotherapy in HPV(+) oropharynx cancer, has completed accrual and should demonstrate how the HPV(+) population responds to cetuximab and radiation. If substitution of EGFR-directed therapy for cisplatin affords comparable DFS and OS (with lower toxicity), there will be a strong argument for its use.

POSTOPERATIVE CHEMORADIATION FOR SQUAMOUS CELL CANCER OF THE HEAD AND NECK
Platinum-Based Adjuvant Chemoradiotherapy

Primary surgical resection of locally advanced SCCHN followed by adjuvant radiotherapy is associated with locoregional recurrence rates as high as 30% and 5-year OS rates as low as 40%.[48] Hence, trials have evaluated the efficacy of chemotherapy administered concomitantly with radiation therapy in the postoperative setting. In the absence of widely adopted criteria defining high-risk disease, Cooper and colleagues[49] recalled observations from RTOG 85-03 and RTOG 88-24 to select disease characteristics associated with a high incidence of locoregional recurrence, high rates of development of distant metastasis, and high risk of death at 5 years. The inclusion criteria for RTOG 95-01,[50] a phase III trial comparing adjuvant radiation alone with adjuvant chemoradiation, therefore included any of: histologically evident invasion of at least 2 regional lymph nodes; extracapsular extension (ECE) of nodal disease; and microscopically involved mucosal margins of resection.

Initial reported results from RTOG 95-01 revealed an improvement in the primary end point of LRC within the adjuvant concurrent CCRT arm (HR 0.61, 95% CI 0.41–0.91; P = .01). DFS was also significantly prolonged with adjuvant CCRT (HR 0.78, 95% CI 0.61–0.99; P = .04). However, at the time of initial study publication in 2004, a trend toward improved OS with combined-modality adjuvant therapy was not considered significant. After a minimum follow-up period of 10 years, the investigators examined long-term outcomes in 2012.[51] This more recent analysis yielded discrepant results, with a loss of the statistically significant benefit to locoregional failure rates (29% vs 22%; P = .10) and a now-insignificant difference in DFS (19% vs 20%; P = .25). The difference in OS remained insignificant.

However, an unplanned subset analysis had been undertaken, which revealed significant benefits of adjuvant CCRT for patients with selected high-risk features. Patients with a history of microscopic disease at the surgical margin, nodal extracapsular spread of disease, or some combination of these 2 findings displayed a locoregional failure rate of only 21% (compared with 33% in the arm that had received adjuvant radiotherapy alone; P = .02). The secondary end point of DFS was also improved with adjuvant CCRT within this same subset (18% vs 12%; P = .05), and the OS benefit bordered on significant (27% vs 19%; P = .07). The subset of patients enrolled only on the basis of histologic nodal invasion ($\geq$2 nodes) did not benefit from the addition of chemotherapy to adjuvant management.

The long-term analysis described aligned the findings of RTOG 95-01 with the initial results of the similarly designed European Organization for Research and Treatment of Cancer (EORTC) 22931 trial, which differed most notably by an alternative definition of "high risk" for the purposes of eligibility. These characteristics included microscopic tumor at the surgical margin, extracapsular extension of nodal disease, clinical involvement of lymph nodes at levels IV or V (for oral or oropharyngeal SCCs), perineural disease, and/or vascular embolism. The criterion of 2 or greater histologically involved lymph nodes was notably absent. The EORTC reported marked improvement in both LRC and DFS, in addition to a significant OS improvement (P = .02).[52] CCRT has significant advantages over radiotherapy alone in the adjuvant setting for high-risk disease (defined as extracapsular extension and microscopic disease at the resection margin).[53] In practice, most head and neck specialists administer CCRT for any involved margin, not simply those of the mucosa.

Non–Platinum-Based Adjuvant Chemoradiotherapy

Recent investigations have focused on incorporation of cetuximab and taxanes into the adjuvant combined-modality setting. The phase II RTOG-0234 study limited enrollment to patients with stage III to IV SCCHN and at least 1 of several specified high-risk features including positive surgical margins, ECE, or 2 or more nodal metastases.[54] Owing to previously identified potent radiosensitizing properties of docetaxel in the primary treatment of SCCHN,[55] the investigators examined the efficacy of radiotherapy concomitant with either combined weekly cetuximab plus docetaxel (15 mg/m^2/wk) or weekly cetuximab plus cisplatin (30 mg/m^2/wk). At a median follow-up of 4.4 years, 2-year OS was 69% for the group receiving cisplatin-based therapy and 79% for the group receiving docetaxel. Reported 2-year DFS also favored the docetaxel arm (56% vs 66%), with both OS and DFS significantly improved over 4-year-old RTOG historical controls.

Failure patterns in RTOG-0234 differed between the two arms. The predominant benefit of docetaxel seems to arise from reduction in the incidence of distant metastasis (13% at 2 years in the docetaxel-containing arm vs 25% in the cisplatin-containing arm). p16-positive (a proxy for HPV-associated) oropharyngeal tumors demonstrated markedly improved survival over p16-negative tumors, which was true regardless of treatment, although the benefit appeared greater in the cisplatin arm. There was a greater incidence of grade 3 or 4 myelosuppression on the cisplatin arm (28%) in comparison with the docetaxel arm (14%), with overall similar rates of high-grade mucositis. This combination is the subject of RTOG-1216, a 3-arm phase II/III clinical trial of surgery and postoperative radiation delivered with concurrent cisplatin versus docetaxel versus docetaxel and cetuximab for high-risk SCCHN. Pending the reporting of phase II/III data, platinum-based adjuvant CCRT remains the standard of care.

Considerations Regarding Induction Chemotherapy

Although chemotherapy has been adopted as a standard component of both definitive CCRT and adjuvant CCRT following primary surgical resection, controversy surrounds its benefit when administered in the induction setting. Cisplatin-based therapy is capable of producing excellent responses (as high as 80%) in treatment-naïve patients with locally advanced SCCHN.[56] The CR rate in this setting has been reported to be as high as 50%. In view of the apparent chemosensitivity of untreated SCCHN, investigation of induction (neoadjuvant) systemic regimens for both tumor downstaging and eradication of distant micrometastases has been undertaken. The Meta-Analysis of Chemotherapy in Head and Neck Cancer (MACH-NC) found no significant increase in OS with the addition of induction chemotherapy to the local modalities of surgery and radiotherapy among 93 randomized trials.[1] On examination of the subset of trials that specifically utilized PF (cisplatin and 5-FU), a 3% improvement in survival was observed (HR 0.88, 95% CI 0.79–0.97). Several phase III trials then investigated the addition of a taxane to cisplatin and 5-FU, ultimately establishing the triple-agent combination of docetaxel, cisplatin, and 5-FU (TPF) as the superior induction regimen.[57]

The TPF induction strategy has been compared with CCRT in several phase III randomized trials, 2 of which have reinforced the current standard of CCRT alone. The DeCIDE trial compared TPF induction followed by concurrent CCRT with multiagent CCRT alone (with concurrent docetaxel, 5-FU, and hydroxyurea) in patients in N2/N3 SCCHN. This study revealed a significant decrease in the incidence of distant failure in the induction arm (HR 0.46, 95% CI 0.23–0.92; $P = .025$), but there was no significant improvement in OS (HR 0.92, 95% CI 0.59–1.42; $P = .70$).[5] This trial was criticized for the lack of platinum in the control arm. The phase III Paradigm trial used single-agent cisplatin-based CCRT and compared this with the same treatment after induction TPF. Accrual was terminated in 2008 because of slow enrollment. Of the 145 patients enrolled, there was no benefit in 3-year OS from the inclusion of induction therapy (HR 1.09, 95% CI 0.59–2.03; $P = .77$), and PFS did not differ.[6] Future perspectives are maintaining focus on the potential eradication of micrometastases with resultant survival benefit. Recent investigational approaches have explored the addition of other agents to platinum-based induction regimens, such as EGFR inhibitors or antiangiogenic therapy. TPF is the regimen of choice if induction therapy is used, but its application is not supported by results of clinical trials.

PALLIATIVE SYSTEMIC THERAPY FOR RECURRENT AND METASTATIC DISEASE
First-Line Treatment

The prognosis for recurrent/metastatic SCCHN is dismal. Historically, the most common regimens for recurrent/metastatic SCCHN included cisplatin plus 5-FU, cisplatin plus a taxane, or single-agent methotrexate, with unproven survival benefits.[58–60] Burtness and colleagues[61] studied the role of cetuximab plus cisplatin in the first-line treatment of incurable advanced SCCHN (E5397). In this study, 117 patients were randomized to either cisplatin (100 mg/m^2 every 4 weeks) with placebo or cisplatin with cetuximab (400 mg/m^2 loading dose followed by 250 mg/m^2 weekly). There was a statistically significant improvement in response rate from 10% to 26% with the addition of cetuximab ($P = .03$) and a trend toward a benefit in OS from 8 to 9.2 months. The 1-year survival rates for the cisplatin plus cetuximab and cisplatin plus placebo arms were 39% and 32%, respectively. This insignificant survival difference was attributed to a lack of power in the study design and permission required to cross over to cetuximab after progressing on the placebo arm.

Subsequently, in the first-line EXTREME trial, 442 patients with recurrent or metastatic SCCHN were randomized to a standard platinum-containing doublet with or without cetuximab; cross-over was not allowed.[46] The chemotherapy regimen used was platinum (cisplatin at 100 mg/m^2 or carboplatin at area under the curve 5 on day 1) in combination with 5-FU 1000 mg/m^2 on days 1 to 4 for a maximum of 6 cycles. Patients who were randomized to cetuximab with chemotherapy could continue with maintenance cetuximab until progression. The chemotherapy with cetuximab combination resulted in a statistically significant improvement in survival from 7.4 to 10.1 months ($P = .036$). In a subset analysis, there was a greater benefit for patients younger than 65 years, with better performance status, and for those who received cisplatin as opposed to carboplatin. These data established the role of cetuximab in first-line therapy for advanced SCCHN when given in combination with cisplatin and 5-FU, and EXTREME was the first trial to show that systemic treatment conferred a survival benefit in the palliative setting.

The equivalence of the doublet regimens, including either platinum plus a taxane or 5-FU, was established by ECOG, so it is considered standard to combine cetuximab with either of these backbones.[62]

Beyond First Line

The antitumor activity of cetuximab in patients with recurrent SCCHN that was evident in early phase I investigations[63,64] provided the impetus to study cetuximab in the platinum-refractory population, which historically had a very poor prognosis. One multicenter phase II trial treated 96 patients with platinum-refractory disease with cetuximab while continuing platinum therapy.[65] This approach resulted in a 10% response rate with a disease control rate of 53%, median time to progression of 2.8 months, and OS of 6 months. In a similar phase II study, 130 patients with stable disease (SD) or progressive disease (PD) on previous platinum therapy received treatment with cetuximab and cisplatin.[66] Again, responses were noted in both groups with median survival of 11.7 months (SD group), and 6.1 months and 4.3 months, respectively in 2 PD cohorts. These studies indicated that cetuximab was an active agent. A landmark phase II study by Vermorken and colleagues[67] enrolled 103 patients who progressed after platinum-based therapies and treated them with single-agent cetuximab as a monotherapy; they reported a response rate of 12.6%, disease control rate of 46%, and median OS of 5.8 months. At the time, the historical response rate to second-line chemotherapy in SCCHN was 2.5%, with an OS of 3.4 months; thus this seemingly modest activity for cetuximab monotherapy was notable.[68,69]

In a phase II trial in the second-line setting, 84 patients received cetuximab and docetaxel (35 mg/m^2 on days 1, 8, and 15 of a 4-week cycle) with a response rate of 12%, PFS of 4 months, and OS of 7 months.[70]

The toxicity of cetuximab in the palliative setting is similar to that in the curative treatment setting. It causes significant grade 4 infusion reactions in a minority (~3%) of patients; the incidence is higher in the southeastern United States.[71,72] The most common toxicity of cetuximab occurs in the skin, with a characteristic acne-like pustular rash often accompanied by xerosis, nail changes, paronychia, and digital fissuring. This rash is routinely managed with emollients, topical glucocorticoids, and oral antibiotics such as doxycycline and minocycline. Hypomagnesemia is another common toxicity related to cetuximab, resulting from inhibition of magnesium reabsorption in the ascending loop of Henle, a direct consequence of EGFR blockade in the kidney. Monitoring and repletion of potassium and magnesium is necessary in patients receiving cetuximab, especially on a long-term basis.

In the third-line setting the prognosis is dismal. For instance, the activity of methotrexate, which is considered to be a standard option, is only documented to be 4% with a median OS of 6.7 months in the advanced population.[73] Oral small-molecule EGFR inhibitors also have been studied, but in the same randomized trial the response rate and OS for gefitinib 250 mg/500 mg were also both unimpressive, at 2.7%/7.6% and 5.6/6 months, respectively. Afatinib, an oral anilino-quinazoline derivative that, unlike gefitinib, binds irreversibly to EGFR, also has activity against the HER2 and ErbB4 receptors.[74,75] In patients with advanced, platinum-refractory SCCHN (n = 121), afatinib 50 mg was shown to have efficacy comparable with that of cetuximab: response rate 8.1% (afatinib) versus 9.7% (cetuximab) by independent review, and PFS 13 weeks (afatinib) versus 15 weeks (cetuximab).[76,77] Cross-over after initial progression provided data regarding the efficacy of these agents in sequence, with a higher disease control rate and stage II PFS in the patients who transitioned from cetuximab to afatinib at progression. A phase III trial comparing afatinib with methotrexate met its primary end point of PFS (2.6 months [afatinib] vs 1.7 months [methotrexate]; $P = .03$).[78] Disease control rate was also greater in the afatinib group, although this did not translate to a significant improvement in OS. Thus, it remains to be seen how afatinib will be used in the treatment of platinum-refractory advanced disease.

CURRENT INVESTIGATIONAL APPROACHES

The advent of immunotherapy and a wider selection of targeted agents with a greater awareness of genetic alterations in SCCHN are fueling clinical trials, in particular for patients with advanced disease. The heterogeneous genomic milieu in SCCHN had few specific oncogenic drivers that are responsive to targeted monotherapy.[79] With greater understanding of the relevant genomic targets in this disease, future trials should be able to incorporate more individualized treatment selection. Several novel therapeutics are currently under development.

Immune Checkpoint Inhibitors

Immune-modulating agents have proved to be an intriguing new approach for the treatment of solid tumors.[80] The immune checkpoint pathway, including the programmed death (PD)-1 receptor on activated T cells and its ligand PD-L1, which is found on tumors and stroma, is thought to facilitate immune suppression by malignancy.[81,82] In a phase I study of nivolumab, an IgG4 monoclonal antibody against PD-1, responses were noted in patients with non–small cell lung cancer, renal cell cancer, and melanoma.[83] This finding prompted further study of this class of agents in additional disease sites, including SCCHN, in light of evidence of tumor-infiltrating T cells in SCCHN. There are ongoing studies in SCCHN of the PD-1 inhibitors nivolumab and pembrolizumab, and a PD-L1 targeting antibody, MEDI14736. In the initial reporting of the activity of pembrolizumab (Keynote-012), 60 HPV(+) and HPV(−) patients were treated with pembrolizumab 10 mg/kg every 2 weeks.[84] PD-L1 positivity, liberally defined as 1% staining, was required for treatment and noted in 78% of patients screened. Treatment was well tolerated; reported toxicities included fatigue, rash, pruritus, and nausea. Low rates of adrenal insufficiency, diarrhea, and transaminitis were also observed. Half of the patients, both HPV(+) and HPV(−), had some degree of tumor response with an overall response rate of 20%. Similarly to other trials involving these agents, tumor flare was noted before responses in a subset of patients. There are also limited preliminary data with MEDI14736, with responses in a subset of patients and expected immune-related toxicities.[85]

Aurora Kinase Inhibitors

Alisertib (MLN8237) is a selective inhibitor of aurora kinase A. Its study for SCCHN is based on preclinical demonstration of greater aurora A expression in SCCHN, which is associated with worse outcomes.[86,87] Single-agent activity of alisertib to date in an advanced pretreated SCCHN population showed a response rate of 9% and PFS of 2.7 months.[88] In addition, there is synergy in preclinical models with combined EGFR and aurora kinase inhibition,[89,90] whish has provided the impetus for a phase I trial of cetuximab and alisertib with radiation for potentially curable patients with SCCHN (NCT01540682).

Biologically Targeted Agents

One of the more prevalent genomic alterations of SCCHN involves the phosphoinositide 3-kinase (PI3K) pathways (31% of cases),[91–93] suggesting a therapeutic role for agents that target either PI3K or its downstream target mTOR.[94] Recent reports on the results of a phase II study of carboplatin, paclitaxel, and temsirolimus for the treatment of unselected recurrent/metastatic SCCHN showed an overall response rate of 43% and OS of 13 months.[95] In an effort to avoid feedback signaling by targeting multiple points in the pathway, PI3K inhibitors are currently being developed.[96] Additional targets of interest include MET,[97] and trials are currently under way to evaluate the clinical activity of MET inhibitors.

SUMMARY

The use of systemic therapy for SCCHN has evolved, and cytotoxic therapy is now an integral component of the combined-modality treatment of locally advanced disease. In addition, an increasing understanding of the molecular basis of SCCHN has led to the development if EGFR-targeting agents such as cetuximab and afatinib. Further advances are required for the treatment HPV(−) disease, which often is associated with a poor prognosis. In addition, while systemic therapy can palliate and extend the survival of patients with recurrent/metastatic disease, the development of novel therapeutics in this setting is an area of ongoing research.

REFERENCES

1. Pignon JP, le Maitre A, Maillard E, et al. Meta-analysis of chemotherapy in head and neck cancer (MACH-NC): an update on 93 randomised trials and 17,346 patients. Radiother Oncol 2009;92:4–14.
2. Posner M. Evolving strategies for combined-modality therapy for locally advanced head and neck cancer. Oncologist 2007;12:967–74.
3. Machtay M, Moughan J, Trotti A, et al. Factors associated with severe late toxicity after concurrent chemoradiation for locally advanced head and neck cancer: an RTOG analysis. J Clin Oncol 2008;26:3582–9.
4. Calais G, Alfonsi M, Bardet E, et al. Randomized trial of radiation therapy versus concomitant chemotherapy and radiation therapy for advanced-stage oropharynx carcinoma. J Natl Cancer Inst 1999;91:2081–6.
5. Cohen EE, Karrison TG, Kocherginsky M, et al. Phase III randomized trial of induction chemotherapy in patients with N2 or N3 locally advanced head and neck cancer. J Clin Oncol 2014;32:2735–43.
6. Haddad R, O'Neill A, Rabinowits G, et al. Induction chemotherapy followed by concurrent chemoradiotherapy (sequential chemoradiotherapy) versus concurrent chemoradiotherapy alone in locally advanced head and neck cancer (PARADIGM): a randomised phase 3 trial. Lancet Oncol 2013;14:257–64.
7. Forastiere AA, Goepfert H, Maor M, et al. Concurrent chemotherapy and radiotherapy for organ preservation in advanced laryngeal cancer. N Engl J Med 2003;349:2091–8.
8. Forastiere AA, Zhang Q, Weber RS, et al. Long-term results of RTOG 91-11: a comparison of three nonsurgical treatment strategies to preserve the larynx in patients with locally advanced larynx cancer. J Clin Oncol 2013;31:845–52.
9. Seiwert TY, Salama JK, Vokes EE. The concurrent chemoradiation paradigm—general principles. Nat Clin Pract Oncol 2007;4:86–100.
10. Vokes EE, Weichselbaum RR, Lippman SM, et al. Head and neck cancer. N Engl J Med 1993;328:184–94.
11. Adelstein DJ, Tan EH, Lavertu P. Treatment of head and neck cancer: the role of chemotherapy. Crit Rev Oncol Hematol 1996;24:97–116.
12. Haselow RE, Warshaw MG, Oken MM. Radiation alone versus radiation with weekly low dose cis-platinum in unresectable cancer of the head and neck. In: Fee WE Jr, Goepfert H, Johns ME, editors. Head and neck cancer. Philadelphia: Lippincott; 1990. p. 279–81.
13. Marcial VA, Pajak TF, Mohiuddin M, et al. Concomitant cisplatin chemotherapy and radiotherapy in advanced mucosal squamous cell carcinoma of the head and neck. Long-term results of the radiation therapy oncology group study 81-17. Cancer 1990;66:1861–8.
14. Adelstein DJ, Li Y, Adams GL, et al. An intergroup phase III comparison of standard radiation therapy and two schedules of concurrent chemoradiotherapy in patients with unresectable squamous cell head and neck cancer. J Clin Oncol 2003;21:92–8.
15. Pfister DG, Spencer S, Brizel DM, et al. Head and neck cancers, Version 2.2014. Clinical practice guidelines in oncology. J Natl Compr Canc Netw 2014;12:1454–87.
16. Beckmann GK, Hoppe F, Pfreundner L, et al. Hyperfractionated accelerated radiotherapy in combination with weekly cisplatin for locally advanced head and neck cancer. Head Neck 2005;27:36–43.
17. Grandis JR, Tweardy DJ. Elevated levels of transforming growth factor alpha and epidermal growth factor receptor messenger RNA are early markers of carcinogenesis in head and neck cancer. Cancer Res 1993;53:3579–84.

18. Chung CH, Zhang Q, Hammond EM, et al. Integrating epidermal growth factor receptor assay with clinical parameters improves risk classification for relapse and survival in head-and-neck squamous cell carcinoma. Int J Radiat Oncol Biol Phys 2011;81:331–8.

19. Huang SM, Bock JM, Harari PM. Epidermal growth factor receptor blockade with C225 modulates proliferation, apoptosis, and radiosensitivity in squamous cell carcinomas of the head and neck. Cancer Res 1999;59:1935–40.

20. Harari PM, Huang SM. Head and neck cancer as a clinical model for molecular targeting of therapy: combining EGFR blockade with radiation. Int J Radiat Oncol Biol Phys 2001;49:427–33.

21. Bonner JA, Harari PM, Giralt J, et al. Radiotherapy plus cetuximab for squamous-cell carcinoma of the head and neck. N Engl J Med 2006;354:567–78.

22. Bonner JA, Harari PM, Giralt J, et al. Radiotherapy plus cetuximab for locoregionally advanced head and neck cancer: 5-year survival data from a phase 3 randomised trial, and relation between cetuximab-induced rash and survival. Lancet Oncol 2010;11:21–8.

23. Ang KK, Zhang Q, Rosenthal DI, et al. Randomized phase III trial of concurrent accelerated radiation plus cisplatin with or without cetuximab for stage III to IV head and neck carcinoma: RTOG 0522. J Clin Oncol 2014;32:2940–50.

24. Giralt J, Fortin A, Mesia R, et al. A phase II, randomized trial (CONCERT-1) of chemoradiotherapy (CRT) with or without panitumumab (pmab) in patients (pts) with unresected, locally advanced squamous cell carcinoma of the head and neck (LASCCHN). J Clin Oncol 2012;30(Suppl 15):5502.

25. Giralt J, Trigo J, Nuyts S, et al. Phase 2, randomized trial (CONCERT-2) of panitumumab (PMAB) plus radiotherapy (PRT) compared with chemoradiotherapy (CRT) in patients (pts) with unresectable SCCHN. ESMO; 2012.

26. Gandhi MD, Agulnik M. Targeted treatment of head and neck squamous-cell carcinoma: potential of lapatinib. Lancet Oncol 2015;16:221–32.

27. Hegde PS, Rusnak D, Bertiaux M, et al. Delineation of molecular mechanisms of sensitivity to lapatinib in breast cancer cell lines using global gene expression profiles. Mol Cancer Ther 2007;6:1629–40.

28. de Souza JA, Davis DW, Zhang Y, et al. A phase II study of lapatinib in recurrent/metastatic squamous cell carcinoma of the head and neck. Clin Cancer Res 2012;18:2336–43.

29. Del Campo JM, Hitt R, Sebastian P, et al. Effects of lapatinib monotherapy: results of a randomised phase II study in therapy-naive patients with locally advanced squamous cell carcinoma of the head and neck. Br J Cancer 2011;105:618–27.

30. Harrington K, Berrier A, Robinson M, et al. Randomised phase II study of oral lapatinib combined with chemoradiotherapy in patients with advanced squamous cell carcinoma of the head and neck: rationale for future randomised trials in human papilloma virus-negative disease. Eur J Cancer 2013;49:1609–18.

31. Radiation Therapy Oncology Group. TRYHARD: Radiation therapy plus cisplatin with or without lapatinib in treating patients with head and neck cancer. In: ClinicalTrials.gov. Bethesda (MD): US National Library of Medicine. Available at: http://clinicaltrials.gov/show/NCT01711658. NLM identifier: NCT01711658. Accessed April 2015.

32. UNC Lineberger Comprehensive Cancer Centre. Multimodality risk adapted tx including induction chemo for SCCHN amenable to transoral surgery. Bethesda (MD): US National Library of Medicine; 2012. ClinicalTrials.gov. NLM identifier: NCT01612351. Available at: http://clinicaltrials.gov/show/NCT01612351.

33. Adelstein DJ, Saxton JP, Rybicki LA, et al. Multiagent concurrent chemoradiotherapy for locoregionally advanced squamous cell head and neck cancer: mature results from a single institution. J Clin Oncol 2006;24:1064–71.
34. Adelstein DJ, Saxton JP, Lavertu P, et al. A phase III randomized trial comparing concurrent chemotherapy and radiotherapy with radiotherapy alone in resectable stage III and IV squamous cell head and neck cancer: preliminary results. Head Neck 1997;19:567–75.
35. Brizel DM, Albers ME, Fisher SR, et al. Hyperfractionated irradiation with or without concurrent chemotherapy for locally advanced head and neck cancer. N Engl J Med 1998;338:1798–804.
36. Denis F, Garaud P, Bardet E, et al. Final results of the 94-01 French Head and Neck Oncology and Radiotherapy Group randomized trial comparing radiotherapy alone with concomitant radiochemotherapy in advanced-stage oropharynx carcinoma. J Clin Oncol 2004;22:69–76.
37. Rodriguez CP, Adelstein JA, Rybicki LA, et al. A phase III randomized trial of two cisplatin-based concurrent chemoradiation regimens for locally advanced head and neck squamous cell carcinoma. Head Neck 2014. http://dx.doi.org/10.1002/hed.23794.
38. Lambin P, Ramaekers BL, van Mastrigt GA, et al. Erythropoietin as an adjuvant treatment with (chemo) radiation therapy for head and neck cancer. Cochrane Database Syst Rev 2009;(8):CD006158.
39. Garden AS, Harris J, Vokes EE, et al. Preliminary results of radiation therapy oncology group 97-03: a randomized phase ii trial of concurrent radiation and chemotherapy for advanced squamous cell carcinomas of the head and neck. J Clin Oncol 2004;22:2856–64.
40. Kies MS, Haraf DJ, Rosen F, et al. Concomitant infusional paclitaxel and fluorouracil, oral hydroxyurea, and hyperfractionated radiation for locally advanced squamous head and neck cancer. J Clin Oncol 2001;19:1961–9.
41. Kao J, Genden EM, Gupta V, et al. Phase 2 trial of concurrent 5-fluorouracil, hydroxyurea, cetuximab, and hyperfractionated intensity-modulated radiation therapy for locally advanced head and neck cancer. Cancer 2011;117:318–26.
42. Seiwert TY, Herchock D, Cohen EE, et al. A phase I study of bevacizumab (B) with fluorouracil (F) and hydroxyurea (H) with concomitant radiotherapy (X) (B-FHX) for poor prognosis head and neck cancer (HNC). Atlanta (GA): ASCO; 2006.
43. Fakhry C, Westra WH, Li S, et al. Improved survival of patients with human papillomavirus-positive head and neck squamous cell carcinoma in a prospective clinical trial. J Natl Cancer Inst 2008;100:261–9.
44. Ang KK, Harris J, Wheeler R, et al. Human papillomavirus and survival of patients with oropharyngeal cancer. N Engl J Med 2010;363:24–35.
45. Marur S, Lee J, Cmelak A, et al. ECOG 1308: A phase II trial of induction chemotherapy followed by cetuximab with low dose versus standard dose IMRT in patients with HPV-associated resectable squamous cell carcinoma of the oropharynx. J Clin Oncol 2012;30(Suppl):5566.
46. Vermorken JB, Mesia R, Rivera F, et al. Platinum-based chemotherapy plus cetuximab in head and neck cancer. N Engl J Med 2008;359:1116–27.
47. Lassen P, Overgaard J, Eriksen JG. Expression of EGFR and HPV-associated p16 in oropharyngeal carcinoma: correlation and influence on prognosis after radiotherapy in the randomized DAHANCA 5 and 7 trials. Radiother Oncol 2013;108:489–94.

48. Laramore GE, Scott CB, al-Sarraf M, et al. Adjuvant chemotherapy for resectable squamous cell carcinomas of the head and neck: report on Intergroup Study 0034. Int J Radiat Oncol Biol Phys 1992;23:705–13.
49. Cooper JS, Pajak TF, Forastiere A, et al. Precisely defining high-risk operable head and neck tumors based on RTOG #85-03 and #88-24: targets for postoperative radiochemotherapy? Head Neck 1998;20:588–94.
50. Cooper JS, Pajak TF, Forastiere AA, et al. Postoperative concurrent radiotherapy and chemotherapy for high-risk squamous-cell carcinoma of the head and neck. N Engl J Med 2004;350:1937–44.
51. Cooper JS, Zhang Q, Pajak TF, et al. Long-term follow-up of the RTOG 9501/intergroup phase III trial: postoperative concurrent radiation therapy and chemotherapy in high-risk squamous cell carcinoma of the head and neck. Int J Radiat Oncol Biol Phys 2012;84:1198–205.
52. Bernier J, Domenge C, Ozsahin M, et al. Postoperative irradiation with or without concomitant chemotherapy for locally advanced head and neck cancer. N Engl J Med 2004;350:1945–52.
53. Bernier J, Cooper JS, Pajak TF, et al. Defining risk levels in locally advanced head and neck cancers: a comparative analysis of concurrent postoperative radiation plus chemotherapy trials of the EORTC (#22931) and RTOG (# 9501). Head Neck 2005;27:843–50.
54. Harari PM, Harris J, Kies MS, et al. Postoperative chemoradiotherapy and cetuximab for high-risk squamous cell carcinoma of the head and neck: Radiation Therapy Oncology Group RTOG-0234. J Clin Oncol 2014;32:2486–95.
55. Glisson BS. The role of docetaxel in the management of squamous cell cancer of the head and neck. Oncology (Williston Park) 2002;16:83–7.
56. Argiris A. Induction chemotherapy for head and neck cancer: will history repeat itself? J Natl Compr Canc Netw 2005;3:393–403.
57. Posner MR, Herchock D, Le Lann L, et al. TAX 324: a phase III trial at TPF vs. PF induction chemotherapy followed chemoradiotherapy in locally advanced SCCHN. Atlanta (GA): ASCO; 2006.
58. Tannock IF. Chemotherapy for head and neck cancer. J Otolaryngol 1984;13:99–104.
59. Al-Sarraf M. Chemotherapy strategies in squamous cell carcinoma of the head and neck. Crit Rev Oncol Hematol 1984;1:323–55.
60. Glick JH, Zehngebot LM, Taylor SG. Chemotherapy for squamous cell carcinoma of the head and neck: a progress report. Am J Otolaryngol 1980;1:306–23.
61. Burtness B, Goldwasser MA, Flood W. Phase II randomized trial of cisplatin plus placebo compared with cisplatin plus cetuximab in metastatic/recurrent head and neck cancer: an Eastern Cooperative Oncology Group study. J Clin Oncol 2005;23:8646–54.
62. Gibson MK, Li Y, Murphy B, et al. Randomized phase III evaluation of cisplatin plus fluorouracil versus cisplatin plus paclitaxel in advanced head and neck cancer (E1395): an intergroup trial of the Eastern Cooperative Oncology Group. J Clin Oncol 2005;23:3562–7.
63. Baselga J, Pfister D, Cooper M, et al. Phase I studies of anti-epidermal growth factor receptor chimeric monoclonal antibody C225 alone and in combination with cisplatin. J Clin Oncol 2000;18:904–14.
64. Robert F, Ezekiel M, Spencer S. Phase I study of anti-epidermal growth factor receptor antibody cetuximab in combination with radiation therapy in patients with advanced head and neck cancer. J Clin Oncol 2001;19:3234–43.

65. Baselga J, Trigo JM, Bourhis J. Phase II multicenter study of the antiepidermal growth factor receptor monoclonal antibody cetuximab in combination with platinum-based chemotherapy in patients with platinum-refractory metastatic and/or recurrent squamous cell carcinoma of the head and neck. J Clin Oncol 2005;23:5568–77.
66. Herbst RS, Arquette M, Shin DM. Phase II multicenter study of the epidermal growth factor receptor antibody cetuximab and cisplatin for recurrent and refractory squamous cell carcinoma of the head and neck. J Clin Oncol 2005;23:5568–77.
67. Vermorken JB, Trigo J, Hitt R. Open-label, uncontrolled, multicenter phase II study to evaluate the efficacy and toxicity of cetuximab as a single agent in patients with recurrent and/or metastatic squamous cell carcinoma of the head and neck who failed to respond to platinum-based therapy. J Clin Oncol 2007;25:2171–7.
68. Leon X, Hitt R, Constenla M, et al. A retrospective analysis of the outcome of patients with recurrent and/or metastatic squamous cell carcinoma of the head and neck refractory to a platinum-based chemotherapy. Clin Oncol (R Coll Radiol) 2005;17:418–24.
69. Vermorken J, Herbst R, Leon X, et al. Overview of the efficacy of cetuximab in recurrent and/or metastatic squamous cell carcinoma of the head and neck in patients who previously failed platinum-based therapies. Cancer 2008;112:2710–9.
70. Knoedler MK, Gauler T, Matzdorff A, et al. Multicenter phase II study of cetuximab plus docetaxel in 84 patients with recurrent or metastatic, platinum-pretreated SCCHN. J Clin Oncol 2009;27(Suppl 15):6048.
71. O'Neil B, Allen R, Spigel D. High incidence of cetuximab-related infusion reactions in Tennessee and North Carolina and the association with atopic history. J Clin Oncol 2007;25:3644–8.
72. Chung C, Mirakhur B, Chan E. Cetuximab-induced anaphylaxis and IgE specific for galactose-alpha-1,3-galactose. N Engl J Med 2008;358:1109–17.
73. Stewart JS, Cohen EE, Licitra L, et al. Phase III study of gefitinib compared with intravenous methotrexate for recurrent squamous cell carcinoma of the head and neck [corrected]. J Clin Oncol 2009;27:1864–71.
74. Minkovsky N, Berezov A. BIBW-2992, a dual receptor tyrosine kinase inhibitor for the treatment of solid tumors. Curr Opin Investig Drugs 2008;9:1336–46.
75. Solca F, Dahl G, Zoephel A, et al. Target binding properties and cellular activity of afatinib (BIBW 2992), an irreversible ErbB family blocker. J Pharmacol Exp Ther 2012;343:342–50.
76. Seiwert TY, Fayette J, Cupissol D, et al. A randomized, open-label, phase II study of afatinib versus cetuximab in recurrent/metastatic head and neck squamous cell carcinoma. 10th Annual Meeting of the Japanese Society of Medical Oncology. Osaka Japan. Ann Oncol 2014;25(9):1813–20.
77. Seiwert TY, Fayette J, Cupissol D, et al. A randomized, phase II study of afatinib versus cetuximab in metastatic or recurrent squamous cell carcinoma of the head and neck. Ann Oncol 2014;25:1813–20.
78. Machiels J, Haddad R, Fayette J, et al. Afatinib versus methotrexate (MTX) as second-line treatment for patients with recurrent and/or metastatic (R/M) head and neck squamous cell carcinoma (HNSCC) who progressed after platinum-based therapy: primary efficacy results of LUX-Head & Neck 1, a phase III trial. Ann Oncol 2014;25.
79. Walter V, Yin X, Wilkerson MD, et al. Molecular subtypes in head and neck cancer exhibit distinct patterns of chromosomal gain and loss of canonical cancer genes. PLoS One 2013;8:e56823.

80. Leach DR, Krummel MF, Allison JP. Enhancement of antitumor immunity by CTLA-4 blockade. Science 1996;271:1734–6.
81. Dong H, Zhu G, Tamada K, et al. B7-H1, a third member of the B7 family, co-stimulates T-cell proliferation and interleukin-10 secretion. Nat Med 1999;5:1365–9.
82. Freeman GJ, Long AJ, Iwai Y, et al. Engagement of the PD-1 immunoinhibitory receptor by a novel B7 family member leads to negative regulation of lymphocyte activation. J Exp Med 2000;192:1027–34.
83. Topalian SL, Hodi FS, Brahmer JR, et al. Safety, activity, and immune correlates of anti-PD-1 antibody in cancer. N Engl J Med 2012;366:2443–54.
84. Seiwert T, Burtness B, Weiss J, et al. A phase Ib study of MK-3475 in patients with human papillomavirus (HPV)-associated and non-HPV–associated head and neck (H/N) cancer. J Clin Oncol 2014;32(Suppl 5):6011.
85. Fury M, Ou S, Balmanoukian A, et al. Clinical activity and safety of MEDI4736, an anti-PD-L1 antibody, in patients with head and neck cancer. Ann Oncol 2014;25(Suppl 4):iv340–56.
86. Mazumdar A, Henderson YC, El-Naggar AK, et al. Aurora kinase A inhibition and paclitaxel as targeted combination therapy for head and neck squamous cell carcinoma. Head Neck 2009;31:625–34.
87. Reiter R, Gais P, Jutting U, et al. Aurora kinase A messenger RNA overexpression is correlated with tumor progression and shortened survival in head and neck squamous cell carcinoma. Clin Cancer Res 2006;12:5136–41.
88. Melichar B, Adenis A, Havel L, et al. Phase (Ph) I/II study of investigational Aurora A kinase (AAK) inhibitor MLN8237 (alisertib): Updated ph II results in patients (pts) with small cell lung cancer (SCLC), non-SCLC (NSCLC), breast cancer (BrC), head and neck squamous cell carcinoma (HNSCC), and gastroesophageal cancer (GE). J Clin Oncol 2013;31(Suppl):605.
89. Astsaturov I, Ratushny V, Sukhanova A, et al. Synthetic lethal screen of an EGFR-centered network to improve targeted therapies. Sci Signal 2010;3:ra67.
90. Hoellein A, Pickhard A, von Keitz F, et al. Aurora kinase inhibition overcomes cetuximab resistance in squamous cell cancer of the head and neck. Oncotarget 2011;2:599–609.
91. Agrawal N, Frederick MJ, Pickering CR, et al. Exome sequencing of head and neck squamous cell carcinoma reveals inactivating mutations in NOTCH1. Science 2011;333:1154–7.
92. Lui VW, Hedberg ML, Li H, et al. Frequent mutation of the PI3K pathway in head and neck cancer defines predictive biomarkers. Cancer Discov 2013;3:761–9.
93. Stransky N, Egloff AM, Tward AD, et al. The mutational landscape of head and neck squamous cell carcinoma. Science 2011;333:1157–60.
94. Amornphimoltham P, Patel V, Sodhi A, et al. Mammalian target of rapamycin, a molecular target in squamous cell carcinomas of the head and neck. Cancer Res 2005;65:9953–61.
95. Fury M, Xiao H, Baxi S, et al. A phase II trial of temsirolimus plus low-dose weekly carboplatin and paclitaxel for recurrent/metastatic HNSCC. J Clin Oncol 2014;32(Suppl 5):6019.
96. Available at: clinicaltrials.gov. Accessed April 2015.
97. Seiwert TY, Jagadeeswaran R, Faoro L, et al. The MET receptor tyrosine kinase is a potential novel therapeutic target for head and neck squamous cell carcinoma. Cancer Res 2009;69:3021–31.

Imaging for Head and Neck Cancer

Jesty Abraham, DO

KEYWORDS

- Head and neck • Anatomy • Neoplasm • Imaging

KEY POINTS

- Imaging facilitates staging, treatment planning, posttreatment evaluation, and detection of recurrent/residual disease and provides prognostic information regarding survival outcomes.
- Primary tumor staging can be adequately performed with either computed tomography (CT) or MRI. MRI is more useful for assessing perineural spread of disease.
- Ultrasound is most useful for evaluating cervical lymphadenopathy and for obtaining specimens through fine-needle aspirations and core biopsies.
- PET/CT is most useful for identifying regional and distant metastatic disease.
- Posttreatment imaging may be performed with CT, MRI, or PET/CT; however, an imaging-free period immediately after treatment is needed to present false-positive studies.

HEAD AND NECK CANCER

Head and neck carcinomas include neoplasms of the nose and nasal cavity, nasopharynx, lips and oral cavity, oropharynx, larynx, hypopharynx, proximal trachea and esophagus, and maxillofacial sinuses. Tumors of the salivary glands, thyroid gland, cervical lymph nodes (lymphoma), and skin cancers can be included in head and neck cancers. Most nonthyroid head and neck neoplasms consist of squamous cell carcinomas of the mucosal lining of the upper respiratory tract and oral cavity.

In order to reduce treatment toxicity, the extent of disease must be assessed efficiently. This assessment includes a combined multidisciplinary effort to examine, image, diagnose, and stage patients properly. Imaging is only one element of the process. Collaboration between specialists in head and neck imaging and treating oncologists is an essential element of multidisciplinary collaboration. Modern imaging methods, including ultrasound (US), computed tomography (CT), MRI, and PET, have dramatically enhanced the process of diagnosis and staging as well as the evaluation for tumor recurrence.[1]

The author has nothing to disclose.
Department of Radiology, Fox Chase Cancer Center, 333 Cottman Avenue, Philadelphia, PA 19111, USA
E-mail address: jesty.abraham@fccc.edu

Surg Oncol Clin N Am 24 (2015) 455–471
http://dx.doi.org/10.1016/j.soc.2015.03.012
surgonc.theclinics.com
1055-3207/15/$ – see front matter © 2015 Elsevier Inc. All rights reserved.

RATIONALE FOR MODALITY SELECTION

How should a clinician determine which imaging modality to use? This decision is complex and multifactorial. Elements include the body part under evaluation, histology of the cancer, stage of disease, and anticipated treatment. Proper modality selection aids the choice of operative approach, potential organ and functional preservation of affected or adjacent tissue, as well as helping to determine the role of surgical, radiation, and medical oncology in treatment. Imaging enhances clinical information beyond examination by assessing the submucosal extent of head and neck tumors and the presence of cervical nodal metastases.[2]

CT and MRI are the primary techniques for evaluating head and neck cancers. CT is superior to MRI because of its speed, easy access, and patient tolerance. The disadvantages of CT include exposure to ionizing radiation and need for iodinated contrast agents. CT is preferable for evaluating metastatic lymph node necrosis. MRI has better soft tissue contrast resolution and multiplanar imaging capability. MRI is superior for evaluating perineural tumor spread along the skull base. However, important disadvantages with MRI include the long time required for imaging acquisition (leading to motion degradation), patient intolerance, metallic implant noncompliance (pacemakers), and gadolinium contrast. In the head and neck, swallowing can cause significant artifact, limiting evaluation of the adjacent soft tissue.[2]

US is especially useful to evaluate cervical nodes and salivary gland tumors. It is particularly helpful for biopsy of small lymph nodes or salivary gland masses (**Figs. 1** and **2**). It provides a ready way to guide the needle to the lesion in real time. Doppler sonography helps avoid vasculature, thus reducing risk of bleeding.[2]

For head and neck malignancies that are deep rooted and challenging to palpate, fine-needle aspiration (FNA) with CT guidance can be a beneficial alternative option to US-guided biopsies. Many different approaches to deep-seated malignancies using CT guidance have been described. These approaches include needle biopsy of lesions of the parotid gland,[3,4] Meckel cave,[5] foramen ovale,[6] middle cranial fossa,[7] nasopharynx,[8,9] sphenoid ridge and maxillary sinus,[9] nasal cavity,[3,10] infratemporal fossa,[3,10] and the parapharyngeal space.[11] CT-guided FNA is safe, well tolerated, and accurate for the diagnosis of head and neck lesions.

MRI has strengths for tumor localization and assessing for tumor extension through T1- and T2-weighted imaging. T1-weighted multiplanar postcontrast fat-suppressed images allow for detection of possible perineural spread of malignancy.

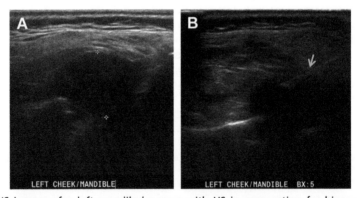

Fig. 1. US images of a left mandibular mass with US in preparation for biopsy (A). The second image (B) demonstrates the tip of the 22-gauge spinal needle (yellow arrow) within the mass during fine-needle aspiration for assignment of diagnosis.

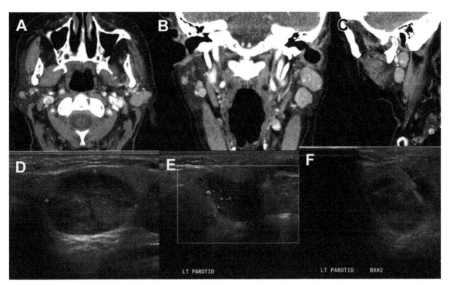

Fig. 2. Axial (*A*), coronal (*B*), and sagittal (*C*) contrast-enhanced images demonstrate well-circumscribed hyperdense lesions in the left parotid gland. US and Doppler images depict the same left parotid gland lesions (*D, E*) with internal vascularity. (*E*) The square refers to the region that was evaluated by ultrasound for vascularity. These images were used to guide the biopsy of this lesion, which proved to be a Warthin tumor (*F*).

Nasopharyngeal malignancy is often best evaluated by PET/CT, MRI, and CT, rather than US, because of its anatomic location and natural history of ready metastatic disease. MRI is the primary imaging tool to image nasopharyngeal malignancy because of its superior anatomic detail in the absence of motion. MRI can detect tumor invasion into the adjacent soft tissues and in particular invasion of the pharyngobasilar fascia, sinus of Morgagni, skull base, intracranial involvement, and perineural invasion. CT is suboptimal compared with MRI for assessing adjacent soft tissue involvement but better for bone. However, PET/CT is better than MRI and CT for evaluating for cervical, supraclavicular, and mediastinal lymph node involvement as well as distant metastases. In patients with nasopharyngeal carcinomas, PET/CT allows for posttreatment functional response assessment. Such a PET/CT should be obtained approximately 3 months following treatment to decrease false-positive results secondary to treatment-related inflammatory changes.[12–14]

CT, MRI, and PET/CT are of benefit in evaluating sinonasal malignancy. CT gives important information regarding possible osseous invasion and extent of the primary tumor, providing the clinician with a detailed anatomic picture when preparing for open or endoscopic sinus surgery. MRI should be used to define the tumor extent (distinguishing the lesion from edema and retained mucus) and assessing orbital and intracranial extension. US has a limited role in the evaluation of sinonasal malignancy. PET/CT is used for cervical lymph node involvement and staging. PET/CT evaluation is usually obtained at 3 months following treatment because this waiting period allows for minimal false-positive fluorodeoxyglucose (FDG) avidity from post-therapy inflammatory changes.[2]

The choice of imaging modality in carcinomas of the oral cavity and oropharynx is also multifactorial. CT is usually the initial imaging modality for tumor staging. Dental hardware artifact may represent a problem if angled maxilla and mandibular views are not obtained. CT can define osseous invasion of the mandible and maxilla. MRI is more useful for evaluating bone marrow invasion and perineural spread. MRI may be superior to CT to evaluate for primary tongue tumor's submucosal extent as well as small tumors.[12–14] The limitations of MRI imaging of the oral cavity and oropharynx are related to artifacts from patient breathing and swallowing. PET/CT is chiefly used for evaluating nodal involvement and systemic metastases in patients with advanced stage. It represents an excellent imaging tool for posttreatment assessment for residual tumor or recurrence in the oral cavity and oropharynx. US again has a limited role in assessment of primary tumors of the oral cavity and oropharynx, though estimation of tumor thickness with US has been studied.[15,16]

CT is the preferred modality for evaluating the primary laryngeal or hypopharyngeal malignancy, including its involvement of adjacent cartilaginous, bony, and soft tissue structures. MRI is suboptimal in evaluating tumors in this region because the long image acquisition time introduces possible swallowing artifact. CT imaging does not suffer this limitation because a study of the neck can be completed in less than a minute.[17]

Detection of nodal metastases is important. It is present in 50% of patients at diagnosis of head and neck cancers and typically reduces survival by half.[18] CT and MRI are used on a wide scale to assess for cervical lymphadenopathy. Studies that have compared the accuracy of CT and MRI for the assessment of cervical lymphadenopathy have found no significant difference between these two modalities. However, as a rule, between 40% and 60% of all occult metastases are identified by using either CT or MRI.[19] US, less commonly used in North America, has a main advantage in that it can readily be used with FNA biopsy, which results in a specificity of 100% for the combined technique. However, US-guided FNA biopsy identifies clinically occult metastases with a sensitivity of no more than 48% to 73%.[19] Diagnostic accuracy for metastatic nodal detection does not seem to improve considerably by the fusion of FDG-PET with CT when compared with just PET. Problems that limit the accuracy are the suboptimal anatomic resolution of PET even after fusion with low-dose noncontrast CT as well as the incapability to reliably find metastatic nodes less than 5 mm. Thus, the sensitivity of PET/PET-CT detection of metastatic node metastases is similar to CT and MRI.[19] There are new technological advances to improve the ability of MRI to distinguish metastatic from benign cervical lymph nodes with diffusion-weighted imaging (DWI), dynamic contrast-enhanced MRI, or the use of new (lymphotropic) contrast agents as enhancers. DWI MRI may be a useful tool to differentiate tumoral from nontumoral signal with a sensitivity and specificity for the detection of nodal metastasis of 98% and 88%.[19]

Malignant cervical lymphadenopathy will demonstrate a heterogeneous internal architecture, central necrosis, and even extracapsular spread.[20,21] Metastatic lymphadenopathy usually demonstrates necrosis when the lesion is greater than 3 cm. These areas of necrosis usually show a characteristic pattern on imaging, which helps the radiologist identify malignant lesions quickly. With MRI they have hypointense signal in T1-weighted imaging as well as hyperintense signal on T2-weighted imaging. Postcontrast CT images display necrosis as a central area without enhancement, usually with peripheral areas of enhancing malignant soft tissue. Necrotic tumor on PET/CT imaging does not show FDG avidity and appears hypometabolic or as a cold defect.[20]

Extracapsular spread (ECS) in cervical lymph node metastases from head and neck squamous cell carcinoma is a poor prognostic factor.[22,23] ECS has been linked with a 50% decrease in survival and about 1.5- to 3.5-fold increase in local relapse.[24–26] Contrast-enhanced CT is the imaging modality that is usually used to assess cervical lymph node for metastatic disease. CT criteria for abnormal lymph nodes include size, if there is central necrosis, and the presence of a cluster of lymph nodes in the expected drainage path of a tumor. However, this may not be precise if patients have had prior surgery, radiation, or infection.[27] On CT or MRI, in the setting of head and neck carcinomas, cervical lymph nodes larger than 1.5 cm with a rounded contour and loss of the fatty hilum are malignant if they are in the nodal drainage path of the primary malignancy. Additionally central nodal necrosis within any size node is an indication of neoplastic involvement. The most accurate radiological predictor of lymph node metastasis is the presence of central lymph node necrosis. Radiologically, lymph node central necrosis is described as a central area of hypodensity with a peripheral irregular rim of enhancing tissue.[27] Lymph node central necrosis has been reported to be almost 100% accurate in identifying metastatic disease.[28,29]

Radiological signs that indicate lymph node ECS include nodal capsular enhancement, infiltration of adjacent fat or muscle planes, and capsular contour irregularity.[30,31] Using CT to evaluate for of ECS has a sensitivity of 81% and a specificity of 72%, compared with 57% to 77% and 57% to 72%, respectively, for MRI.[32] With regard to MRI, precontrast T1- and T2-weighted images are more sensitive than gadolinium-enhanced T1-weighted images.[31] US has demonstrated to be acceptably sensitive, but less specific, for the detection of ECS.[33] On US imaging, abnormal cervical lymph nodes will demonstrate rounded contour with loss of hilar echogenicity, and power Doppler may demonstrate loss of normal hilar flow and increased peripheral vascularity. Nodal matting and soft tissue edema can be seen in pretreatment and posttreatment nodes.[34]

Perineural Spread

A significant predictive element of treatment outcome is perineural spread of tumor in patients with suprahyoid neoplasms. CT imaging can be dependably used to localize perineural spread of malignancy by looking for clues, such as enlargement of the neural foramina at the skull base, degeneration of the muscles that are innervated by the trigeminal nerve (cranial nerve V), or even fatty infiltration of the pterygopalatine fossa.[35] However, perineural spread of malignancy on MRI is usually denoted by irregular thickening and postcontrast abnormal enhancement of the affected nerve.[35] Adenoid cystic carcinomas usually demonstrate more perineural spread than squamous cell carcinomas.[35]

DIAGNOSTIC IMAGING TECHNIQUE

Patients are usually supine for CT and MRI head and neck imaging. Artifacts are common in CT, and they may obscure or mimic pathology. CT artifacts include noise, beam hardening, scatter, pseudoenhancement, and motion, cone beam, helical, ring, and metal artifacts. For head and neck imaging, metal streak artifacts from dental fillings or surgical hardware are the main concern.[36] The artifacts are triggered by many mechanisms, some of which are related to the metal itself and others related to the metal edges. Metal causes beam hardening, scatter effects, and Poisson noise. Beam hardening and scatter cause dark streaks with surrounding bright streaks. The metal edges cause streaks because of undersampling, motion, cone beam, and windmill artifacts.[37] Metal artifacts are usually seen with higher atomic number materials, such as iron or platinum, and less so with lower atomic number metals, such as titanium. In most head and neck cases with dental fillings, patient positioning or gantry tilt may be used to angle the metal outside of the axial slices of interest.[38]

For contrast-enhanced CT and MRI, the patients should have blood tests within approximately 2 weeks of the examination to evaluate renal function. Diabetic patients who are having intravenous contrast for their CT or MRI scans must stop taking the following medications for 48 hours: metformin hydrochloride (Glucophage), glyburide and metformin (Glucovance), metformin hydrochloride, and metformin or its derivatives. Noncontrast imaging does not require prior preparation.[39] During the MRI examination metallic items must be removed. Individuals with metallic implants, pacemakers, metallic clips, and stents must disclose their presence before the study to prevent excessive heating (burns that have been associated with implants and metallic devices). Additionally, ferromagnetic implants may move or even dislodge causing pain and injury to the patients.[40–42]

INTERPRETATION/ASSESSMENT OF CLINICAL IMAGES

A radiologist must have a strong knowledge of anatomy when interpreting images of the head and neck. General features specific to each imaging modality allow a radiologist to discern benign from malignant tumors.

Benign Tumors

Benign lesions on US may appear hypoechoic or hyperechoic but typically demonstrate well-circumscribed, lobulated margins with posterior acoustic enhancement, internal homogeneity, as well as peripheral calcification. Soft tissue lesions that are hypodense (or even cystic) with intact muscle borders and osseous cortex on CT are also usually benign. On MRI, lesions that are homogenous in signal intensity with hypointense signal on T1 and hyperintense signal on T2 are also mostly benign. With regard to PET/CT, low level of FDG activity compared with blood pool activity is usually benign.[1]

Malignant Tumors

Malignant lesions on US usually demonstrate an irregular shape, border, and margin. The lesion may also have increased vascularity. On CT, cancers typically demonstrate soft tissue thickening or a bulky mass with surrounding infiltration and stranding of the adjacent tissues (with or without osseous invasion). Malignant tumors generally may have a suboptimally defined border and may also demonstrate heterogeneous internal signal with possible cystic change and necrosis on MRI. Aggressive lesions on MRI may show heterogeneous enhancement on postcontrast imaging. On PET/CT, malignant lesions often demonstrate increased FDG avidity when compared with blood pool or liver pool uptake images.[1]

Nasopharyngeal Masses

Approximately 80% of neoplastic nasopharyngeal masses are of squamous cell carcinoma origin. The other nasopharyngeal masses are adenocarcinoma, minor salivary gland tumors, and lymphoma.[20] The lateral pharyngeal recess is the most common location for nasopharyngeal carcinomas. As individuals age, the fat content increases and lymphoid and muscular tissue content decreases over time.[43] MRI and CT are used in concert for the initial evaluation of the primary tumor. However, PET/CT is more useful to detect recurrence as well as lymph node and metastatic disease. T1-weighted imaging without contrast is best used for assessing skull base invasion and involvement of the different fat-containing spaces in the skull base. T2-weighted fast spin echo imaging is an additional imaging tool that is helpful when evaluating for parapharyngeal, paranasal, or cervical lymph node involvement. In order to assess intracranial tumor extension or perineural spread, the most useful MRI sequence is T1-weighted contrast-enhanced imaging with fat suppression. Some calculate the choline/creatine ratio using magnetic resonance spectroscopy. The choline/creatine ratio is usually elevated in cases of metastatic lymphadenopathy.[44]

Nasopharyngeal carcinomas may present as infiltration of adjacent soft tissues with little mass effect. Infiltration of the adjacent tissue then leads to effacement of the margins of the muscular tissues. MRI allows for better delineation of the soft tissue infiltration and discerns lymphoid tissue from adjacent soft tissue and muscle.[42–44] For example, tumor infiltration of the region between the tensor and levator veli palatini muscles (part of the parapharyngeal space) or even fatty infiltration of the region between the nasopharyngeal mucosa and longus capitis muscle (which is known as the retropharyngeal region) will be depicted as an area of fatty infiltration or even obliteration of the usually seen normal hyperintense signal on T1-weighted imaging.[21]

In patients with nasopharyngeal carcinomas, tumors begin in the fossa of Rosenmüller and have local extension with initial metastases to the retropharyngeal lymph nodes of Rouvière.[18] This extension can usually be seen in the region between the skull base to the level of C3 vertebral body. Lymph node involvement usually progresses laterally in nasopharyngeal carcinomas. Nodal spread starts in the retropharyngeal region, and then it moves to the spinal accessory chain (Va/Vb), internal jugular chain (level III-IV), and lastly supraclavicular lymph nodes. Nodal involvement in the region posterior to the jugular vein (IIa/b) is not considered retropharyngeal nodal involvement.[34]

Parapharyngeal Space Masses

The parapharyngeal space contains fat, the V3 segment of the trigeminal nerve, the internal maxillary artery, as well as the ascending pharyngeal artery and veins. This space is divided into a prestyloid compartment (about 80% of lesions occurring there are pleomorphic adenomas) and the poststyloid compartment. The lesions that arise in the poststyloid compartment are of neurogenic origin and paragangliomas. Squamous cell carcinomas may arise from the adjacent pharyngeal mucosa and invade the pharyngeal space.[35]

Parotid Space Masses

The parotid space contains the parotid glands, lymph nodes, retromandibular vein, facial nerve, and external carotid artery. Although surgeons use the facial nerve to divide the gland into the deep and superficial lobes, the retromandibular vein divides the gland into superficial and deep lobes on imaging studies. The most common lesion in this space is a benign tumor, such as a pleomorphic adenoma (about 80% of parotid neoplasms are benign). The second most common lesion in this location is a Warthin tumor. These lesions are usually seen in elderly men who smoke and may be bilateral. Malignant lesions include mucoepidermoid carcinomas, adenoid cystic carcinomas, other primary parotid cancers, metastases, and lymphoma. With respect to imaging by MRI, the benign lesions are usually hyperintense on T2-weighted imaging, whereas malignant neoplasms are hypointense on T2-weighted imaging. DWI will demonstrate restricted diffusion with malignant lesions.[45–47]

Sublingual and Submandibular Space Masses

Sublingual space is in the superior/medial region to the mylohyoid muscle and houses the tongue, lingual neurovascular plexus, sublingual glands/ducts, and Wharton ducts. The most common malignancy to occur in this region is squamous cell carcinoma. However, the sublingual gland tumors, cellulitis, abscesses, calculi, ranulas, lymphangioma, epidermoid/dermoid cysts, ectopic thyroid, and hemangioma produce masses there. The submandibular space is inferior/lateral to the mylohyoid muscle and superior to the hyoid bone as well as medial to the horizontal ramus of the mandible. This region houses the submandibular gland, nodes, anterior belly of the digastric muscle, as well as the facial vein and artery. The most common malignant masses to occur in this region are metastatic squamous cell carcinoma spread from the mouth. Submandibular gland tumors, lipoma, epidermoid/dermoid cysts, ranulas, infections, second branchial cleft cyst, and lymphangioma are seen.[48,49]

Salivary Gland Tumors

The benign and malignant features of salivary gland tumors on imaging demonstrate moderate similarities, and it may be difficult to distinguish between them. MRI has been shown to be superior in imaging salivary gland tumors. US uses irregular morphology of the lesion and its margin as well as the lesion's internal architecture to help differentiate between malignant and begin salivary gland tumors, but characteristic features may not always be present in a lesion.[50] Highly malignant lesions of the salivary glands may demonstrate rapid uptake of contrast on MRI images as well as slow washout. Additional features that are helpful when assessing for salivary gland tumors is perineural spread and (for large lesions) infiltration within the parapharyngeal space and adjacent musculature as well as osseous involvement. Perineural spread associated with salivary gland tumors on MRI will appear as fatty replacement in the neural foramina at the skull base with thickening of the nerve root with enhancement on postcontrast imaging.[51]

CT imaging of salivary gland tumors may underestimate the malignant potential because of a lack of contrast enhancement. Lesions such as adenoid cystic carcinoma do not demonstrate enhancement on CT postcontrast imaging. CT is an excellent adjunct to MRI if there is clinical concern for invasion of adjacent osseous structures as well as to assess for malignant cervical lymphadenopathy. PET/CT is accurate for assessing the extent of high-grade lesions and their nodal metastasis, but differentiating benign and low-grade malignant salivary tumors may be a challenge.[18,52] Hence, with regard to salivary gland tumors, PET/CT is mainly used to detect nodal involvement or distant metastasis.

Oral Cavity and Oropharyngeal Space Masses

Approximately 90% of oral cavity and oropharyngeal tumors are of squamous cell origin, followed by lymphoma and minor salivary gland tumors.[35]

Most oral cavity as well as oropharyngeal malignancies can be initially evaluated by contrast-enhanced CT imaging. MRI may be used to aid in revealing small tongue lesions and to delineate submucosal extension that cannot be detected by physical examination. Oral cavity lesions may benefit from multi-modality imaging: CT/MRI to assess tumor invasion in the soft tissue and mandible (**Fig. 3**) and PET/CT and US to search for lymph node metastasis.[53] The maximum accuracy of PET/CT is still relativity low at approximately 76%. PET/CT has demonstrated the highest specificity for staging oral cavity/oropharyngeal carcinomas, and US-guided FNA has shown the highest sensitivity.[16,54] For oral cavity cancers, imaging is of great benefit for surgical planning regarding the tongue and mandible. Squamous cell carcinomas invading the mandible usually do so through the alveolar crest, and mandibular involvement may need marginal resection or segmental mandibulectomy.[55] Osseous involvement of the mandible or maxilla is usually evaluated through CT or fused CT images and PET images (**Fig. 4**).[56]

MRI can also demonstrate osseous involvement, detected because malignancies replace the hypointense cortical bone and hyperintense medullary bone with hypointense bone marrow signal on T1-weighted imaging and hyperintense bone marrow signal on fat-suppressed T2-weighted imaging.[57,58] If imaging demonstrates neoplastic involvement of the prevertebral fascia, which is depicted as hyperintense

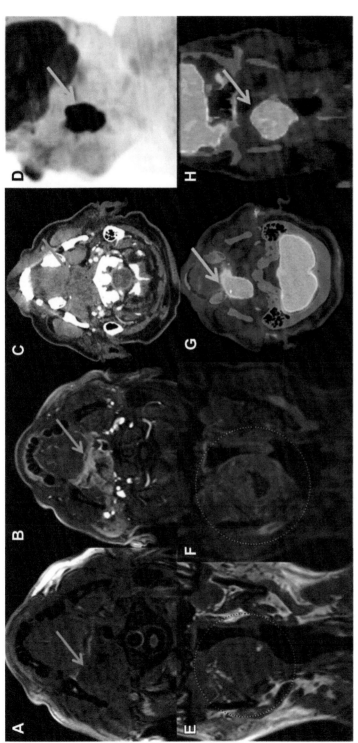

Fig. 3. Illustrating combining imaging modalities in evaluating clinical stage III-IV T3-T4 right tonsillar adenoid cystic carcinoma in 55-year-old man. Precontrast axial T1-weighted image (WI) (*A*), postcontrast axial T2WI (*B*), contrast-enhanced axial CT image (*C*), coronal PET (*D*), precontrast coronal T1WI (*E*), postcontrast coronal T1WI (*F*), as well as (*G*) axial and (*H*) coronal fused PET/CT demonstrates abnormal enhancing mass (*green arrow*) in the right tonsil, which causes mass effect and narrowing of the oropharynx with invasion of the adjacent tissues at the skull base. Radiographically, this is stage IV T4. The yellow *arrow* refers to the abnormal mass which represents the lesion on the axial CT imaging. The circles in (*E*) and (*F*) also show the abnormal mass which also represents the lesion on the coronal CT imaging.

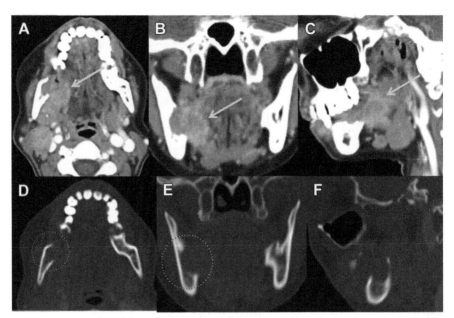

Fig. 4. Contrast-enhanced axial (*A, D*), coronal (*B, E*), as well as sagittal (*C, F*) soft tissue and bone windows demonstrate abnormally enhancing lesion (*arrows*) adjacent to the right mandible with invasion and osseous destruction of the right lingual mandible. The circles in (*D, E*) and F refer to the osseous destruction of the lingual mandible.

signal on T2-weighted imaging, then the lesion is often unresectable. Thus, it is important to examine the retropharyngeal fat plane and its preservation.[14,59] Lesions exceeding 2 cm with sublingual involvement are associated with involvement of the neurovascular bundle in the floor of the mouth.[60–62]

Masticator Space Masses

The masticator space contains the vertical mandibular ramus, masseter muscle, temporalis muscle, medial/lateral pterygoid muscles, V3 of cranial nerve V (trigeminal nerve), and inferior alveolar artery/vein. The superficial layer of the deep cervical fascia surrounds these areas. **Fig. 5** demonstrates recurrent squamous cell carcinoma eroding the left mandibular ramus. The most common lesions in the masticator space are odontogenic infections, osseous malignancies, neurogenic neoplasms, lymphoma, leukemia, or extensive squamous cell carcinomas that arise from the retromolar trigone.[62]

Buccal Space Masses

The buccal space is located posterolateral to the lower maxilla and is mostly fatty in nature. However, it also carries the facial artery and vein as well as the distal parotid duct. The buccinator muscle forms the buccal space's lateral margin. The processes affecting this region are similar to those that affect the masticator space.[63]

Laryngeal Masses

The larynx extends from the vallecula to the region between the cricoid and first tracheal ring. The supraglottic larynx starts with the tip of the epiglottis and terminates in the laryngeal ventricle. The glottic larynx runs from the true vocal cords to a centimeter below the vibrating surface. The infraglottic larynx extends from there to the

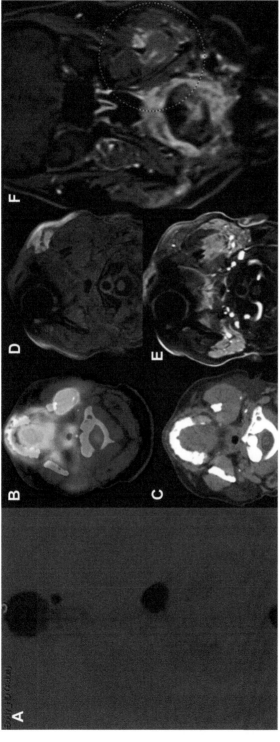

Fig. 5. Coronal maximum-intensity projection (*A*) and axial fused PET/CT (*B*) image demonstrates an FDG avid lesion with significant metabolic activity. This lesion corresponds to a masticator space mass with osseous invasion involving the left mandible (axial noncontrast CT image [*C*]). Image (*D*) is the precontrast fat-suppressed image, which also demonstrated lysis of the left mandible. This lesion demonstrated abnormal enhancement of postcontrast axial and coronal MRI fat-suppressed T1-weighted imaging (*E*, *F*). The circles in (*F*) refer to the abnormal enhancing left masticator mass.

inferior aspect of the cricoid. The most common malignant lesion in this region is squamous cell carcinoma. Other laryngeal masses include small cell tumors, adenocarcinoma, minor salivary gland tumors, and sarcomas. It is important to report nodal metastases, cartilage invasion, infraglottic extension, pre-epiglottic and paraglottic invasion, as well as extension to midline, which are staging criteria.[64] **Fig. 6** demonstrates the normal anatomy of the larynx.

Laryngeal carcinomas are best evaluated with contrast-enhanced CT imaging, which can accurately stage the primary tumor, informing decisions regarding larynx preservation. PET/CT can be used to assess metastatic disease **(Fig. 7)**.[1] Invasion of paraglottic space, laryngeal cartilage, and base of the tongue can be adequately assessed by either contrast-enhanced CT or MRI studies. MRI images in laryngeal carcinomas can show cervical esophageal invasion by assessing for esophageal wall thickening, evaluating the integrity of the adjacent fat planes, as well as T2 signal abnormality.[65,66] Early cartilage involvement can sometimes be detected by hyperintense signal on T1- and T2-weighted contrast-enhanced MRI.[67]

Hypopharyngeal Masses

Hypopharyngeal carcinomas may invade the prevertebral space and cause effacement of the retropharyngeal fat plane on CT and MRI images. These carcinomas usually present at an advanced stage with nodal involvement at initial diagnosis. Thus, PET/CT is usually recommended to evaluate regional as well as distant metastasis.

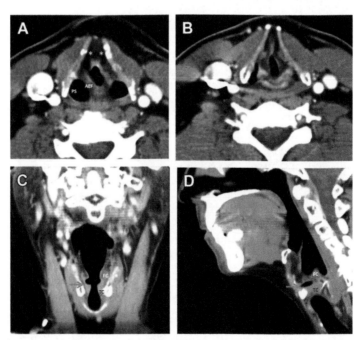

Fig. 6. False cord and true vocal cords: (A) Contrast-enhanced axial CT image demonstrates the false vocal cords (FC), which are characterized by the low-density fat (*asterisk*) in the paraglottic space. (B) The true vocal cords (TC) are located at the lower cricoarytenoid joint. The thyroarytenoid muscle makes up the paraglottic tissue, and this muscle attaches to the vocal process of arytenoid. The *arrows* point to the laryngeal ventricle, which is located between the FC and TC. (C, D) demonstrate the true and false vocal cords in the coronal and sagittal planes. PS, pyriform sinus; AEF, aryepiglottic fold.

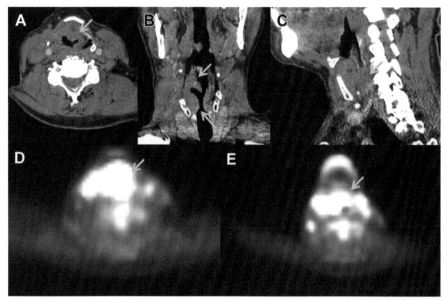

Fig. 7. Contrast-enhanced axial (*A*), coronal (*B*), and sagittal images (*C*) as well as axial PET images (*D*, *E*) demonstrate a significantly avid lesion with the supraglottic larynx (*arrows*). This lesion is a stage IVA (T3N2c) squamous cell carcinoma of the supraglottic larynx.

A standardized uptake value less than 9.0 in the primary mass has been linked to a decreased incidence of relapse and an increased chance of disease-free survival. Additionally, the metabolic tumor volume before treatment has also been implicated as an independent prognostic factor in patients with local or regionally advanced squamous cell carcinoma of the hypopharynx.[68,69]

Restaging After Treatment

Posttreatment imaging is used to detect residual, recurrent, or distant metastatic disease. Surgery and radiation therapy significantly alter the anatomy of the head and neck, creating great challenge for the interpreting radiologist. PET/CT is frequently used for posttreatment evaluation of suprahyoid malignancy because it can alter patient management significantly. All imaging modalities are subject to false-positive results. Thus, it is imperative that abnormal imaging findings should be paired with clinical findings and possible tissue sampling to increase diagnostic accuracy. Imaging immediately after treatment is generally not advised because of the elevated false-positive rates from surrounding inflammatory changes. Most institutions recommend an imaging-free interval after treatment ranging through 1 week after needle biopsy, 3 weeks after chemotherapy, 6 weeks after surgery, and up to 3 months after radiation therapy.[70]

CT and MRI are superior in evaluating treatment response and residual or recurrent local and regional tumor in infrahyoid head and neck neoplasms. Tumor volume, vocal cord mobility, and laryngeal cartilage sclerosis on CT as well as abnormal signal within the laryngeal cartilage on MRI are all important signs suggesting recurrence and have predictive value.[67,68] However, PET/CT is also a valuable tool in evaluating laryngeal and hypopharyngeal carcinomas when used for treatment response, residual, recurrent, or metastatic disease. As discussed earlier, these imaging studies are best performed about 3 months after radiation treatment. Local and regional imaging with CT or MRI is not usually undertaken in asymptomatic patients unless examination suggests recurrent disease.

SUMMARY

Imaging is an essential tool in the management of head and neck cancer. Oral, oropharyngeal, laryngeal, and hypopharyngeal lesions are usually initially imaged with CT because the modality allows rapid image acquisition and reduces artifacts related to respiration and swallowing, which can significantly degrade image quality and limit evaluation. Sinonasal, nasopharyngeal, and salivary gland tumors are better approached with MRI because it allows for better delineation of tumor extent. PET/CT is usually reserved for advanced disease to evaluate for distant metastatic disease as well as to evaluate posttreatment residual and recurrent disease. Imaging overall is best used in combination with expert clinical and physical examination.

REFERENCES

1. Antoniou AJ, Marcus C, Subramaniam RM. Value of imaging in head and neck tumors. Surg Oncol Clin N Am 2014;23:685–707.
2. Alberico RA, Husain SH, Sirotkin I. Imaging in head and neck oncology. Surg Oncol Clin N Am 2004;13:13–35.
3. Ljung BM, Larsson SG, Hanafee W. Computed tomography guided aspiration cytology examination in head and neck lesions. Arch Otolaryngol 1984;110: 604–7.
4. Cameron RH, Mann CH. Fine needle aspiration and computed tomographic scanning in the evaluation of parotid lesions. Ear Nose Throat J 1989;68: 226–36.
5. Dresel SH, Mackey JK, Lufkin RB, et al. Meckel cave lesions: percutaneous fine-needle-aspiration biopsy cytology. Radiology 1991;179:579–82.
6. Barakos JA, Dillon WP. Lesions of the foramen ovale: CT-guided fine-needle aspiration. Radiology 1992;182:573–5.
7. Stechison MT, Bernstein M. Percutaneous transfacial needle biopsy of a middle cranial fossa mass: case report and technical note. Neurosurgery 1989;25:996–9.
8. Mukherji SK, Turetsky D, Tart RP, et al. A technique for core biopsies of head and neck masses. AJNR Am J Neuroradiol 1994;15:518–20.
9. Gatenby RA, Mulhern CB, Richter MP, et al. CT-guided biopsy for the detection and staging of tumors of the head and neck. AJNR Am J Neuroradiol 1984;5: 287–9.
10. Abemayor E, Ljung BM, Larsson S, et al. CT directed fine needle aspiration biopsies of masses in the head and neck. Laryngoscope 1985;95:1382–6.
11. Yousem DM, Sack MJ, Scanlan KA. Biopsy of parapharyngeal space lesions. Radiology 1994;193:619–22.
12. Kim SY, Roh JL, Kim JS, et al. Utility of FDG PET in patients with squamous cell carcinomas of the oral cavity. Eur J Surg Oncol 2008;34(2):208–15.
13. Ng SH, Yen TC, Chang JT, et al. Prospective study if [18F] fluorodeoxyglucose positron emission tomography and computed tomography and magnetic resonance imaging in oral cavity squamous cell carcinoma with palpably negative neck. J Clin Oncol 2006;24(27):4371–6.
14. Hsu WC, Loevner LA, Karpati R, et al. Accuracy of magnetic resonance imaging in predicting absence of fixation of head and neck cancer to the prevertebral space. Head Neck 2005;27(2):95–100.

15. Baatenburg de Jong RJ, Rongen RJ, Verwoerd CD, et al. Ultrasound-guided fine-needle aspiration biopsy of neck nodes. Arch Otolaryngol Head Neck Surg 1991; 117(4):402–4.
16. Van den Brekel MW, Castelijns JA, Stel HV, et al. Modern imaging techniques and ultrasound-guided aspiration cytology for the assessment of neck node metastases: a prospective comparative study. Eur Arch Otorhinolaryngol 1993;250:11–7.
17. Kerberle M, Kenn W, Hahn D. Current concepts in imaging of laryngeal and hypopharyngeal cancer. Eur Radiol 2002;12(7):1672–83.
18. Chong VF, Khoo JB, Fan YF. Imaging of the nasopharynx and skull base. Magn Reson Imaging Clin N Am 2002;10:547–71.
19. Genden GM, Alfio F, Silver CM, et al. Contemporary management of cancer of the oral cavity. Eur Arch Otorhinolaryngol 2010;267(7):1001–17.
20. Ettl T, Schwarz-Furlan S, Gosau M, et al. Salivary gland carcinomas. Oral Maxillofac Surg 2012;16(3):267–83.
21. Lee YY, Wong KT, King A, et al. Imaging of salivary gland tumours. Eur J Radiol 2008;66(3):267–83.
22. Johnson JT, Barnes EL, Myers EN, et al. The extracapsular spread of tumors in cervical node metastasis. Arch Otolaryngol 1981;107:725–9.
23. Ferlito A, Rinaldo A, Devaney KO, et al. Prognostic significance of microscopic and macroscopic extracapsular spread from metastatic tumor in the cervical lymph nodes. Oral Oncol 2002;38:747–51.
24. Johnson JT, Myers EN, Bedetti CD, et al. Cervical lymph node metastases: incidence and implications of extracapsular carcinoma. Arch Otolaryngol 1985;111:534–7.
25. Snyderman NL, Johnson JT, Schramm VL, et al. Extracapsular spread of carcinoma in cervical lymph nodes: impact upon survival in patients with carcinoma of the supraglottic larynx. Cancer 1985;56:1597–9.
26. Carvalho BM. Quantitative analysis of the extent of extra-capsular invasion and its prognostic significance: a prospective study of 170 cases of carcinoma of the larynx and hypopharynx. Head Neck 1998;20:16–21.
27. Som PM. Detection of metastasis in cervical lymph nodes: CT and MR criteria and differential diagnosis. AJR Am J Roentgenol 1992;158:961–9.
28. Van den Brekel MW, Stel HV, Castelijins JA, et al. Cervical lymph node metastases: assessment of radiological criteria. Radiology 1990;177:379–84.
29. Steinkamp HJ, van der Hoeck E, Böck JC, et al. The extracapsular spread of cervical lymph node metastases: the diagnostic value of computed tomography. Rofo 1999;170:457–62 [in German].
30. Van den Brekel MW, van der Waal I, Meijer CJ, et al. The incidence of micrometastases in neck dissection specimens obtained from elective neck dissections. Laryngoscope 1996;106:987–91.
31. Yousem DM, Som PM, Hackney DB, et al. Central nodal necrosis and extracapsular neoplastic spread in cervical lymph nodes: MR imaging versus CT. Radiology 1992;182:753–9.
32. Steinkamp HJ, Hosten N, Richter C, et al. Enlarged cervical lymph nodes at helical CT. Radiology 1994;191:795–8.
33. Tartaglione T, Summaria V, Medoro A, et al. Metastatic lymphadenopathy from ENT carcinoma: role of diagnostic imaging. Rays 2000;25:429–46.
34. Hudgins PA, Kingdom TT, Weissler MC, et al. Selective neck dissection: CT and MR imaging findings. AJNR Am J Neuroradiol 2005;26(5):1174–7.
35. Yousem DM, Chalian AA. Oral cavity and pharynx. Radiol Clin North Am 1998; 36(5):967–81.

36. Boas FE, Fleischmann D. Evaluation of two iterative techniques for reducing metal artifacts in computed tomography. Radiology 2011;259(3):894–902.
37. De Man B, Nuyts J, Dupont P, et al. Metal streak artifacts in X-ray computed tomography: a simulation study. IEEE Trans Nucl Sci 1999;46(3):691–6.
38. Boas FE, Fleischmann D. CT artifacts: causes and reduction techniques. Imaging Med 2012;4(2):229–40.
39. American College of Radiology. ACR manual on contrast media. Available at: http://www.acr.org/Quality -Safety/Resources/Contrast-Manual, v9; http://www.acr.org/~/media/ACR/Documents/PDF/QualitySafety/Resources/Contrast%20Manual/2013_Contrast_Media.pdf/#2013_Contrast_Media_Manual.indd:.27730:10177. Accessed January 10, 2015.
40. Bottomley PA, Kumar A, Edelstein WA, et al. Designing passive MRI-safe implantable conducting leads with electrodes. Med Phys 2010;37:3828–43.
41. Shellock FG, Kanal E, Gilk T. Regarding the value reported for the term "spatial gradient 5magnetic field" and how this information is applied to labeling of medical implants and devices. Am J Roentgenol 2011;12:30–6.
42. Shellock FG, Begnaud J, Inman DM. System: in vitro evaluation of MRI-related heating and function at 1.5- and 3-Tesla. Neuromodulation 2006;9:204–13.
43. Yamashiro I, Souza RP. Imaging diagnosis of nasopharyngeal tumors. Radiol Bras 2007;40(1):45–52.
44. Chan JY, Wei WI. Current management strategy of hypopharyngeal carcinoma. Auris Nasus Larynx 2013;40(1):2–6.
45. Kato H, Kanematsu M, Mizuta K, et al. Carcinoma ex pleomorphic adenoma of the parotid gland. Radiology-pathologic correlation with MR imaging including diffusion-weighted imaging. AJNR Am J Neuroradiol 2008;29:865–7.
46. Moonis G, Patel P, Koshkareva Y, et al. Imaging characteristics of recurrent pleomorphic adenoma of the parotid gland. AJNR Am J Neuroradiol 2007;28:1532–6.
47. Shah GV. MR imaging of the salivary glands. Magn Reson Imaging Clin N Am 2002;10:631–62.
48. Kaneda T, Minami M, Ozawa K, et al. MR of the submandibular gland: normal and pathologic states. AJNR Am J Neuroradiol 1996;17:1575–81.
49. Laine FJ, Smoker WR. Oral cavity: anatomy and pathology. Semin Ultrasound CT MR 1995;16:527–45.
50. Bialek EJ, Jakubowski W, Zajkowski P, et al. US of the major salivary glands: anatomy and spatial relationships, pathologic conditions, and pitfalls. Radiographics 2006;26(3):745–63.
51. Thoeny HC. Imaging of salivary gland tumors. Cancer Imaging 2007;7:52–62.
52. Hadiprodjo D, Ryan T, Truong MT, et al. Parotid gland tumors: preliminary data for the value of FDG PET/CT diagnostic parameters. AJR Am J Roentgenol 2012;198(2):W185–90.
53. Tahari AK, Alluri KC, Quon H, et al. FDG PET/CT imaging of oropharyngeal squamous cell carcinoma: characteristics of human papillomavirus-positive and-negative tumors. Clin Nucl Med 2014;39(3):225–31.
54. Stuckensen T, Kovascs AF, Adams S, et al. Staging of the neck in patients with oral cavity squamous cell carcinomas: a prospective comparison of PET, ultrasound, CT and MRI. J Craniomaxillofac Surg 2000;28(6):319–24.
55. Huntley TA, Busmanis I, Desmond P, et al. Mandibular invasion by squamous cell carcinoma: a computed tomographic and histological study. Br J Oral Maxillofac Surg 1996;34(1):69–74.
56. Babin E, Desmonts C, Hamon M, et al. PET/CT for assessing mandibular invasion by intraoral squamous cell carcinomas. Clin Otolaryngol 2008;33(1):47–51.

57. Bolzoni A, Cappiello J, Piazza C, et al. Diagnostic accuracy of magnetic resonance imaging in the assessment of mandibular involvement in oral-oropharyngeal squamous cell carcinoma: a prospective study. Arch Otolaryngol Head Neck Surg 2004;130(7):837–43.

58. Vidiri A, Guerrisi A, Pellini R, et al. Multi-detector row computed tomography (MDCT) and magnetic resonance imaging (MRI) in the evaluation of the mandibular invasion by squamous cell carcinomas (SCC) of the oral cavity. Correlation with pathological data. J Exp Clin Cancer Res 2010;29:73.

59. Lam P, Au-Yeung KN, Cheng PW, et al. Correlating MRI and histologic tumor thickness in assessment of oral tongue cancer. AJR Am J Roentgenol 2004; 182(3):803–8.

60. Miller FR, Karnad AB, Eng T, et al. Management of the unknown primary carcinoma: long-term follow-up on a negative PET scan and negative panendoscopy. Head Neck 2008;30(1):28–34.

61. Minn H, Paul R, Ahonen A. Evaluation of treatment response to radiotherapy in head and neck cancer with fluorin-18 fluorodeoxyglucose. J Nucl Med 1988; 29(9):1521–5.

62. Connor SE, David SM. Masticator space masses and pseudomasses. Clin Radiol 2004;59:237–45.

63. Tart RP, Kotzyr IM, Mancuso AA, et al. CT and MR imaging of the buccal space and buccal space masses. Radiographics 1995;15:531–50.

64. Yousem DM, Tufano RP. Laryngeal imaging. Neuroimaging Clin N Am 2004;14: 611–24.

65. Hermanas R. Staging of laryngeal and hypopharyngeal cancer: value of imaging studies. Eur Radiol 2006;16(11):2386–400.

66. Rumbolt Z, Gordon L, Gordon L, et al. Imaging in head and neck cancer. Curr Treat Options Oncol 2006;7(1):23–34.

67. Becker M, Burkhardt K, dulquerov P, et al. Imaging of the larynx and hypopharynx. Eur J Radiol 2008;66(3):460–79.

68. Joshi VM, Wadhwa V, Mukheriji SK, et al. Imaging in laryngeal cancers. Indian J Radiol Imaging 2012;22(3):209–26.

69. Park GC, Kim JS, Roh JL, et al. Prognostic value of metabolic tumor volume measured by 18F-FDG PET/CT in advanced-stage squamous cell carcinoma of the larynx and hypopharynx. Ann Oncol 2013;24(1):208–14.

70. Goerres GW, von Schulthless GK, Hany TF. Positron emission tomography and PET/CT of the head and neck: FDG uptake in normal anatomy, in benign lesions, and in changes resulting from treatment. AJR Am J Roentgenol 2002;179: 1337–43.

Principles and Practice of Reconstructive Surgery for Head and Neck Cancer

Sameer A. Patel, MD*, Eric I. Chang, MD

KEYWORDS

- Head and neck reconstruction • Tongue reconstruction • Pharyngeal reconstruction
- Mandible reconstruction • Oral cavity reconstruction • Free flap • Microsurgery

KEY POINTS

- Goals for head and neck reconstruction include optimal functional and aesthetic outcomes.
- Free flaps are often the first choice of reconstructive options in head and neck reconstruction.
- Appropriate flap selection optimizes functional outcomes.
- When possible, replace tissue with similar tissue.
- Early referral to physical therapy, occupational therapy, and speech and swallow therapy helps to optimize outcomes.

PATIENT EVALUATION OVERVIEW

Evaluation of the patient needing reconstructive surgery is multifaceted but can be simplified based on the anatomic site of the cancer and the anticipated defect, evaluation of the potential donor sites for reconstruction, and whether adjuvant therapies are required. Attention to these domains during patient evaluation helps produce the best reconstructive result for each patient. Replacing like with like is an important principle in reconstructive surgery.

SOFT TISSUE RECONSTRUCTION

Soft tissue reconstruction of the head and neck stems largely from the extirpation of cutaneous malignancies, including basal cell carcinoma, squamous cell carcinoma, and melanoma. Based on the size of the residual defect after wide local excision of the malignancies with clear margins, reconstruction can pose a formidable challenge (**Table 1**).[1] This observation is especially true in sites where full-thickness defects

The authors have nothing to disclose.
Division of Plastic and Reconstructive Surgery, Department of Surgical Oncology, Fox Chase Cancer Center, 333 Cottman Avenue, Philadelphia, PA 19111, USA
* Corresponding author.
E-mail address: sameer.patel@fccc.edu

Table 1
Surgical margins of resection for skin malignancies

Type of Cancer	Recommended Margins of Resection
Basal cell carcinoma	1–2 mm
Squamous cell carcinoma	2–4 mm
Melanoma	
Melanoma in situ	5 mm
<1 mm	5 mm
1–2 mm	1 cm
>2 mm	2 cm

involve components such as cartilage or mucosa in addition to the overlying skin. With the advent of Mohs micrographic surgery, the size of these defects can be decreased to facilitate closure and reconstruction. Healing by second intention, primary closure for small defects, or skin grafts for larger defects are the simplest options. They may produce inferior cosmetic outcomes. Here, the principal techniques for soft tissue reconstruction are presented by anatomic site.[2]

Eye

Reconstruction of the periorbital region can usually be achieved with skin grafts for partial-thickness defects or local tissue rearrangement for full-thickness defects. Large, full-thickness defects of the eyelids require lid switch procedures such as Fricke or Tripier flaps.[3,4] If an orbital exenteration is necessary, reconstruction with cervicofacial flaps or free tissue transfer (such as a radial forearm flap) may be needed.[5,6] If a prosthesis is planned, reconstruction with less bulky soft tissue is preferable. A bulkier flap is necessary to fill the cavity if prostheses are not used.[7]

Ear

Because the ear is composed of cartilage as well as overlying soft tissue, reconstruction largely depends on whether a full-thickness or partial-thickness defect is created. If the perichondrium has been preserved, skin grafting or primary closure is the best option. However, if the defect encompasses the perichondrium or cartilage, conversion to a full-thickness wedge resection and primary closure or Antia-Buch helical advancement may be preferable.[8] Another option is to use a cartilage graft from the contralateral ear or rib, which requires flap coverage with retroauricular skin or temporoparietal fascia. This approach requires a second stage to divide and inset the flap as well as additional skin grafting.[9,10]

Mouth

The lips are composed of mucosa as well as the wet and dry vermilion overlying the orbicularis oris muscles. The upper lip has several distinct anatomic subunits, including the philtral columns, the Cupid bow, the white roll, and the tubercle.[2] Lip reconstruction depends strongly on the amount of vermilion remaining. Partial-thickness defects may be reconstructed with vermilion switch procedures or vermilion and mucosal advancement flaps. Reconstruction of full-thickness defects also depends on the amount of residual lip tissue (**Table 2**).[11–14]

Table 2 Surgical options for lip reconstruction	
Size of Defect	**Reconstruction**
<30%	Primary closure
Central lip defect 30%–50%	Abbé flap
30%–50%	Schuchardt procedure
Subtotal lip defect 50%–80%	Karapandzic flap
Subtotal lip defect involving commissure	Estlander flap
Total lip defect	Radial forearm free flap

Nose

The nose can be divided into 9 distinct cosmetic zones, including the nasal tip, dorsum, columella, and the paired nasal sidewalls, ala, and soft triangles.[15] Primary closure is difficult because of absence of soft tissue laxity and skin grafts are prone to contour irregularities and pin-cushioning. Full-thickness defects can be particularly challenging because of the need to reconstruct the nasal mucosa. The primary options for nasal reconstruction include the bilobed flap, nasolabial flap, and paramedian forehead flap (**Table 3**).[16–22]

Cheek

The cheek is the largest surface of the face and can be divided in 3 anatomic zones: suborbital, preauricular, and buccomandibular.[23] Primary closure of most cheek defects is recommended if possible. Local advancement, transposition, and rotation flaps are helpful for closure of smaller defects.[24] For defects too large for local maneuvers, cervicofacial and cervicopectoral flaps are recommended.[25,26]

Scalp

The scalp is composed of 5 distinct layers, including skin, subcutaneous fat, galea aponeurotica, loose areolar tissue, and pericranium.[2] The blood supply is excellent. Although skin grafting can be performed whenever the pericranium is preserved, reconstruction of the scalp is determined largely by the size of the defect (**Table 4**).[27–29] If calvarial reconstruction is needed in addition to soft tissue coverage, concurrent cranioplasty with an implant can be performed without increased risk of complications (**Fig. 1**).[30]

Major Soft Tissue Defects of the Neck

In some instances, soft tissue reconstruction of the neck may be necessary when treating patients with head and neck cancers. These defects may be caused by primary extirpation of malignancies (large skin malignancies, combined laryngopharyngeal and skin defects) or secondary to complications attributable to previous surgery

Table 3 Surgical options for nasal reconstruction		
Type of Flap	**Size (cm)**	**Location**
Bilobed flap	<1	Ala, sidewall
Nasolabial flap	<1.5	Ala
Paramedian forehead flap	>2	All

Table 4
Surgical options for scalp reconstruction

Size of Defect (cm)	Reconstruction
<3	Primary closure with or without galeal scoring
3–6	Scalp rotation flap
6–9	Scalp rotation flap with skin grafting
>9	Free tissue transfer

(pharyngocutaneous or orocutaneous fistulas, exposure of mandibular hardware, skin flap necrosis). The pectoralis or deltopectoral flaps may be useful in these scenarios.[31–33] Once considered workhorse flaps for head and neck reconstruction for a multitude of defects (pharyngeal, mandibular, oral cavity), these 2 regional flaps are now more commonly used for soft tissue reconstruction of the oral cavity and neck in patients not deemed good candidates for free tissue transfer and for management of complications arising from previous resection and reconstruction. The pectoralis flap can transpose muscle alone or as a myocutaneous paddle. Based on the thoracoacromial blood supply, it provides ample muscle with a robust vascular supply to resurface neck defects, aid in healing orocutaneous or pharyngocutaneous fistulas (PCFs), or coverage of exposed mandible or mandibular hardware. The arc of rotation

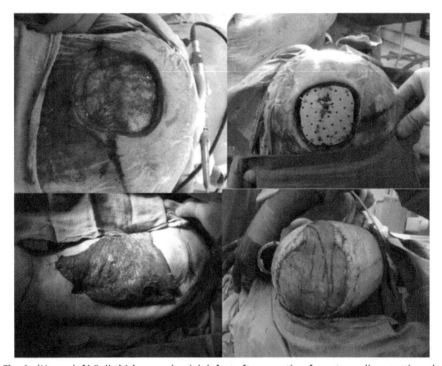

Fig. 1. (*Upper left*) Full-thickness calvarial defect after resection for osteoradionecrotic scalp secondary to skin cancer treatment. (*Upper right*) Polyether-ether ketone implant for calvarial reconstruction. (*Lower left*) Latissimus dorsi flap elevated at the donor site. (*Lower right*) Latissimus flap coverage of implant and scalp reconstruction with superficial temporal vessels as recipient vessels.

limits its scope and may place tension on the superior aspect of the suture line. In addition, fibrosis and contracture may result from rotation of the flap from the chest wall to the neck, limiting range of motion. Bulk may limit its usefulness for applications related to tracheostomal revisions. To avoid problems with neck and shoulder function, attention to rehabilitation is imperative after pectoralis flap reconstruction. The deltopectoral flap is an axial pattern skin flap based on perforators arising from the internal mammary vessels. It may be used in 1 stage, but transposed tissue survival is improved by delaying it before transfer. Skin grafting to the donor site may leave a prominent scar at the donor site. The pectoralis and deltopectoral flaps, although less important in the era of microsurgery, should remain in the armamentarium of the reconstructive head and neck surgeon.

MAXILLA RECONSTRUCTION

Although resection of palatomaxillary malignancies is uncommon, the resulting defect can cause substantial functional and cosmetic problems, because of the need to replace the mucosa, bony framework, and sometimes, the overlying soft tissue.[29,34] Reconstruction of the three-dimensional framework of the midface must restore form as well as function. Reconstruction should enable the patient to speak and eat and should provide support for the orbital contents, maintaining separation of the oral and nasal cavities. In most centers, the most common approach is the placement of an obturator. However, they impose limitations in terms of maintenance, fitting, and comfort.[35,36] Even when prosthetic rehabilitation is a reasonable option, free flap reconstruction of maxillary defects provides the patient with an excellent alternative.[37–39]

To assess the extent of the maxillectomy defect and therefore select the appropriate reconstructive option, various classification systems have been proposed. The most common was proposed by Cordeiro and Santamaria in 2000[40] to address the anatomy of palatal and maxillary defects (**Table 5**). A more elaborate classification system was proposed by Brown and colleagues,[41] which defines the extent of the maxillary defect based on horizontal and vertical components.

The largest reported series of maxillectomy reconstructions included 246 patients over a 10-year period; the investigators[42] proposed an algorithm based on the defect classification noted earlier. For partial maxillectomy defects that preserve both canine teeth, a prosthetic obturator is a reasonable option. However, if a large portion of the palate is resected, an obturator may not prove possible to retain. For suprastructure, premaxillary, and unilateral posterior defects, the investigators recommend a soft tissue flap to deliver adequate bulk and volume within the cheek as well as obliterate the maxillary sinus. Osteocutaneous flaps were reserved for unilateral and bilateral palatomaxillectomy defects to restore structure to the midface and provide the option for

Table 5 Classification of maxillectomy defects	
Type	**Extent of Defect**
I	Limited maxillectomy without palatal involvement
II	Subtotal maxillectomy with preservation of orbital floor
IIIA	Total maxillectomy with preservation of the orbit
IIIB	Total maxillectomy with orbital exenteration
IV	Orbitomaxillectomy with preservation of the palate

dental rehabilitation.[43] Orbital floor reconstruction is certainly recommended and can be performed with a variety of materials, including titanium mesh, bone graft, or allo-plastic materials. In the setting of orbital exenteration with palatomaxillectomy de-fects, large soft tissue flaps with multiple skin paddles are necessary to fill the orbital cavity, decrease the incidence of fistula, and to maintain the contour of the midface.

TONGUE RECONSTRUCTION

Reconstruction of the tongue after tumor resection is challenging, because of the high-ly specialized and important functions of the tongue. The tongue plays a major role in speech as well as the oral and pharyngeal phases of swallowing. The aim of recon-struction is to minimize the impact of resection on these crucial functions.

Classically, small defects of the tongue have been treated with primary closure, healing by second intention, or skin grafting. Although these approaches work well for defects isolated to the lateral tongue, larger glossectomies involving the oral tongue, anterior tongue, the base of tongue, or a combination of these (with or without involvement of the floor of mouth) often require more sophisticated microsurgical reconstructions.[44–46]

The radial forearm free flap (RFFF) and the anterolateral thigh (ALT) free flap are the 2 most commonly used free flaps for tongue reconstruction, although others have been described.[47–50] Use of vascularized flaps minimizes tethering of the tongue (thereby preserving mobility), provides bulk when needed, and allows for initiation of adjuvant radiation in a timely manner.

Selection of the appropriate flap requires nuanced judgment and should be made on an individual basis. For instance, hemiglossectomy defects isolated to the oral tongue are best suited for reconstruction with a thin, pliable flap such as an RFFF **(Fig. 2)**.[51–53] In contrast, large defects involving the oral tongue and base of tongue or total glossectomy are best suited for reconstruction with more bulky tissue such as an ALT flap.[54,55] There is no accepted classification in terms defining the nature of tongue defects, which significantly limits the ability to evaluate outcomes related to the type of flap used. Flap selection is important: the use of an overly bulky ALT flap for an oral tongue defect, or a thin RFFF flap for a large combined defect of the oral and base of tongue, would adversely affect the functional outcome.

Lam and Samman[56] provide a systematic review of speech and swallowing function after glossectomy with free flap reconstruction. For defects involving the oral tongue or base of tongue (alone) reconstructed with free flaps, sentence intelligibility returned to normal or near normal in most patients within 6 months to a year. However, those patients with involvement of both oral and base of tongue (total or subtotal glossec-tomy) had significant impairment in speech rehabilitation. In this group, more than 60% had speech that was only occasionally understood, unintelligible, or could be un-derstood only when the context was known to the listener. Factors influencing speech outcomes included tumor size, preservation of the tongue tip, and adjuvant radiation therapy.[57–59] In addition, lateral defects with flap reconstruction had better outcomes in speech than anterior defects.[60]

In the same review by Lam and Samman, swallowing function after glossectomy with flap reconstruction was evaluated. For oral tongue defects, although spillage and an increased number of attempts to clear liquid bolus may be seen in the short postoperative follow-up, these functions seem to return to normal or near normal at 1 year in most patients. For defects involving the base of tongue, bulk seems to be more important for swallowing to allow for contact with the pharyngeal wall

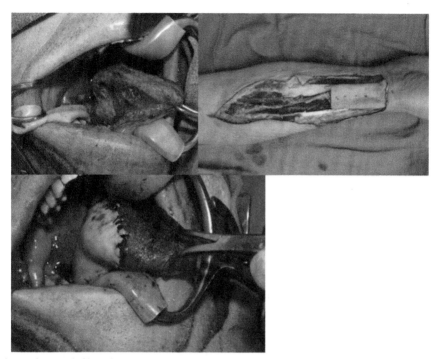

Fig. 2. (*Upper left*) Right hemiglossectomy defect. (*Upper right*) RFFF elevated in preparation for tongue reconstruction. (*Lower left*) Radial forearm flap reconstruction of the tongue.

(to enhance the pharyngeal phase of swallowing). For these defects, a more bulky flap such as an ALT flap should be considered. Problems include aspiration as well as pharyngeal residue for liquids and pudding consistencies. Most are able to resume pureed and solid food within a year. In the short-term, patients undergoing subtotal or total glossectomy as well as those with a combined oral and base of tongue resection have worse functional recovery despite free flap reconstruction than those undergoing resection of either oral tongue or base of tongue with a higher incidence of aspiration. However, these patients are also often able to return to a solid or soft diet within 2 years.[61,62]

Postoperative radiation therapy has been shown to decrease functional recovery after free tissue transfer. This decrease is likely related to the fibrosis and decreased mobility of the reconstructed tongue. Aggressive speech and swallow therapy should be implemented to maximize function.

Attempts at sensory and motor reinnervation of flaps to restore sensation and motor function have been reported.[49,51,54,63,64] Although various types of sensory recovery can be obtained (eg, 2-point discrimination, temperature), no functional improvement in terms of speech or swallowing has been demonstrated.

MANDIBLE RECONSTRUCTION

Defects involving the mandible may involve only an edge (marginal) or a complete segment (segmental). Small marginal mandibulectomy defects may be covered with local flaps or skin grafts if postoperative radiation therapy is not anticipated. However, for most larger marginal mandibulectomy defects, the RFFF is ideal given the thin, pliable nature of the tissue.[65–67] If dental rehabilitation is planned, an osteocutaneous radial forearm flap or a free fibula osteocutaneous flap can be used to augment mandibular height.

Segmental defects of the mandible after ablative surgery are best reconstructed with microsurgical free flaps. Bone grafts in this setting (in which postoperative radiation is likely) lead to high rates of complications, including bone resorption, osteoradionecrosis, orocutaneous fistula, and infection.[68,69] Reconstruction with a spanning titanium plate alone (without bony reconstruction) has also been described, but complication rates. including plate fracture, orocutaneous fistula, and need for plate removal. are high.[70,71] Pedicled osteomyocutaneous flaps such as sternocleidomastoid with clavicle and pectoralis with rib have also been described,[72,73] but the perfusion and quality of the bone stock in these flaps is low and does not allow for osteotomies for shaping. Free tissue transfer has supplanted these approaches.

Free osteocutaneous flaps provide optimal current outcomes for reconstruction of segmental defects of the mandible. The fibula, scapula, iliac crest, and radial forearm are the most commonly used; the free fibula flap is the workhorse for mandible reconstruction. These osteocutaneous flaps have characteristics that make them more or less suited to mandibular reconstruction, depending on the specific clinical situation (**Table 6**). First described and popularized by Hidalgo in the 1980s,[74] the free fibula flap can provide more than 20 cm of bicortical bone with excellent blood supply and good pedicle length to allow for reconstruction of most mandibular defects (**Fig. 3**). Simultaneous elevation of the flap and extirpation of the cancer using a 2-team approach allow for shorter operative time (when compared with sequential tumor resection followed by flap harvesting and reconstruction). The investigators recommend preoperative computed tomography angiography for evaluation of vascular runoff to the foot as well as assessment of the quality of the pedicle (peroneal artery).

Swartz and colleagues[75] first described the use of the scapula osteocutaneous free flap for mandible and maxillary reconstruction, and it is still widely used for mandible reconstruction. Using the lateral border of the scapula as the source of bone, and allowing for harvest of greater amounts of soft tissue, including the scapular and parascapular skin paddles (**Fig. 4**), this flap is based on the circumflex scapular vessels. Additional bone and muscle can be harvested by including the thoracodorsal system (latissimus dorsi muscle and tip of the scapula).[76] A 2-team approach is not feasible, and therefore, operative times are typically longer. However, this arteriovenous pedicle is usually spared from atherosclerotic disease and may represent a good option for those whose severe peripheral vascular disease precludes use of the fibula flap. Because of the limited blood supply to the lateral border of the bone, the number of osteotomies in a scapula flap should be limited to 2 or 3.

Table 6
Comparison of osteocutaneous free flaps for mandible reconstruction

Flap Type	Bone Stock	Soft Tissue	Pedicle Length	Donor Site Morbidity	Simultaneous Harvest (2-Team Approach)
Fibula	Excellent	Good	Good	Good	Yes
Scapula	Good	Excellent	Poor	Excellent	No
Iliac crest	Good	Good	Good	Poor	Yes
Radial forearm	Poor	Good	Excellent	Good	Yes

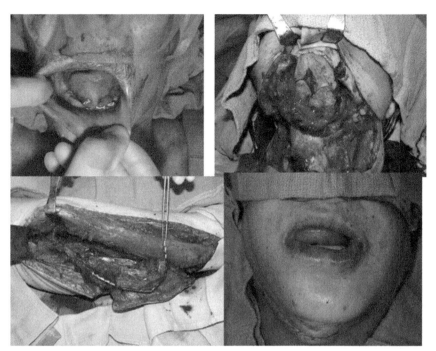

Fig. 3. (*Upper left*) Preoperative view of biopsy sites of intraoral squamous cell carcinoma. (*Upper right*) Intraoperative view of mandibular and intraoral defect. (*Lower left*) Free fibula flap harvest with multiple osteotomies mounted on reconstruction plate. (*Lower right*) Final intraoperative view.

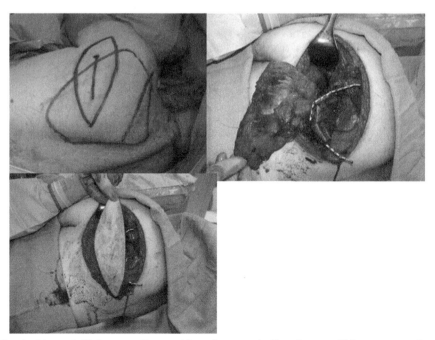

Fig. 4. (*Upper left*) Preoperative markings for scapula flap for mandible reconstruction. (*Upper right and lower left*) Intraoperative view of the scapula flap demonstrating generous amount of soft tissue that can be harvested from this donor site.

The deep circumflex iliac artery (DCIA) flap and radial forearm osteocutaneous flap (RFOF) have also been used for mandibular reconstruction.[77,78] However, because of significant donor site morbidity (gait disturbances and hernias with the DCIA flap and pathologic fracture of the radius with the RFOF flap), most centers frequently performing mandibular reconstruction reserve these flaps for settings in which the free fibula or scapula flaps are not available.

Several classification systems describe segmental defects of the mandible,[79–81] but that of Boyd and colleagues[79] is useful when discussing reconstruction of the mandible. This system describes the defects as central (c, including all 4 incisors and 2 canines), lateral (l, condyle is preserved), and hemimandible defect (h, lateral defects including the condyle). It also classifies the soft tissue involvement as skin (s), mucosa (m), and no soft tissue involvement (o).

For defects of the central and lateral type with mucosal loss, osteocutaneous free tissue transfer (such as the free fibula flap) is the preferred method of reconstruction. This situation is true of h-type defects that encroach on or include the central segment as well. Although condyle and temporomandibular joint reconstruction with prostheses or vascularized tissue can be considered, erosion into the skull base and ankylosis are potential and serious drawbacks. In this scenario, the lateral fibula segment can be left free floating, with good functional outcomes.[82,83] For h-type defects, which do not approach the central segment, good functional outcomes can be derived with either an osteocutaneous flap or a soft tissue flap alone (eg, ALT flap).[83]

Computer-assisted preoperative surgical planning with medical modeling is a new tool that can be applied to mandibular reconstruction with free osteocutaneous flaps. Templates for performing osteotomies on the mandible as well as the bone flap can reduce operative time, enhance bone contact, and reduce cost.[84] This technology is particularly useful when direct intraoperative plate contouring to the native mandible would not be possible (such as with exophytic tumors,[85] or in those patients whose preoperative occlusion has been lost as a result of pathologic fracture, osteoradionecrosis, or previous segmental resection without reconstruction).

Computer-assisted planning improves outcomes. Bony union at sites of osteotomies as well as the fibula-mandible junction is more than 90%, with good long-term maintenance of bone height.[86,87] Resumption of an oral diet can be expected in most patients with good speech intelligibility.[88] Risk of osteoradionecrosis is significantly reduced (compared with bone graft reconstruction), but should this late complication transpire, optimal treatment often involves the use of an additional bone flap.[89,90] Dental rehabilitation can also be performed in appropriately selected patients, with low risk of complications.[91] A fibula flap adds height to the reconstructed mandible to minimize cantilevering of dental implants.[92] For those patients who are not candidates for implants, dentures may be more practical, but limited by the absence of an alveolus on the bone flap.

PHARYNGEAL RECONSTRUCTION

Squamous cell carcinomas of the hypopharynx and larynx often result in either subtotal or circumferential hypopharyngeal defects. Initial efforts at organ preservation with definitive radiation often complicate the management of these defects. Primary closure is an important consideration for patients who have ample residual pharyngeal mucosa that can be reapproximated under no tension. In most other cases, free fasciocutaneous flaps (primarily the radial forearm and ALT flaps) have become the preferred method of reconstruction. In general, defects of two-thirds or less of the pharyngeal mucosa can be reconstructed with an RFFF in a patchlike fashion (**Fig. 5**). Larger

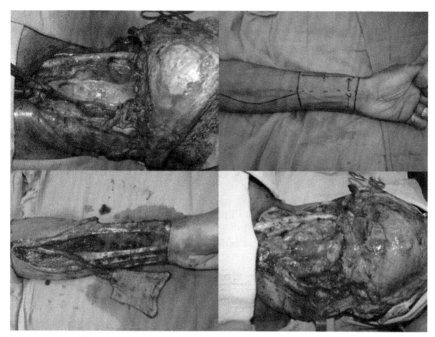

Fig. 5. (*Upper left*) Partial pharyngeal defect. (*Upper right and lower left*) Intraoperative harvest of radial forearm flap. (*Lower right*) Patchlike reconstruction of the pharyngeal defect.

and circumferential defects are better suited for reconstruction with a tubularized ALT flap. Yu and colleagues[93] reported the use of the ALT for total laryngopharyngectomy defects with low rates of PCF (9%), stenosis (6%), and flap failure (2%). Their technique includes harvesting of additional fascia to cover the anastomotic suture lines, preserving a small strip of posterior mucosa when possible, and spatulation of the distal cervical esophageal anastomosis. For partial defects of the hypopharynx, Disa and colleagues[94] reported comparable outcomes in terms of fistula rates, stenosis rates, and flap loss rates using the RFFF. Other teams have reported similar results with low mortality, PCF, and stricture rates with use of the radial forearm and ALT flaps for pharyngoesophageal reconstructions.[95–98]

The free jejunum flap provides another option for reconstruction of near circumferential or circumferential defects. Some debate exists as to whether PCF and stenosis rates are better with a jejunal flap or ALT flap for reconstruction of circumferential defects. Disa and colleagues[94] reported PCF and stenosis rates of 10% and 7%, and Chan and colleagues[99] reported rates of 5% and 2%, respectively, which are comparable with the ALT flap incidence. However, the possible donor site complications associated with the free jejunum flap (bowel obstruction, ileus, and intra-abdominal anastomotic leak) carry more morbidity than those of the ALT, rendering the jejunal flap less favorable. Hospital costs are also lower when using an ALT flap compared with the free jejunal flap with shorter postoperative ventilator support, time in intensive care unit, and hospital stay.[100]

The pedicled pectoralis myocutaneous flap is used for reconstruction of pharyngeal defects in some institutions, but this approach has lost favor. Studies have highlighted the increased rate of PCF as well as distal stricture, with reported rates as high as 57% and 43%, respectively.[96] This situation is related to the bulkiness of the flap, resulting in poor suture approximation to the residual mucosa, particularly at the cervical esophageal anastomosis. The weight of the flap may also place constant tension at the proximal suture line.

Swallowing function has been evaluated with respect to the reconstruction type. Fasciocutaneous flaps have shown superior feeding tube independence with return to regular diet in most patients when compared with the other flaps discussed earlier.[101–104] Peristalsis associated with the jejunum may lead to discoordinated swallowing, dysphagia, and regurgitation.[105] Restoration of good-quality, intelligible voice with either primary or secondary tracheoesophageal puncture is better with free fasciocutaneous flaps compared with the pectoralis or jejunal flaps.[103,106,107] The issue has been thoroughly reviewed.[108]

SUMMARY

Reconstruction after cancer surgery of the head and neck requires a wide variety of reconstructive techniques, ranging from simple to advanced. Attention to selection of the reconstructive procedure yields optimal aesthetic and functional recovery.

REFERENCES

1. National Comprehensive Cancer Network Clinical Practice Guidelines for Basal and Squamous Cell Skin Cancers and Melanoma. 2013.
2. Thorne CH, editor. Grabb and Smith's plastic surgery. 6th edition. Philadelphia: Lippincott Williams & Wilkins; 2007.
3. Spinelli HM, Jelks GW. Periocular reconstruction: a systematic approach. Plast Reconstr Surg 1993;91(6):1017–24.
4. Mustarde JC. Reconstruction of eyelids. Ann Plast Surg 1983;11(2):149–69.
5. Weizman N, Horowitz G, Gil Z, et al. Surgical management of tumors involving the orbit. JAMA Otolaryngol Head Neck Surg 2013;139(8):841–6.
6. Rabey N, Abood A, Gillespie P, et al. Reconstruction of complex orbital exenteration defects: a single center's experience with a five-year follow-up. Ann Plast Surg 2014;73(2):158–63.
7. Hanasono MM, Lee JC, Yang JS, et al. An algorithmic approach to reconstructive surgery and prosthetic rehabilitation after orbital exenteration. Plast Reconstr Surg 2009;123(1):98–105.
8. Antia NH, Buch MS. Chondocutaneous advancement flap for the marginal defect of the ear. Plast Reconstr Surg 1967;39:472.
9. Harris PA, Ladhani K, Das-Gupta R, et al. Reconstruction of acquired sub-total ear defects with autologous costal cartilage. Br J Plast Surg 1999;52(4):268.
10. Thorne CH, Brecht LE, Bradley JP, et al. Auricular reconstruction: indications for autogenous and prosthetic techniques. Plast Reconstr Surg 2001;107(5):1241.
11. Dupin C, Metzinger S, Rizzuto R. Lip reconstruction after ablation for skin malignancies. Clin Plast Surg 2004;31(1):69.
12. Langstein HN, Robb GL. Lip and perioral reconstruction. Clin Plast Surg 2005; 32(3):431.
13. Lubek JE, Ord RA. Lip reconstruction. Oral Maxillofac Surg Clin North Am 2013; 25(2):203–14.
14. Harris L, Higgins K, Enepekides D. Local flap reconstruction of acquired lip defects. Curr Opin Otolaryngol Head Neck Surg 2012;20(4):254–61.
15. Burget GC, Menick FJ. Subunit principle in nasal reconstruction. Plast Reconstr Surg 1985;76:239.
16. Elliots RA. Rotation flaps of the nose. Plast Reconstr Surg 1969;44:47.

17. Menick FJ. Ten-year experience in nasal reconstruction with the three-stage forehead flap. Plast Reconstr Surg 2002;109:1839.
18. Santos Stahl A, Gubisch W, Fischer H, et al. A cohort study of paramedian forehead flap in 2 stages (87 flaps) and 3 stages (100 flaps). Ann Plast Surg 2014. [Epub ahead of print].
19. Jellinek NJ, Nguyen TH, Albertini JG. Paramedian forehead flap: advances, procedural nuances, and variations in technique. Dermatol Surg 2014;40:S30–42.
20. Hubbard TJ. Leave the fat, skip the bolster: thinking outside the box in lower third nasal reconstruction. Plast Reconstr Surg 2004;114(6):1427–35.
21. Yotsuyanagi T, Yamashita K, Urushidate S, et al. Reconstruction of large nasal defects with a combination of local flaps based on the aesthetic subunit principle. Plast Reconstr Surg 2001;107(6):1358–62.
22. Svedman P. Advancement flaps for alar reconstruction. Ann Plast Surg 1990; 25(6):502–7.
23. Chadawarkar R, Cervino A. Subunits of the cheek: an algorithm for the reconstruction of partial thickness defects. Br J Plast Surg 2003;56:135–9.
24. Jowett N, Mlynarek AM. Reconstruction of cheek defects: a review of current techniques. Curr Opin Otolaryngol Head Neck Surg 2010;18(4):244–54.
25. Kroll SS, Reece GP, Robb GL, et al. Deep-plane cervicofacial rotation-advancement flap for reconstruction of large cheek defects. Plast Reconstr Surg 1994;94:88–93.
26. Rapstine ED, Knaus WJ, Thornton JF. Simplifying cheek reconstruction: a review of 400 cases. Plast Reconstr Surg 2012;129(6):1291–9.
27. Hoffman JF. Management of scalp defects. Otolaryngol Clin North Am 2001; 34(3):571–81.
28. Molnar JA, DeFranzo AJ, Marks MW. Single-stage approach to skin grafting the exposed skull. Plast Reconstr Surg 2000;105(1):174–7.
29. Wei FC, Dayan JH. Scalp, skull, orbit, and maxilla reconstruction and hair transplantation. Plast Reconstr Surg 2013;131(3):411e–24e.
30. Chao AH, Yu P, Skoracki RJ, et al. Microsurgical reconstruction of composite scalp and calvarial defects in patients with cancer: a 10-year experience. Plast Reconstr Surg 2012;34(12):1759–64.
31. Hanasono MM, Matros E, Disa JJ. Important aspects of head and neck reconstruction. Plast Reconstr Surg 2014;134(6):968e–80e.
32. Schneider DS, Wu V, Wax MK. Indications for pedicled pectoralis major flap in a free tissue transfer practice. Head Neck 2012;34(8):1106–10.
33. Mortensen M, Genden EM. Role of the island deltopectoral flap in contemporary head and neck reconstruction. Ann Otol Rhinol Laryngol 2006;115(5):361–4.
34. Neligan PC. Head and neck reconstruction. Plast Reconstr Surg 2013;131(2): 260e–9e.
35. Moreno MA, Skoracki RJ, Hanna EY, et al. Microvascular free flap reconstruction versus palatal obturation for maxillectomy defects. Head Neck 2010;32(7):860–8.
36. Rieger JM, Tang JA, Wolfaardt J, et al. Comparison of speech and aesthetic outcomes in patients with maxillary reconstruction versus maxillary obturators after maxillectomy. J Otolaryngol Head Neck Surg 2011;40(1):40–7.
37. Andrades P, Militsakh O, Hanasono MM, et al. Current strategies in reconstruction of maxillectomy defects. Arch Otolaryngol Head Neck Surg 2011;137(8): 806–12.
38. Corderio PG, Chen CM. A 15-year review of midface reconstruction after total and subtotal maxillectomy: Part I. Algorithm and outcomes. Plast Reconstr Surg 2012;129(1):124–36.

39. Corderio PG, Chen CM. A 15-year review of midface reconstruction after total and subtotal maxillectomy: Part II. Technical modifications to maximize aesthetic and functional outcomes. Plast Reconstr Surg 2012;129(1):139–47.

40. Cordeiro PG, Santamaria E. A classification system and algorithm for reconstruction of maxillectomy and midfacial defects. Plast Reconstr Surg 2000; 105(7):2331–46.

41. Brown JS, Rogers SN, McNally DN, et al. A modified classification for the maxillectomy defect. Head Neck 2000;22(1):17–26.

42. Hanasono MM, Silva AK, Yu P, et al. A comprehensive algorithm for oncologic maxillary reconstruction. Plast Reconstr Surg 2013;131(1):47–60.

43. Hanasono MM, Skoracki RJ. The omega-shaped fibula osteocutaneous free flap for reconstruction of extensive midfacial defects. Plast Reconstr Surg 2010; 125(4):160e–2e.

44. Urken ML, Moscoso JF, Lawson W, et al. A systematic approach to functional reconstruction of the oral cavity following partial and total glossectomy. Arch Otolaryngol Head Neck Surg 1994;120(6):589–601.

45. Engel H, Huang JJ, Lin CY, et al. A strategic approach for tongue reconstruction to achieve predictable and improved functional and aesthetic outcomes. Plast Reconstr Surg 2010;126(6):1967–77.

46. Hurvitz KA, Kobayashi M, Evans GR. Current options in head and neck reconstruction. Plast Reconstr Surg 2006;118(5):122e–33e.

47. Lyos AT, Evans GR, Perez D, et al. Tongue reconstruction: outcomes with the rectus abdominis flap. Plast Reconstr Surg 1999;103(2):442–7.

48. Thankappan K, Kuriakose MA, Chatni SS, et al. Lateral arm free flap for oral tongue reconstruction: an analysis of surgical details, morbidity, and functional and aesthetic outcome. Ann Plast Surg 2011;66(3):261–6.

49. Yousif NJ, Dzwierzynski WW, Sanger JR, et al. The innervated gracilis musculocutaneous flap for total tongue reconstruction. Plast Reconstr Surg 1999;104(4): 916–21.

50. Huang JJ, Wu CW, Lam WL, et al. Anatomical basis and clinical application of the ulnar forearm free flap for head and neck reconstruction. Laryngoscope 2012;122(12):2670–6.

51. Santamaria E, Wei FC, Chen IH, et al. Sensation recovery on innervated radial forearm flap for hemiglossectomy reconstruction by using different recipient nerves. Plast Reconstr Surg 1999;103(2):450–7.

52. Brown L, Rieger JM, Harris J, et al. A longitudinal study of functional outcomes after surgical resection and microvascular reconstruction for oral cancer: tongue mobility and swallowing function. J Oral Maxillofac Surg 2010;68(11):2690–700.

53. Bokhari WA, Wang SJ. Tongue reconstruction: recent advances. Curr Opin Otolaryngol Head Neck Surg 2007;15(4):202–7.

54. Yu P. Reinnervated anterolateral thigh flap for tongue reconstruction. Head Neck 2004;26(12):1038–44.

55. Ali RS, Bluebond-Langner R, Rodriguez ED, et al. The versatility of the anterolateral thigh flap. Plast Reconstr Surg 2009;124(6 Suppl):e395–407.

56. Lam L, Samman N. Speech and swallowing following tongue cancer surgery and free flap reconstruction–a systematic review. Oral Oncology 2013;49:507–24.

57. Sun J, Weng Y, Li J, et al. Analysis of determinants on speech function after glossectomy. J Oral Maxillofac Surg 2007;65(10):1944–50.

58. Shin YS, Koh YW, Kim SH, et al. Radiotherapy deteriorates postoperative functional outcome after partial glossectomy with free flap reconstruction. J Oral Maxillofac Surg 2012;70(1):216–20.

59. Nicoletti G, Soutar DS, Jackson MS, et al. Objective assessment of speech after surgical treatment for oral cancer: experience from 196 selected cases. Plast Reconstr Surg 2004;113(1):114–25.

60. Matsui Y, Ohno K, Yamashita Y, et al. Factors influencing postoperative speech function of tongue cancer patients following reconstruction with fasciocutaneous/myocutaneous flaps–a multicenter study. Int J Oral Maxillofac Surg 2007; 36(7):601–9.

61. Yun IS, Lee DW, Lee WJ, et al. Correlation of neotongue volume changes with functional outcomes after long-term follow-up of total glossectomy. J Craniofac Surg 2010;21(1):111–6.

62. Yanai C, Kikutani T, Adachi M, et al. Functional outcome after total and subtotal glossectomy with free flap reconstruction. Head Neck 2008;30(7):909–18.

63. Yamamoto Y, Sugihara T, Furuta Y, et al. Functional reconstruction of the tongue and deglutition muscles following extensive resection of tongue cancer. Plast Reconstr Surg 1998;102(4):993–8.

64. Uwiera T, Seikaly H, Rieger J, et al. Functional outcomes after hemiglossectomy and reconstruction with a bilobed radial forearm free flap. J Otolaryngol 2004; 33(6):356–9.

65. Deleyiannis FW, Dunklebarger J, Lee E, et al. Reconstruction of the marginal mandibulectomy defect: an update. Am J Otolaryngol 2007;28(6):363–6.

66. Alvi A, Myers EN. Skin graft reconstruction of the composite resection defect. Head Neck 1996;18(6):538–43.

67. Shaha AR. Marginal mandibulectomy for carcinoma of the floor of the mouth. J Surg Oncol 1992;49(2):116–9.

68. Tidstrom KD, Keller EE. Reconstruction of mandibular discontinuity with autogenous iliac bone graft: report of 34 consecutive patients. J Oral Maxillofac Surg 1990;48(4):336–46.

69. Foster RD, Anthony JP, Sharma A, et al. Vascularized bone flaps versus nonvascularized bone grafts for mandibular reconstruction: an outcome analysis of primary bony union and endosseous implant success. Head Neck 1999;21(1): 66–71.

70. Klotch DW, Prein J. Mandibular reconstruction using AO plates. Am J Surg 1987;154:384–8.

71. Gullane PJ. Primary mandibular reconstruction: analysis of 64 cases and evaluation of interface radiation dosimetry on bridging plates. Laryngoscope 1991; 101:1–24.

72. Conley J. Use of composite flaps containing bone for major repairs in the head and neck. Plast Reconstr Surg 1972;49(5):522–6.

73. Cuono CB, Ariyan S. Immediate reconstruction of a composite mandibular defect with a regional osteomusculocutaneous flap. Plast Reconstr Surg 1980; 65(4):477–84.

74. Hidalgo DA. Fibula free flap: a new method of mandible reconstruction. Plast Reconstr Surg 1989;84(1):71–9.

75. Swartz WM, Banis JC, Newton ED, et al. The osteocutaneous scapular flap for mandibular and maxillary reconstruction. Plast Reconstr Surg 1986;77(4): 530–45.

76. Coleman JJ, Sultan MR. The bipedicled osteocutaneous scapula flap: a new subscapular system free flap. Plast Reconstr Surg 1991;87:682–92.

77. Urken ML, Vickery C, Weinberg H, et al. The internal oblique-iliac crest osseomyocutaneous free flap in oromandibular reconstruction. Report of 20 cases. Arch Otolaryngol Head Neck Surg 1989;115:339–49.

78. Soutar DS, Scheker LR, Tanner NS, et al. The radial forearm flap: a versatile method for intra-oral reconstruction. Br J Plast Surg 1983;36:1–8.
79. Boyd JB, Gullane PJ, Rotstein LE, et al. Classification of mandibular defects. Plast Reconstr Surg 1993;92(7):1266–75.
80. Urken ML, Weinberg H, Vickery C, et al. Oromandibular reconstruction using microvascular composite free flaps. Report of 71 cases and a new classification scheme for bony, soft-tissue, and neurologic defects. Arch Otolaryngol Head Neck Surg 1991;117(7):733–44.
81. Jewer DD, Boyd JB, Manktelow RT, et al. Orofacial and mandibular reconstruction with the iliac crest free flap: a review of 60 cases and a new method of classification. Plast Reconstr Surg 1989;84(3):391–403.
82. Chao JW, Rohde CH, Chang MM, et al. Oral rehabilitation outcomes after free fibula reconstruction of the mandible without condylar restoration. J Craniofac Surg 2014;25(2):415–7.
83. Hanasono MM, Zevallos JP, Skoracki RJ, et al. A prospective analysis of bony versus soft-tissue reconstruction for posterior mandibular defects. Plast Reconstr Surg 2010;125(5):1413–21.
84. Toto JM, Chang EI, Agag R, et al. Improved operative efficiency of free fibula flap mandible reconstruction with patient-specific, computer-guided preoperative planning. Head Neck 2014. [Epub ahead of print].
85. Hanasono MM, Skoracki RJ. Computer-assisted design and rapid prototype modeling in microvascular mandible reconstruction. Laryngoscope 2013;123(3):597–604.
86. Disa JJ, Hidalgo DA, Cordeiro PG, et al. Evaluation of bone height in osseous free flap mandible reconstruction: an indirect measure of bone mass. Plast Reconstr Surg 1999;103(5):1371–7.
87. Disa JJ, Winters RM, Hidalgo DA. Long-term evaluation of bone mass in free fibula flap mandible reconstruction. Am J Surg 1997;174(5):503–6.
88. Hidalgo DA, Pusic AL. Free-flap mandibular reconstruction: a 10-year follow-up study. Plast Reconstr Surg 2002;110(2):438–49.
89. Chang DW, Oh HK, Robb GL, et al. Management of advanced mandibular osteoradionecrosis with free flap reconstruction. Head Neck 2001;23(10):830–5.
90. Baumann DP, Yu P, Hanasono MM, et al. Free flap reconstruction of osteoradionecrosis of the mandible: a 10-year review and defect classification. Head Neck 2011;33(6):800–7.
91. Urken ML, Buchbinder D, Weinberg H, et al. Primary placement of osseointegrated implants in microvascular mandibular reconstruction. Otolaryngol Head Neck Surg 1989;101(1):56–73.
92. Chang YM, Wallace CG, Tsai CY, et al. Dental implant outcome after primary implantation into double-barreled fibula osteoseptocutaneous free flap-reconstructed mandible. Plast Reconstr Surg 2011;128(6):1220–8.
93. Yu P, Hanasono MM, Skoracki RJ, et al. Pharyngoesophageal reconstruction with the anterolateral thigh flap after total laryngopharyngectomy. Cancer 2010;116(7):1718–24.
94. Disa JJ, Pusic AL, Hidalgo DA, et al. Microvascular reconstruction of the hypopharynx: defect classification, treatment algorithm, and functional outcome based on 165 consecutive cases. Plast Reconstr Surg 2003;111(2):652–60.
95. Selber JC, Xue A, Liu J, et al. Pharyngoesophageal reconstruction outcomes following 349 cases. J Reconstr Microsurg 2014;30(9):641–54.

96. Hong JW, Jeong HS, Lew DH, et al. Hypopharyngeal reconstruction using remnant narrow pharyngeal wall as omega-shaped radial forearm free flap. J Craniofac Surg 2009;20(5):1334–40.
97. Yang CC, Lee JC, Wu KC, et al. Voice and speech outcomes with radial forearm free flap-accompanied phonation tube after total pharyngolaryngectomy of hypopharyngeal cancer. Acta Otolaryngol 2011;131(8):847–51.
98. Genden EM, Jacobson AS. The role of the anterolateral thigh flap for pharyng-oesophageal reconstruction. Arch Otolaryngol Head Neck Surg 2005;131: 796–9.
99. Chan YW, Ng RW, Liu LH, et al. Reconstruction of circumferential pharyngeal defects after tumour resection: reference or preference. J Plast Reconstr Aesthet Surg 2011;64:1022–9.
100. Yu P, Lewin JS, Reece GP, et al. Comparison of clinical and functional outcomes and hospital costs following pharyngoesophageal reconstruction with the anterolateral thigh free flap versus the jejunal flap. Plast Reconstr Surg 2006;117(3): 968–74.
101. Harii K, Ebihara S, Ono I, et al. Pharyngoesophageal reconstruction using a fabricated forearm free flap. Plast Reconstr Surg 1985;75(4):463–76.
102. Azizzadeh B, Yafai S, Rawnsley JD, et al. Radial forearm free flap pharyngoeso-phageal reconstruction. Laryngoscope 2001;111(5):807–10.
103. Anthony JP, Singer MI, Deschler DG, et al. Long-term functional results after pharyngoesophageal reconstruction with the radial forearm free flap. Am J Surg 1994;168(5):441–5.
104. Murray DJ, Novak CB, Neligan PC. Fasciocutaneous free flaps in pharyngolaryngo-oesophageal reconstruction: a critical review of the literature. J Plast Reconstr Aesthet Surg 2008;61(10):1148–56.
105. Lewin JS, Barringer DA, May AH, et al. Functional outcomes after circumferential pharyngoesophageal reconstruction. Laryngoscope 2005;115(7):1266–71.
106. Alam DS, Vivek PP, Kmiecik J. Comparison of voice outcomes after radial forearm free flap reconstruction versus primary closure after laryngectomy. Otolaryngol Head Neck Surg 2008;139(2):240–4.
107. Robb GL, Lewin JS, Deschler DG, et al. Speech and swallowing outcomes in reconstructions of the pharynx and cervical esophagus. Head Neck 2003; 25(3):232–44.
108. Piazza C, Taglietti V, Nicolai P. Reconstructive options after total laryngectomy with subtotal or circumferential hypopharyngectomy and cervical esophagec-tomy. Curr Opin Otolaryngol Head Neck Surg 2012;20(2):77–88.

Cancer of the Oral Cavity

Pablo H. Montero, MD, Snehal G. Patel, MD*

KEYWORDS

- Oral cavity cancer • Oral cancer • Squamous cell carcinoma
- Head and neck cancer

KEY POINTS

- Cancer of the oral cavity is a common malignancy in the United States and around the world.
- The standard of care is primary surgical resection with or without postoperative adjuvant therapy.
- Multidisciplinary treatment is crucial to improve the oncologic and functional results in patients with oral cancer.
- Primary and secondary prevention of oral cancer requires education about lifestyle-related risk factors, and improved awareness and tools for early diagnosis.

INTRODUCTION

Cancer of the oral cavity is one of the most common malignancies,[1] especially in developing countries but also in the developed world.[2] Squamous cell carcinoma (SCC) is the most common histology, and the main etiologic factors are tobacco and alcohol use.[3] Although early diagnosis is relatively easy, presentation with advanced disease is not uncommon. The standard of care is primary surgical resection with or without postoperative adjuvant therapy. Improvements in surgical techniques combined with the routine use of postoperative radiation or chemoradiation therapy have resulted in improved survival statistics over the past decade.[4] Successful treatment of patients with oral cancer is predicated on multidisciplinary treatment strategies to maximize oncologic control and minimize impact of therapy on form and function.

ANATOMY OF THE ORAL CAVITY

The oral cavity extends from the vermilion border of the lips to the circumvallate papillae of the tongue inferiorly and the junction of the hard and soft palate superiorly.

The authors have nothing to disclose.
Head and Neck Surgery Service, Department of Surgery, Memorial Sloan-Kettering Cancer Center, 1275 York Avenue, New York, NY 10065, USA
* Corresponding author.
E-mail address: patels1@mskcc.org

Surg Oncol Clin N Am 24 (2015) 491–508
http://dx.doi.org/10.1016/j.soc.2015.03.006
1055-3207/15/$ – see front matter © 2015 Elsevier Inc. All rights reserved.

surgonc.theclinics.com

The oral cavity is divided into several anatomic subsites: lip, oral tongue, floor of the mouth, buccal mucosa, upper and lower gum, retromolar trigone, and hard palate (**Fig. 1**). Despite their proximity, these subsites have distinct anatomic characteristics that need to be taken into account in planning oncologic therapy.

EPIDEMIOLOGY AND ETIOLOGY

Worldwide, 405,000 new cases of oral cancer are anticipated each year, the countries with the highest rates being Sri Lanka, India, Pakistan, Bangladesh, Hungary, and France (**Fig. 2**).[5] In the European Union there are an estimated 66,650 new cases each year. The American Cancer Society estimates that there will be 45,780 new cancers of the oral cavity and pharynx in the United States in 2015, causing 8,650 deaths.[6]

Tobacco smoking and alcohol are the main etiologic factors in SCC of the oral cavity (SCCOC).[3,7] Other habits such as chewing of betel nuts and tobacco have been implicated in the Asian population. Tobacco contains many carcinogenic molecules, especially polycyclic hydrocarbons and nitrosamines. A directly proportional effect exists between the pack-years of tobacco used and the risk of SCCOC.[8] This risk can be reduced after tobacco cessation, but does not fully abate (30% in the first 9 years and 50% for more than 9 years).[9,10] A decreased incidence of oral cavity cancer has been reported in the last 15 years, widely attributed to a reduction in tobacco use.[11]

Alcohol and tobacco seem to have a synergistic effect in the etiology of oral and oropharyngeal SCC.[3,12,13] However, alcohol is linked to an increased risk of cancer even in nonsmokers.[14] Other factors such as poor oral hygiene,[15] wood dust exposure,[16] dietary deficiencies,[17] and consumption of red meat and salted meat[18,19] have been reported as etiologic factors. The herpes simplex virus (HSV) has been suspected but has not been implicated in the etiology of SCCOC.[20] Despite the emerging evidence supporting the role of the human papillomavirus (HPV) in the etiology of oropharyngeal cancer, it has not been conclusively linked to SCCOC.[21] Host factors

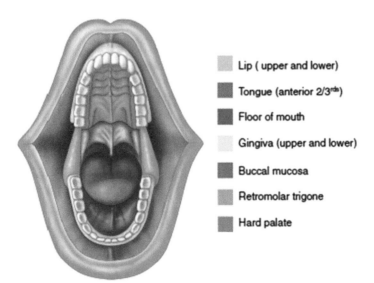

Lip (upper and lower)

Tongue (anterior 2/3rds)

Floor of mouth

Gingiva (upper and lower)

Buccal mucosa

Retromolar trigone

Hard palate

Fig. 1. Anatomic sites of the oral cavity. (*From* Shah JP, Patel SG, Singh B, et al. Jatin Shah's head and neck surgery and oncology. 4th edition. Philadelphia: Elsevier/Mosby; 2012; with permission. Copyright © 2012 by Jatin P. Shah, Snehal G. Patel, Bhuvanesh Singh.)

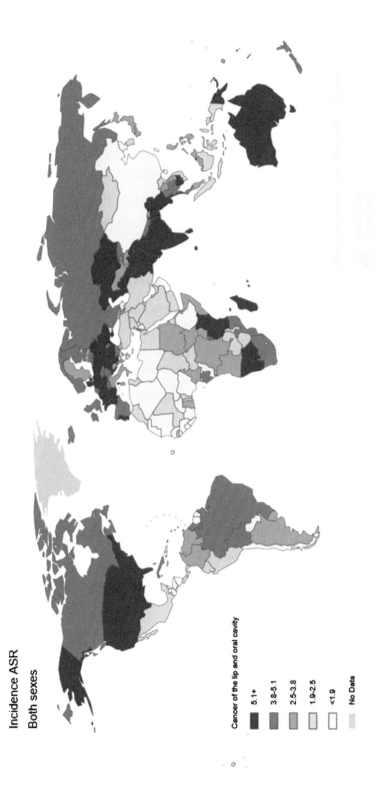

Fig. 2. Incidence of oral cavity cancer among both sexes expressed by level of age-standardized rate (ASR) in countries of the world. (*From* GLOBOCAN 2012. International Agency for Research on Cancer. Available at: http://globocan.iarc.fr/Pages/Map.aspx.)

such as immune-system alterations in transplant patients[22,23] and human immunode-ficiency virus–infected patients with AIDS,[24] and genetic conditions such as xero-derma pigmentosum, Fanconi anemia, and ataxia-telangiectasia are associated with an increased incidence of head and neck cancer.[25–28]

Oral cancer is more common in men and usually occurs after the fifth decade of life. Approximately 1.5% will have another synchronous primary in the oral cavity or the aerodigestive tract (larynx, esophagus, or lung).[29] Metachronous tumors develop in 10% to 40% in the first decade after treatment of the index primary[30,31]; therefore, reg-ular post-therapy surveillance and lifestyle alteration are important strategies for sec-ondary prevention.

PATHOLOGY

SCCs constitute more than 90% of all oral cancers. Other malignant tumors can arise from the epithelium, connective tissue, minor salivary glands, lymphoid tissue, and melanocytes, or metastasis from a distant tumor.

A variety of premalignant lesions have been associated with development of SCC.[32] The more common premalignant lesions including leukoplakia, erythroplakia, oral lichen planus, and oral submucous fibrosis have varying potential for malignant trans-formation.[33] The 2005 classification of the World Health Organization categorizes pre-malignant lesions according to degree of dysplasia into mild, moderate, severe, and carcinoma in situ.

Leukoplakia is a clinical term defined as a "white patch or plaque that cannot be characterized clinically or pathologically as any other disease."[34] This lesion is usually associated with smoking and alcohol use. The prevalence of leukoplakia worldwide is about 2%. Dysplastic changes are seen in only 2% to 5% of patients. The annual rate of malignant transformation for leukoplakia is 1%. Risk factors for malignant transfor-mation include presence of dysplasia, female gender, long duration of leukoplakia, location on the tongue or floor of the mouth, leukoplakia in nonsmokers, size greater than 2 cm, and nonhomogeneous type. In addition to lifestyle alteration to avoid to-bacco and alcohol use, excision constitutes the only definitive modality for accurate diagnosis and treatment.

Erythroplakia is a "bright red velvety patch that cannot be characterized clinically or pathologically as being caused by any other condition."[34] Surgical excision is recom-mended, as these lesions have higher malignant potential than leukoplakia and are commonly associated with dysplasia and carcinoma in situ.

Nonsquamous cell carcinomas of the oral cavity are uncommon. Minor salivary gland carcinomas, representing less than 5% of the oral cavity cancers, frequently arise on the hard palate (60%), lips (25%), and buccal mucosa (15%).[35] Mucoepider-moid carcinoma is the most common type (54%), followed by low-grade adenocarci-noma (17%) and adenoid cystic carcinoma (15%).[36,37]

Mucosal melanomas are rare but usually present as locally aggressive tumors, mainly of the hard palate and gingiva. Bony tumors, including osteosarcoma of the mandible or maxilla and odontogenic tumors such as ameloblastoma, can present within the oral cavity and may be mistaken for a mucosal lesion if there is surface ulceration.

CLINICAL PRESENTATION AND EVALUATION

Despite easy self-examination and physical examination, patients often present with advanced-stage disease. A comprehensive head and neck examination is mandatory in patients with suspected oral cavity cancer. Visual inspection and palpation allow an accurate impression of the extent of the disease, the third dimension of tumor, the presence of bone invasion, or skin breakdown. Appropriate documentation with draw-ings and photographic records of the tumor are useful in staging, decision making, and further follow-up. The clinical TNM stage should be recorded at first encounter and modified as evaluation progresses.

The initial workup consists of diagnosis by biopsy. Accessible lesions may be adequately biopsied in the clinic using punch forceps, core needle biopsy, or fine-needle aspiration. Some patients will require examination under general anes-thesia to access posteriorly located lesions or complete a physical examination limited by pain and trismus. Radiographic imaging is crucial for evaluation of the relation of the tumor to adjacent bone and for assessing regional lymph nodes. Computed to-mography (CT) is the method of choice for evaluation of bone and neck nodes, espe-cially early cortical involvement and extracapsular nodal spread. MRI provides complementary information about the extent of soft tissue and perineural invasion, and is also helpful for evaluating the extent of medullary bone involvement because adult marrow is normally replaced by fat. Most patients with oral cancer are not at risk for distant metastases, and therefore the role of positron emission tomography (PET) in initial assessment is debatable. However, a preoperative PET scan may be useful as a baseline if adjuvant treatment is anticipated, and a PET scan will be used for radiation therapy planning (although this is undertaken differently from a diag-nostic PET scan). Patients with locally advanced tumors require appropriate multidis-ciplinary consultations with the reconstructive surgeon, medical specialists for presurgical optimization, dental professionals, speech and swallowing pathologists, and behavioral therapists for smoking cessation and other lifestyle alterations.

The TNM system is the most widely accepted prognostic system, owing to its rela-tively simple design and user-friendliness. The clinical staging of the oral cavity tumors consists of primary tumor characteristics, the neck, and assessment for distant metastases (**Table 1**). This information allows TNM stage grouping for the tumor (**Table 2**).[38] The basic elements in staging of the primary site are the tumor size and invasion of deep structures. Advanced disease is defined by invasion of structures such as medullary bone, deep muscle of the tongue, maxillary sinus, and skin for T4a disease, or masticator space, pterygoid plates, or skull base and/or encasement of the internal carotid artery for T4b disease. Lymphatic spread into the neck generally occurs in a stepwise, orderly, and predictable fashion. The lymph node echelons of the neck are described using the terminology standardized by the American Head and Neck Society Guidelines (**Fig. 3**).[39]

Knowledge of the patterns of nodal metastasis has practical implications in the design of neck dissection for patients with oral cancer. The patient with a clinically negative neck is at highest risk of metastasis to levels I to III.[40] Skip metastases to level IV do occur, especially in cancer of the anterior tongue. Metastases to level V are extremely rare (1%), even in patients with clinically positive neck. Oral tongue tumors have the greatest propensity of all oral cancers for metastasis to the neck, and tumor thickness (**Fig. 4**) is a major predictor of the risk of nodal metastasis.[41]

TREATMENT

Surgical resection is the treatment of choice for SCCOC. Resection allows accurate pathologic staging, with information about the status of margins, tumor spread, and histopathologic characteristics, which can then be used to inform subsequent man-agement based on assessment of risk versus benefit. Adjuvant radiotherapy with or without chemotherapy is used for specific indications in locoregionally advanced tu-mors. A multidisciplinary team is essential to ensuring a favorable outcome. Multiple

Table 1 TNM classification of carcinomas of the oral cavity[73]	
T	**Primary Tumor**
TX	Primary tumor cannot be assessed
T0	No evidence of primary tumor
Tis	Carcinoma in situ
T1	Tumor 2 cm or less in greatest dimension
T2	Tumor more than 2 cm but not more than 4 cm in greatest dimension
T3	Tumor more than 4 cm in greatest dimension
T4a (lip)	Tumor invades through cortical bone, inferior alveolar nerve, floor of mouth, or skin (chin or nose)
T4a (oral cavity)	Tumor invades through cortical bone, into deep/extrinsic muscle of tongue (genioglossus, hyoglossus, palatoglossus, and styloglossus), maxillary sinus, or skin of face
T4b (lip and oral cavity)	Tumor invades masticator space, pterygoid plates, or skull base; or encases internal carotid artery
N	**Regional Lymph Nodes**
NX	Regional lymph nodes cannot be assessed
N0	No regional lymph node metastasis
N1	Metastasis in a single ipsilateral lymph node, 3 cm or less in greatest dimension
N2	Metastasis as specified in N2a, 2b, 2c below
N2a	Metastasis in a single ipsilateral lymph node, more than 3 cm but not more than 6 cm in greatest dimension
N2b	Metastasis in multiple ipsilateral lymph nodes, none more than 6 cm in greatest dimension
N2c	Metastasis in bilateral or contralateral lymph nodes, none more than 6 cm in greatest dimension
N3	Metastasis in a lymph node more than 6 cm in greatest dimension
M	**Distant Metastasis**
MX	Distant metastasis cannot be assessed
M0	No distant metastasis
M1	Distant metastasis

Superficial erosion alone of bone/tooth socket by gingival primary is not sufficient to classify a tumor as T4.

Midline nodes are considered ipsilateral nodes.

Used with the permission of the American Joint Committee on Cancer (AJCC), Chicago, Illinois. The original source for this material is the AJCC Cancer Staging Manual, Seventh Edition (2010) published by Springer Science and Business Media LLC, www.springer.com.

factors are taken into account in selecting treatment for an individual patient. The risk of treatment-related complications should be assessed based on physiologic age, comorbid conditions (eg, cardiopulmonary status), lifestyle (smoking or alcohol), surgical resectability, and patient expectations.

Surgical Management

A detailed description of surgical technique for the management of oral cavity cancers is beyond the scope of this article, and the reader is referred to specialized texts for this information.[42] Broad principles of surgical management are discussed, including

Table 2 Oral cancer staging[73]			
Stage	T	N	M
0	Tis	N0	M0
I	T1	N0	M0
II	T2	N0	M0
III	T3	N0	M0
	T1	N1	M0
	T2	N1	M0
	T3	N1	M0
IVA	T4a	N0	M0
	T4a	N1	M0
	T1	N2	M0
	T2	N2	M0
	T3	N2	M0
	T4a	N2	M0
IVB	Any T	N3	M0
	T4b	Any N	M0
IVC	Any T	Any N	M1

Used with the permission of the American Joint Committee on Cancer (AJCC), Chicago, Illinois. The original source for this material is the AJCC Cancer Staging Manual, Seventh Edition (2010) published by Springer Science and Business Media LLC, www.springer.com.

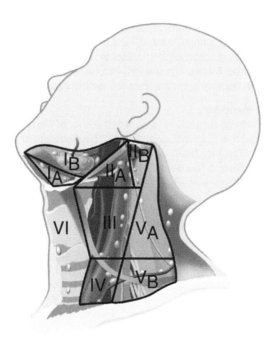

Fig. 3. Cervical lymph node level classification. (*From* Shah JP, Patel SG, Singh B, et al. Jatin Shah's head and neck surgery and oncology. 4th edition. Philadelphia: Elsevier/Mosby; 2012; with permission. Copyright © 2012 by Jatin P. Shah, Snehal G. Patel, Bhuvanesh Singh.)

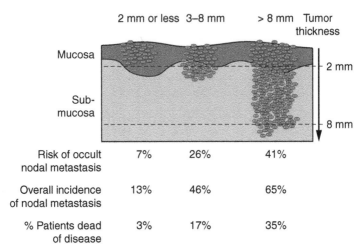

Fig. 4. Incidence of lymph node metastasis and survival stratified by the thickness of the primary tumor. (*From* Shah JP, Patel SG, Singh B, et al. Jatin Shah's head and neck surgery and oncology. 4th edition. Philadelphia: Elsevier/Mosby; 2012; with permission. Copyright © 2012 by Jatin P. Shah, Snehal G. Patel, Bhuvanesh Singh.)

access to the oral cavity, management of the mandible, management of neck nodes, and reconstruction of oral cavity surgical defects.

Surgical access
The transoral approach is usually used for premalignant lesions and small, superficial tumors of the anterior floor of the mouth, alveolus, and tongue. A more invasive approach becomes necessary for posteriorly located tumors or if there are limitations resulting from trismus or inadequate surgical exposure (**Fig. 5**). The lip-splitting paramedian mandibulotomy approach is used for larger posteriorly located tumors of the tongue. The upper cheek flap and midfacial degloving approaches are useful for gaining access to the maxilla.

Management of the mandible
Mandibular invasion can occur early in tumors of the floor of the mouth, the ventral surface of the tongue, and the gingivobuccal sulcus. The mechanism of invasion of these tumors into the mandible has been well studied.[43–45] Tumors invade the mandible through the dental sockets in the dentate mandible, and through the dental pores of the alveolar process in the edentulous mandible.

Early cortical invasion of the mandible is difficult to assess with plain radiography or orthopantomograms, but CT scans are more sensitive. On a practical level, tumors that are in close juxtaposition to the mandibular cortex will require consideration for marginal mandibulectomy to achieve an adequate margin of resection irrespective of radiographically demonstrable early cortical invasion. The role of marginal resection might be limited in patients with reduced vertical height of the body of the mandible because of the higher risk of early involvement of the body of mandible and the risk of pathologic fracture if a marginal resection is performed. Adequate tumor clearance in edentulous patients may therefore necessitate a segmental mandibulectomy. The indications for segmental resection are listed in **Box 1**.

Management of the neck
Sixty percent of patients with early-stage oral cancer will present with a clinically negative neck (cN0). Approximately 20% to 30% will have microscopically evident nodal

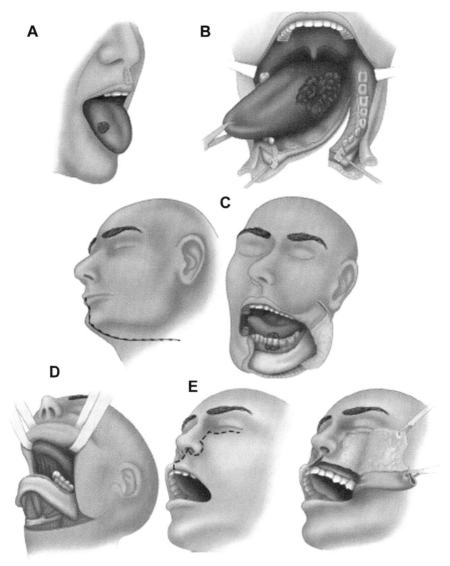

Fig. 5. Various surgical approaches. (*A*) Peroral. (*B*) Mandibulotomy. (*C*) Lower cheek flap. (*D*) Visor flap. (*E*) Upper cheek flap. (*From* Shah JP, Patel SG, Singh B, et al. Jatin Shah's head and neck surgery and oncology. 4th edition. Philadelphia: Elsevier/Mosby; 2012; with permission. Copyright © 2012 by Jatin P. Shah, Snehal G. Patel, Bhuvanesh Singh.)

metastasis on histologic examination after elective neck dissection (END). The risk of nodal metastasis is related to several factors (**Box 2**).[46,47] Cervical lymph node metastasis is the single most important prognostic factor in oral cancer: survival chances are reduced by 50% in comparison with those with similar primary tumors without neck metastases.[48,49] SCC of the oral tongue and the floor of the mouth are more likely to metastasize to the neck, and these patients should be offered END, even for early-stage tumors, if they are thicker than approximately 4 mm.[50] The hard palate and the upper gum have a relatively lower rate of occult nodal metastasis, and END may not be indicated.[51]

Box 1
Indications for segmental mandibulectomy

- Gross invasion of the of the mandible
- Tumor fixation to most of the vertical height of the occlusal surface of the mandible in hypoplastic edentulous mandible, with significant loss of vertical height precluding safe performance of rim resection
- Tumor fixed to the mandible following prior radiotherapy to the mandible

---

Sentinel node biopsy is an alternative to END for staging the cN0 neck in early-stage (T1–T2) SCCOC. The technique was first reported in 2001 by Shoaib and colleagues,[52] and has been analyzed in several single-institutional studies and two prospective multicenter trials, one in Europe[53,54] and the other in the United States.[55] The procedure is technically challenging, and successful identification of sentinel nodes and detecting occult metastasis depends on expertise and experience. Therefore, it should be undertaken only in centers with the necessary proficiency and the appropriate volume of cases.[56]

In patients with clinically or radiographically involved neck nodes, a therapeutic comprehensive neck dissection is indicated (**Table 3**). This approach involves dissection of levels I to V. The need to sacrifice other structures such as the spinal accessory nerve, sternocleidomastoid muscle, or internal jugular vein depends on the location of the metastasis and its characteristics. The most common type of comprehensive neck dissection is the modified radical neck dissection type I. Radical neck dissection is rarely performed unless there is direct infiltration of the relevant structures by gross extranodal extension of disease (see **Table 3**).

In a patient with a clinically negative neck, the risk of occult metastasis is mainly to levels I through III. Potential compromise of levels IV and V is very rare. For these reasons, a supraomohyoid neck dissection (SOHND) (see **Table 3**) is usually adequate to stage the cN0 neck. In patients with primary oral tongue SCCOC, dissection of level IV may be indicated owing to the possibility of skip metastasis. For patients with positive nodes on END, neck recurrence is observed in 10% to 24%.[57] Appropriately selected patients benefit from postoperative radiation therapy.[58,59] For cN0 patients who are proven pathologically N0, failure rates of less than 10% have been reported.[60]

Reconstructive surgery

Restoration of form and function after ablative cancer surgery is the ultimate goal of treatment, and is achieved by choosing the appropriate reconstructive procedure. Surgical defects after resection of early-stage tumors can usually be reconstructed with primary closure or the use of skin graft or skin substitutes. Reconstruction of

---

Box 2
Risk factors for nodal metastasis in oral cancer

- Tumor size
- Histologic grade
- Depth of invasion
- Perineural invasion
- Vascular invasion

Table 3
Types of neck dissections

	Lymph Nodes Excised	Other Structures Excised	Structures Preserved
Radical neck dissection	Levels I–V	Sternocleidomastoid muscle, internal jugular vein, spinal accessory nerve, submandibular gland	
Modified radical neck dissection (MRND) type I	Levels I–V	Sternocleidomastoid muscle, internal jugular vein, submandibular gland	Spinal accessory nerve
MRND type II	Levels I–V	Internal jugular vein, submandibular gland	Sternocleidomastoid muscle, spinal accessory nerve
MRND type III	Levels I–V	Submandibular gland	Sternocleidomastoid muscle, internal jugular vein, spinal accessory nerve
Supraomohyoid neck dissection	Levels I–III	Submandibular gland	Sternocleidomastoid muscle, internal jugular vein, spinal accessory nerve

larger and more complex defects that result from resection of advanced tumors requires participation from an expert reconstructive surgeon. Microvascular free tissue transfer is the technique of choice.[61,62] For example, in patients with soft-tissue defects of the oral tongue, floor of the mouth, and retromolar trigone, the free radial forearm flap results in excellent functional results (**Fig. 6**). In addition to soft-tissue cover, free flaps are also a reliable source for bone reconstruction. The fibula free flap is currently the workhorse in reconstruction of defects following segmental mandibulectomy (see **Fig. 6**). Other composite microvascular flaps include the radial forearm osteocutaneous flap, iliac crest, and scapula free flaps. Several studies have demonstrated the reliability and low morbidity of microvascular free flap reconstruction techniques.[63] The ability reliably to reconstruct large surgical defects has contributed to improved oncologic outcomes in patients with locally advanced cancers by enabling more complete resections.[64] Pedicled myocutaneous flaps such as pectoralis major,

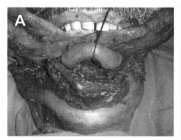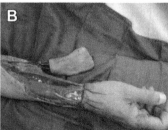

Fig. 6. Fibular (*A*) and radial forearm (*B*) free flaps are 2 of the most common flaps used in oral cavity reconstruction after major resections.

latissimus dorsi, or trapezius flaps are reliable alternatives if surgical expertise is not available or if the patient is not a good candidate for microvascular reconstruction.

Adjuvant Treatment

Adjuvant postoperative treatment is indicated in patients with a high risk of locoregional recurrence. This population includes patients with large primary tumors (pT3 or pT4), bulky nodal disease (pN2 or pN3), metastases to nodal levels IV or V, positive surgical margins, lymphovascular invasion, perineural invasion, and extracapsular spread. External beam radiation therapy has been the traditional modality for postoperative adjuvant treatment, and doses of 66 to 70 Gy result in good locoregional control.[65,66] Two clinical trials have shown that administration of cisplatin chemotherapy concurrently with postoperative radiotherapy improves locoregional control and survival (vs radiotherapy alone) in patients with head and neck cancer with extracapsular spread and/or positive surgical margins.[67,68] However, concurrent chemoradiation can result in significant morbidity, and is best used at centers where appropriate expertise and infrastructure is available.

OUTCOMES OF TREATMENT

The results of treatment of SCCOC in recently published major series are shown in **Table 4**. The overall 5-year survival in a recently analyzed cohort of patients at Memorial Sloan Kettering Cancer Center is 63%. This figure represents a significant improvement over historical cohorts (**Fig. 7**), and may be related to wider use of microvascular free flaps with enhanced ability to resect large tumors and reconstruct large

Table 4
Outcomes of patients treated for squamous carcinoma of the oral cavity in major series worldwide

Series, Year	Country	Total No. of Patients	5-y OS All Patients (%)	5-y DSS All Patients (%)	Stage I (%)	Stage II (%)	Stage III (%)	Stage IV (%)
Loree and Strong,[74] 1990	USA	398	57.0	—	—	—	—	—
Chen et al,[75] 1999	Taiwan	7032	36.1	—	72.0	38.9	26.7	11.8
Funk et al,[76] 2002	USA	30803	43.5	—	—	—	—	—
Carvalho et al,[77] 2002	Brazil	3642	43.0	—	74.0		33.0	
Yeole et al,[78] 2000	India	15051	45.9	—	68.9		26.6	9.5
Rogers et al,[79] 2009	UK	541	56.0	74.0	—	—	—	—
Listl et al,[80] 2013	Germany	15792	54.6	—	—	—	—	—
MSKCC, 2014	USA	1816	62.5	—	78.5	68.4	64.5	34.5

Abbreviations: DSS, disease-specific survival; MSKCC, Memorial Sloan Kettering Cancer Center; OS, overall survival.

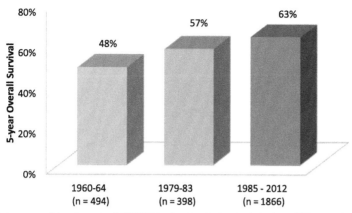

Fig. 7. Outcomes of treatment of SCCOC in 3 cohorts treated during different time periods at Memorial Sloan Kettering Cancer Center (1960–2005). (*Courtesy of* Memorial Sloan Kettering database, New York, NY.)

and complex defects, more aggressive regional therapy including increasing use of elective selective neck dissections, and the use of postoperative adjuvant therapy.

Approximately one-third of patients are treated for SCCOC relapse, and locoregional recurrence is the most common pattern of failure. The clinical stage at presentation is an important predictor of survival (**Fig. 8**), but the most powerful predictor of outcome is the presence of metastatic lymph nodes (**Fig. 9**). Other clinical signs of

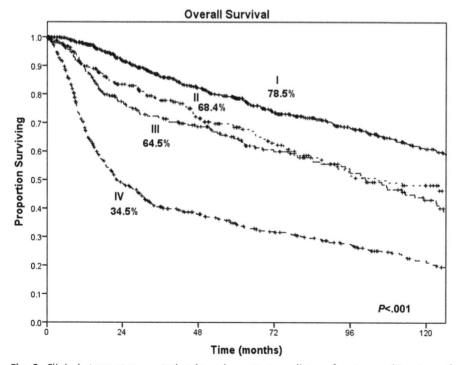

Fig. 8. Clinical stage at presentation is an important predictor of outcome. (*Courtesy of* Memorial Sloan Kettering database, New York, NY.)

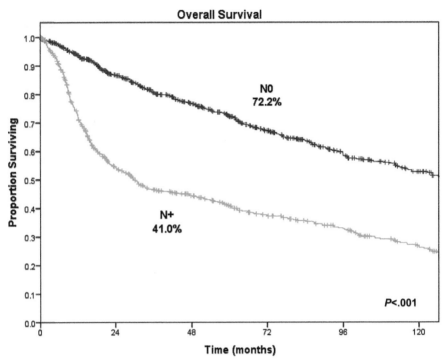

Fig. 9. Impact of clinically palpable lymph node metastasis on disease-specific survival in SCCOC. (*Courtesy of* Memorial Sloan Kettering database, New York, NY.)

locally advanced disease and poor prognosis include trismus, which indicates invasion of the pterygoid, temporalis, or masseter muscle; reduced tongue mobility, which indicates invasion of the extrinsic musculature of the tongue or the hypoglossal nerve; and skin invasion with dermal lymphatic infiltration. Significant histopathologic predictors of outcome include depth of invasion of the primary tumor, positive margins of surgical resection, perineural invasion, and major extracapsular nodal extension.

Follow-up

Patients with oral cancer have a high risk of locoregional recurrence and developing subsequent new primary cancers, but the risk of distant recurrence is low.[69] The possibility of a second head and neck primary is about 4% to 7% per year, and comprehensive clinical examination and a high suspicion are the cornerstones of early diagnosis.[70] Control of lifestyle-related risk factors, such as tobacco and alcohol consumption, is a priority in these patients because of the higher risk of treatment failure and second primaries.[71] Unfortunately there is no effective chemoprevention, and close follow-up remains the most important tool in secondary prevention.[72] Baseline imaging studies are often obtained about 3 to 6 months following completion of treatment and then as needed based on clinical suspicion. Chest imaging is not routinely needed but may be beneficial in patients with a significant smoking history. Other ancillary measures include speech and swallowing rehabilitation as indicated, monitoring of thyroid-stimulating hormone levels if the neck has been treated with radiation therapy, and regular dental evaluation.

SUMMARY

Treatment results for patients with oral cancer have improved considerably over the last several decades, owing to improvements in reconstruction and adjuvant treatment. Further improvements in survival have been hampered by attrition from second and subsequent primary tumors in long-term survivors. Primary and secondary prevention of oral cancer requires better education about lifestyle-related risk factors, improved awareness, and tools for early diagnosis.

REFERENCES

1. Jemal A, Bray F, Center MM, et al. Global cancer statistics. CA Cancer J Clin 2011;61(2):69–90.
2. Siegel R, Naishadham D, Jemal A. Cancer statistics, 2013. CA Cancer J Clin 2013;63(1):11–30.
3. Blot WJ, McLaughlin JK, Winn DM, et al. Smoking and drinking in relation to oral and pharyngeal cancer. Cancer Res 1988;48(11):3282–7.
4. Pulte D, Brenner H. Changes in survival in head and neck cancers in the late 20th and early 21st century: a period analysis. Oncologist 2010;15(9):994–1001.
5. Ferlay J, Shin HR, Bray F, et al. Estimates of worldwide burden of cancer in 2008: GLOBOCAN 2008. Int J Cancer 2010;127(12):2893–917.
6. Siegel RL, Miller KD, Jemal A. Cancer statistics, 2015. CA Cancer J Clin 2015; 65(1):5–29.
7. Blot WJ. Alcohol and cancer. Cancer Res 1992;52(7 Suppl):2119s–23s.
8. Spitz MR, Fueger JJ, Goepfert H, et al. Squamous cell carcinoma of the upper aerodigestive tract. A case comparison analysis. Cancer 1988;61(1):203–8.
9. Macfarlane GJ, Zheng T, Marshall JR, et al. Alcohol, tobacco, diet and the risk of oral cancer: a pooled analysis of three case-control studies. Eur J Cancer B Oral Oncol 1995;31B(3):181–7.
10. Samet JM. The health benefits of smoking cessation. Med Clin North Am 1992; 76(2):399–414.
11. Howlader NN, Krapcho M, Neyman N, et al, editors. SEER Cancer statistics review, 1975–2008, National Cancer Institute. Bethesda (MD). 2011. Available at: http://seercancergov/csr/1975_2008/, based on November 2010 SEER data submission, posted to the SEER web site 2011. Accessed November 1, 2014.
12. McCoy GD, Wynder EL. Etiological and preventive implications in alcohol carcinogenesis. Cancer Res 1979;39(7 Pt 2):2844–50.
13. Brugere J, Guenel P, Leclerc A, et al. Differential effects of tobacco and alcohol in cancer of the larynx, pharynx, and mouth. Cancer 1986;57(2):391–5.
14. Kato I, Nomura AM. Alcohol in the aetiology of upper aerodigestive tract cancer. Eur J Cancer B Oral Oncol 1994;30B(2):75–81.
15. Maier H, Zoller J, Herrmann A, et al. Dental status and oral hygiene in patients with head and neck cancer. Otolaryngol Head Neck Surg 1993;108(6):655–61.
16. Schildt EB, Eriksson M, Hardell L, et al. Occupational exposures as risk factors for oral cancer evaluated in a Swedish case-control study. Oncol Rep 1999;6(2):317–20.
17. La Vecchia C, Tavani A, Franceschi S, et al. Epidemiology and prevention of oral cancer. Oral Oncol 1997;33(5):302–12.
18. Tavani A, Gallus S, La Vecchia C, et al. Diet and risk of oral and pharyngeal cancer. An Italian case-control study. Eur J Cancer Prev 2001;10(2):191–5.
19. De Stefani E, Boffetta P, Ronco AL, et al. Processed meat consumption and risk of cancer: a multisite case-control study in Uruguay. Br J Cancer 2012;107(9): 1584–8.

20. Larsson PA, Edstrom S, Westin T, et al. Reactivity against herpes simplex virus in patients with head and neck cancer. Int J Cancer 1991;49(1):14–8.
21. Sturgis EM, Cinciripini PM. Trends in head and neck cancer incidence in relation to smoking prevalence: an emerging epidemic of human papillomavirus-associated cancers? Cancer 2007;110(7):1429–35.
22. Lishner M, Patterson B, Kandel R, et al. Cutaneous and mucosal neoplasms in bone marrow transplant recipients. Cancer 1990;65(3):473–6.
23. Shah AT, Wu E, Wein RO. Oral squamous cell carcinoma in post-transplant patients. Am J Otolaryngol 2013;34(2):176–9.
24. Ficarra G, Eversole LE. HIV-related tumors of the oral cavity. Crit Rev Oral Biol Med 1994;5(2):159–85.
25. Berkower AS, Biller HF. Head and neck cancer associated with Bloom's syndrome. Laryngoscope 1988;98(7):746–8.
26. Hecht F, Hecht BK. Cancer in ataxia-telangiectasia patients. Cancer Genet Cytogenet 1990;46(1):9–19.
27. Snow DG, Campbell JB, Smallman LA. Fanconi's anaemia and post-cricoid carcinoma. J Laryngol Otol 1991;105(2):125–7.
28. Kutler DI, Auerbach AD, Satagopan J, et al. High incidence of head and neck squamous cell carcinoma in patients with Fanconi anemia. Arch Otolaryngol Head Neck Surg 2003;129(1):106–12.
29. Jones AS, Morar P, Phillips DE, et al. Second primary tumors in patients with head and neck squamous cell carcinoma. Cancer 1995;75(6):1343–53.
30. Leon X, Ferlito A, Myer CM 3rd, et al. Second primary tumors in head and neck cancer patients. Acta Otolaryngol 2002;122(7):765–78.
31. Liao CT, Kang CJ, Chang JT, et al. Survival of second and multiple primary tumors in patients with oral cavity squamous cell carcinoma in the betel quid chewing area. Oral Oncol 2007;43(8):811–9.
32. Silverman S Jr, Gorsky M, Lozada F. Oral leukoplakia and malignant transformation. A follow-up study of 257 patients. Cancer 1984;53(3):563–8.
33. Warnakulasuriya S, Johnson NW, van der Waal I. Nomenclature and classification of potentially malignant disorders of the oral mucosa. J Oral Pathol Med 2007; 36(10):575–80.
34. Neville BW, Day TA. Oral cancer and precancerous lesions. CA Cancer J Clin 2002;52(4):195–215.
35. Waldron CA, el-Mofty SK, Gnepp DR. Tumors of the intraoral minor salivary glands: a demographic and histologic study of 426 cases. Oral Surg Oral Med Oral Pathol 1988;66(3):323–33.
36. Pires FR, Pringle GA, de Almeida OP, et al. Intra-oral minor salivary gland tumors: a clinicopathological study of 546 cases. Oral oncology 2007;43(5):463–70.
37. Buchner A, Merrell PW, Carpenter WM. Relative frequency of intra-oral minor salivary gland tumors: a study of 380 cases from northern California and comparison to reports from other parts of the world. J Oral Pathol Med 2007;36(4):207–14.
38. Sobin LH, Wittekind C, editors. International Union against Cancer. TNM classification of malignant tumours. 6th edition. New York: Wiley-Liss; 2002.
39. Robbins KT, Medina JE, Wolfe GT, et al. Standardizing neck dissection terminology. Official report of the Academy's Committee for Head and Neck Surgery and Oncology. Arch Otolaryngol Head Neck Surg 1991;117(6):601–5.
40. Shah JP, Candela FC, Poddar AK. The patterns of cervical lymph node metastases from squamous carcinoma of the oral cavity. Cancer 1990;66(1):109–13.
41. Fakih AR, Rao RS, Borges AM, et al. Elective versus therapeutic neck dissection in early carcinoma of the oral tongue. Am J Surg 1989;158(4):309–13.

42. Shah JP, Patel SG, Singh B, et al. Jatin Shah's head and neck surgery and oncology. 4th edition. Philadelphia: Elsevier/Mosby; 2012.

43. McGregor AD, MacDonald DG. Routes of entry of squamous cell carcinoma to the mandible. Head Neck Surg 1988;10(5):294–301.

44. Brown JS, Lowe D, Kalavrezos N, et al. Patterns of invasion and routes of tumor entry into the mandible by oral squamous cell carcinoma. Head Neck 2002;24(4): 370–83.

45. McGregor AD, MacDonald DG. Patterns of spread of squamous cell carcinoma within the mandible. Head Neck 1989;11(5):457–61.

46. Woolgar JA, Scott J. Prediction of cervical lymph node metastasis in squamous cell carcinoma of the tongue/floor of mouth. Head Neck 1995;17(6):463–72.

47. Spiro RH, Huvos AG, Wong GY, et al. Predictive value of tumor thickness in squamous carcinoma confined to the tongue and floor of the mouth. Am J Surg 1986; 152(4):345–50.

48. Shah JP, Andersen PE. Evolving role of modifications in neck dissection for oral squamous carcinoma. Br J Oral Maxillofacial Surg 1995;33(1):3–8.

49. Robbins KT, Ferlito A, Shah JP, et al. The evolving role of selective neck dissection for head and neck squamous cell carcinoma. Eur Arch Otorhinolaryngol 2013;270(4):1195–202.

50. Huang SH, Hwang D, Lockwood G, et al. Predictive value of tumor thickness for cervical lymph-node involvement in squamous cell carcinoma of the oral cavity: a meta-analysis of reported studies. Cancer 2009;115(7):1489–97.

51. Farr HW, Arthur K. Epidermoid carcinoma of the mouth and pharynx 1960-1964. J Laryngol Otol 1972;86(3):243–53.

52. Shoaib T, Soutar DS, MacDonald DG, et al. The accuracy of head and neck carcinoma sentinel lymph node biopsy in the clinically N0 neck. Cancer 2001;91(11): 2077–83.

53. Ross GL, Soutar DS, MacDonald G, et al. Sentinel node biopsy in head and neck cancer: preliminary results of a multicenter trial. Ann Surg Oncol 2004;11(7): 690–6.

54. Alkureishi LW, Ross GL, Shoaib T, et al. Sentinel node biopsy in head and neck squamous cell cancer: 5-year follow-up of a European multicenter trial. Ann Surg Oncol 2010;17(9):2459–64.

55. Civantos FJ, Zitsch RP, Schuller DE, et al. Sentinel lymph node biopsy accurately stages the regional lymph nodes for T1-T2 oral squamous cell carcinomas: results of a prospective multi-institutional trial. J Clin Oncol 2010; 28(8):1395–400.

56. Ross GL, Shoaib T, Soutar DS, et al. The First International Conference on sentinel node biopsy in mucosal head and neck cancer and adoption of a multicenter trial protocol. Ann Surg Oncol 2002;9(4):406–10.

57. Tupchong L, Scott CB, Blitzer PH, et al. Randomized study of preoperative versus postoperative radiation therapy in advanced head and neck carcinoma: long-term follow-up of RTOG study 73-03. Int J Radiat Oncol Biol Phys 1991;20(1):21–8.

58. Spiro JD, Spiro RH, Shah JP, et al. Critical assessment of supraomohyoid neck dissection. Am J Surg 1988;156(4):286–9.

59. Huang SF, Kang CJ, Lin CY, et al. Neck treatment of patients with early stage oral tongue cancer: comparison between observation, supraomohyoid dissection, and extended dissection. Cancer 2008;112(5):1066–75.

60. Andersen PE, Shah JP, Cambronero E, et al. The role of comprehensive neck dissection with preservation of the spinal accessory nerve in the clinically positive neck. Am J Surg 1994;168(5):499–502.

61. Hidalgo DA, Disa JJ, Cordeiro PG, et al. A review of 716 consecutive free flaps for oncologic surgical defects: refinement in donor-site selection and technique. Plast Reconstr Surg 1998;102(3):722–32 [discussion: 733–4].
62. Schusterman MA, Miller MJ, Reece GP, et al. A single center's experience with 308 free flaps for repair of head and neck cancer defects. Plast Reconstr Surg 1994;93(3):472–8 [discussion: 479–80].
63. Urken ML, Buchbinder D, Weinberg H, et al. Functional evaluation following microvascular oromandibular reconstruction of the oral cancer patient: a comparative study of reconstructed and nonreconstructed patients. Laryngoscope 1991; 101(9):935–50.
64. Hanasono MM, Friel MT, Klem C, et al. Impact of reconstructive microsurgery in patients with advanced oral cavity cancers. Head Neck 2009;31(10):1289–96.
65. Zelefsky MJ, Harrison LB, Fass DE, et al. Postoperative radiation therapy for squamous cell carcinomas of the oral cavity and oropharynx: impact of therapy on patients with positive surgical margins. Int J Radiat Oncol Biol Phys 1993; 25(1):17–21.
66. Bartelink H, Breur K, Hart G, et al. The value of postoperative radiotherapy as an adjuvant to radical neck dissection. Cancer 1983;52(6):1008–13.
67. Cooper JS, Pajak TF, Forastiere AA, et al. Postoperative concurrent radiotherapy and chemotherapy for high-risk squamous-cell carcinoma of the head and neck. N Engl J Med 2004;350(19):1937–44.
68. Bernier J, Domenge C, Ozsahin M, et al. Postoperative irradiation with or without concomitant chemotherapy for locally advanced head and neck cancer. N Engl J Med 2004;350(19):1945–52.
69. Lin K, Patel SG, Chu PY, et al. Second primary malignancy of the aerodigestive tract in patients treated for cancer of the oral cavity and larynx. Head Neck 2005;27(12):1042–8.
70. Leon X, Martinez V, Lopez M, et al. Second, third, and fourth head and neck tumors. A progressive decrease in survival. Head Neck 2012;34(12):1716–9.
71. Silverman S Jr, Rankin KV. Oral and pharyngeal cancer control through continuing education. J Cancer Educ 2010;25(3):277–8.
72. Foy JP, Bertolus C, William WN Jr, et al. Oral premalignancy: the roles of early detection and chemoprevention. Otolaryngol Clin North Am 2013;46(4):579–97.
73. Edge SB. American Joint Committee on Cancer. AJCC cancer staging manual. 7th edition. New York: Springer; 2010.
74. Loree TR, Strong EW. Significance of positive margins in oral cavity squamous carcinoma. Am J Surg 1990;160(4):410–4.
75. Chen YK, Huang HC, Lin LM, et al. Primary oral squamous cell carcinoma: an analysis of 703 cases in southern Taiwan. Oral Oncol 1999;35(2):173–9.
76. Funk GF, Karnell LH, Robinson RA, et al. Presentation, treatment, and outcome of oral cavity cancer: a National Cancer Data Base report. Head Neck 2002;24(2): 165–80.
77. Carvalho AL, Ikeda MK, Magrin J, et al. Trends of oral and oropharyngeal cancer survival over five decades in 3267 patients treated in a single institution. Oral Oncol 2004;40(1):71–6.
78. Yeole BB, Sankaranarayanan R, Sunny MS, et al. Survival from head and neck cancer in Mumbai (Bombay), India. Cancer 2000;89(2):437–44.
79. Rogers SN, Brown JS, Woolgar JA, et al. Survival following primary surgery for oral cancer. Oral Oncol 2009;45(3):201–11.
80. Listl S, Jansen L, Stenzinger A, et al. Survival of patients with oral cavity cancer in Germany. PLoS One 2013;8(1):e53415.

Cancer of the Oropharynx

David A. Clump, MD, PhD[a], Julie E. Bauman, MD[b],
Robert L. Ferris, MD, PhD[a,c],*

KEYWORDS

- Head and neck squamous cell carcinoma • Oropharynx • Pathogenesis
- Chemoradiation • Transoral surgery • Human papillomavirus

KEY POINTS

- The oropharynx has a crucial role in swallowing because of the surrounding constrictor musculature, need for mobility and pliability, and proximity of the base of tongue to the larynx.
- Human papilloma virus (HPV) infection as a cause of oropharyngeal squamous cell carcinoma (OPSCC) has increased dramatically in proportion and overall numbers of OPSCC cases.
- Better clinical response to therapy and younger age of the HPV+ OPSCC patients has caused functional and quality-of-life considerations to become much more important endpoints in evaluating efficacy of therapeutic options; "deintensification" to ameliorate toxicity is under investigation for this population.
- Poor survival continues to be a problem for patients with HPV– cancers, despite best current chemoradiation treatment; in the future, surgical resection may play a role in intensification of local therapy for these patients.

INTRODUCTION

There are approximately 41,000 cases of squamous cell carcinoma of the head and neck (SCCHN) diagnosed annually in the United States, of which approximately one-third will arise within the oropharynx.[1] Located posterior to the oral cavity and between the nasopharynx and larynx, the oropharynx is critical in maintaining normal speech and swallowing because of the surrounding constrictor musculature, need for mobility and pliability, and proximity of the base of tongue to the larynx. Its main components include the soft palate, posterior and lateral pharyngeal walls, faucial arches, tonsillar fossa, as well as the base of tongue. Its nonrestraining soft tissue boundaries as well as

The authors have nothing to disclose.
[a] Department of Radiation Oncology, University of Pittsburgh Cancer Institute, 5150 Centre Avenue, Pittsburgh, PA 15232, USA; [b] Division of Hematology/Oncology, Department of Internal Medicine, University of Pittsburgh Cancer Institute, 5150 Centre Avenue, Pittsburgh, PA 15232, USA; [c] Department of Otolaryngology/Head and Neck Surgery, University of Pittsburgh Eye and Ear Institute, Suite 500, 200 Lothrop Street, Pittsburgh, PA 15213, USA
* Corresponding author. Suite 500, 200 Lothrop Street, Pittsburgh, PA 15213.
E-mail address: ferrrl@upmc.edu

its rich lymphatic supply allow the escape of malignant cells, resulting in most patients presenting with advanced disease (stage III or IV).[1] With limited surgical exposure and the refinement of radiation therapy (RT) techniques or the use of combination chemo-radiotherapy (CRT),[2] nonsurgical strategies have become standard practice in treating cancer of the oropharynx. Recently, however, the introduction of minimally invasive techniques has rekindled interest in surgical therapy.

This article focuses on how an increased understanding of the pathogenesis and prognosis of oropharyngeal malignancies has transformed therapeutic approaches as well as how technological advancements aim not only to improve oncologic outcomes but also maintain functional integrity of the oropharynx and patient-reported quality of life (QoL).

PATHOGENESIS AND PROGNOSIS FOR OROPHARYNGEAL MALIGNANCIES

Current evidence suggests that improvement in oncologic outcomes for SCCHN not only have coincided with refinement of treatment techniques but also reflect a shift in the cause and pathogenesis of oropharyngeal malignancies.[3] Converging clinical, molecular, and epidemiologic evidence now confirm that human papilloma virus (HPV) status is the single most important determinant of prognosis in oropharyngeal squamous cell carcinoma (SCC). HPV is an epitheliotropic, double-stranded DNA virus with greater than 100 characterized genotypes; HPV16, with its predilection for oropharyngeal mucosa, is the most common genotype isolated from the oropharynx.[4] HPV-initiation underlies the epidemiologic observation that both incidence and survival of oropharyngeal SCC are increasing, in contrast with cancers associated with tobacco and alcohol, whose incidence is decreasing, with survival essentially stable.[5]

The improved prognosis associated with HPV in oropharyngeal SCCHN is related to substantially different responsiveness to treatment. The carcinogenic process in HPV-related malignancies is primarily attributed to the viral oncoproteins, E6 and E7, which bind and inactivate tumor suppressors, p53 and pRb, respectively. Deficiency of p53 and Rb results in loss of cell cycle checkpoints and physiologic apoptosis. HPV-infected cells demonstrate unbridled progression through the cell cycle, a pro-proliferative state that benefits the HPV life cycle in early infection. HPV-related oropharyngeal malignancies more frequently appear in younger men with a good performance status and are associated with small primary tumors yet advanced nodal stage, often with cystic nodes. When compared with patients with HPV-negative (HPV−) disease, HPV-positive (HPV+) tumors are consistently associated with a 50% reduction in risk of death.[6] This association is exhibited in multiple secondary analyses of recent institutional as well as cooperative group prospective studies that examined RT alone or in combination with various chemotherapy regimens.[7]

In the first prospective trial designed to investigate HPV-related cancers, Eastern Cooperative Oncology Group (ECOG) investigators (in ECOG 2399) used an induction regimen of paclitaxel and carboplatin and reported a higher response rate in those that were HPV+.[7] In addition, after a median follow-up of 40 months, progression-free survival (PFS) and overall survival (OS) were superior in HPV+ patients when compared with those that were HPV−.[7] This significant response to CRT led to the first national cooperative group trial testing a deintensification strategy for HPV+ oropharynx cancer. In this recently completed trial (ECOG 1308), patients with resectable HPV+ oropharyngeal cancers were treated with 3 cycles of induction chemotherapy, including cisplatin, paclitaxel, and cetuximab. Complete clinical response at the primary site was used as a dynamic response biomarker; complete responders were treated with a radiation dose reduced by 20% (54.0 Gy vs 69.3 Gy). For those receiving reduced-dose RT, PFS at 23 months was 84%, primary site local control was

94%, nodal control was 95%, and distant control was 92%.[8] The Danish Head and Neck Cancer Group (DAHANCA) reported improved outcomes in those with HPV-related oropharyngeal malignancies. In the DAHANCA 5 trial, patients in which samples were analyzed for p16 (an HPV surrogate) demonstrated improved locoregional control (LRC) as well as disease-free survival (DFS) after adjustment for tumor and nodal stage.[9]

In addition, an unplanned subset analysis of another trial, RTOG 0129, identified an association between tumor HPV status and survival among patient with stage III and IV SCCHN. Here, 64% of enrolled patients were HPV+ and were found to have improved 3-year survival (82%) versus that of HPV− tumors (57%).[10] Using a recursive-partitioning analysis examining increased risk of death between HPV− status and pack-years of smoking identified patients at low, intermediate, and high risk of dying from their cancers.[10] With improved patient risk stratification, future trials will aim at maintaining excellent survival in the HPV+, nonsmoking cohort, while reducing late toxicities associated with current CRT regimens. In contrast, high-risk cohorts will be the focus of intensification strategies as both local and distant relapses continue to affect a significant portion of patients (**Table 1**).

RISK-ADAPTED TREATMENT STRATEGIES FOR OROPHARYNGEAL SQUAMOUS CELL CARCINOMA
Surgical Approaches to the Oropharynx

With the sharp increase in the prevalence of HPV-associated oropharyngeal SCC, there has been a corresponding shift in the affected population to younger, nonsmoking patients.[11] As discussed, the recent treatment paradigm largely consisted of intensive CRT protocols, just as for HPV− cancers, but with dramatically improved OS; this was a result of late recognition that a substantial portion of patients entered into trials had a new, more treatable form of SCCHN—caused by HPV. The increased risk for these younger patients of long-term sequelae, such as xerostomia, osteoradionecrosis, dysphagia, fibrosis, aspiration, and radiation-induced malignancy, in conjunction with newly available technology, led head and neck surgeons to explore minimally invasive surgical techniques in an effort to diminish the morbidity of surgical resection and reduce the need for high-dose CRT.

Minimally invasive surgical techniques have greatly expanded the scope of transoral approaches for oropharyngeal resections. Traditionally, transoral surgery was reserved for cancers of the tonsil, soft palate, and posterior pharyngeal wall less than 2 cm in greatest dimension. Larger neoplasms or tumors of the base of tongue were difficult to expose, especially at the deep margins. The development of endoscopes greatly improved transoral inspection of the oropharynx by magnification, tissue distention, and angled optics. In addition, advances in laser delivery systems and the wristed technology of the da Vinci robot have allowed increased freedom of motion in previously inaccessible (or intractable) subsites. These innovations have enabled surgeons to remove much larger neoplasms from the oropharynx with excellent oncologic control and functional outcomes.

Although most of the supporting evidence for transoral surgery is in early glottic cancer, there have been promising results with oropharyngeal cancer over the last decade.[12] In 2003, Steiner and colleagues[13] reported on a cohort of 48 patients with oropharyngeal cancers treated with transoral laser microsurgery (TLM), of which 94% were stage III/IV. Only 23 of the 48 patients required RT for either deep extension into the tongue base or positive resection margins. The 5-year local control for all T stages was 85% with no local recurrences in the T1 or T2 group and a 20% local recurrence rate for T3/T4 tumors. OS and DFS were 52% and 73%, respectively.

Table 1
Risk-stratified prospective trials

Trial Name	Design	Eligibility	Intervention	Primary Endpoint
ECOG 1308	Phase 2	HPV+ stage III, IV oropharynx	Induction Cisplatin, Paclitaxel, Cetuximab followed by Cetuximab + risk-adapted IMRT (54.0/33fx Gy vs 69.3 Gy/33fx)	2-y PFS
RTOG 1016	Phase 3	HPV+ stage III/IV oropharynx	Cisplatin-IMRT vs Cetuximab-IMRT	5-y OS
RTOG 1333	Randomized phase 2	HPV+ nonsmoking stage III/IV oropharynx	Accelerated-IMRT vs Cisplatin-IMRT	2-y PFS
ECOG 3311	Randomized phase 2	HPV+ stage III/IV oropharynx	TORS followed by risk-adapted (C)RT (Obs, 50.0 Gy/25fx, 60.0 Gy/30fx, 66.0/33fx) + cisplatin if high risk	2-y PFS
RTOG 1221	Randomized phase 2	HPV− stage III/IV oropharynx	Cisplatin-IMRT ± TORS	2-y PFS

A recent, multicenter, prospective study of primary, TLM-resected, stage III/IV oropharyngeal cancers reported 204 patients.[14] Two- and 5-year estimates demonstrated an OS of 89% and 78%, disease-specific survival of 91% and 84%, and DFS of 85% and 74%, respectively. The survival results are comparable to those expected using CRT as the primary treatment modality, with improved functional outcomes. A recent CRT study (n = 71) with 32% of the tumors staged T3 and T4 showed a 3-year OS of 83% and an LRC rate of 90%.[15] In the TLM study, with 34% T3 and T4 tumors, the OS was 86% at 3 years and LRC of 93%. The matched CRT group in this report had a long-term G-tube rate of 35% compared with 3.4% in the TLM study.

Publications also indicate that TLM-based surgical treatment without adjuvant therapy can be used with excellent oncologic control for early T-stage oropharyngeal cancer. In 2009, Grant and colleagues[16] reported 69 cases of oropharyngeal SCC staged T1–T4 (T1 = 25, T2 = 30, T3 = 12, T4 = 2) treated with TLM and a neck dissection, if indicated. None of the patients received adjuvant RT, either because it was not indicated or because the patient declined. Five-year OS was 86% with LRC of 90% for T1 and 94% for T2. None of the T3 or T4 patients had a local recurrence. In terms of functional outcomes, none of the patients required a long-term feeding tube and 98% reported normal or near normal swallowing, using the Salassa scale.[16]

In addition to TLM, the feasibility of transoral robotic surgery (TORS) was investigated, first using a human cadaver,[17] followed by a supraglottic laryngectomy in a canine model.[18] Protocols were then established for positioning, use of 5-mm instruments, and hemostasis.[18,19] The first documented oropharyngeal TORS series reported 3 patients with early T stage, base of tongue squamous cell carcinoma. En bloc resection with clear margins was achieved in all cases with no complications or measured change in swallowing function.[20]

In a 2007 case series of 27 patients with tonsillar SCC who underwent primary resection with TORS,[21] 24 patients were stage III/IVa. Neck dissections were performed on 26 of the 27 patients and 24 had at least one positive node. The cervical lymphadenectomy was performed 1 to 3 weeks after the TORS procedure in an effort to reduce lymphedema in the oropharynx after TORS. Tumor-free margins were achieved in all of the cases and there were no locoregional recurrences during the 2-year study period (with a minimum of 6-month follow-up). All of the patients who returned for evaluation (26 of 27) tolerated a regular diet without the need for a gastrostomy tube. One patient, with preexisting sleep apnea, required a tracheostomy due to its exacerbation by the surgical procedure.

Since 2007, several institutions have published series highlighting the efficacy of TORS for oropharyngeal SCC.[16,22–26] These reports document excellent oncologic outcomes in series of 20 to 47 patients. Moore and coworkers[27] reported that 12 of 45 patients (27%) needed no adjuvant RT, and at 1-year follow-up no local recurrences were detected. Weinstein and coworkers[28] reported a series of 47 patients with stage III/IV oropharyngeal SCC. One patient had tumor at a margin of 2%. Disease-specific survival was 98% at 1 year and 90% at 2 years. After the TORS procedure, 18 of 47 patients (38%) needed no chemotherapy, and 5 patients (11%) did not require any adjuvant therapy. In a prospective, phase I single-arm study,[28] 31 patients underwent TORS with selective neck dissection with a 100% disease-control rate and a 2-year gastrostomy dependency rate of 0%. Seven patients required no adjuvant therapy and 15 of the remaining 24 (63%) received RT alone (60 Gy to the primary site and dissected neck, 54 Gy to the contralateral neck and retropharyngeal nodes) based on the lack of nodal ECE. After recommended postoperative adjuvant therapy using contemporary practice standards, a substantial number of these patients were managed without adjuvant CRT, and sometimes without any RT whatsoever. Such results are contingent on appropriate case selection for transoral resection.

Functional outcome studies in patients with oropharyngeal cancer undergoing TORS resections have reported superior swallowing results when compared with published, nonsurgical protocols.[24,25,27,29,30] In a direct comparison of TORS versus CRT with a matched group of patients with oropharyngeal cancer at a single institution, TORS was associated with better short-term eating ability (swallowing score 72 vs 43, $P = .008$), diet tolerance (43 vs 25, $P = .01$), and functional oral intake score (FOIS) (5.5 vs 3.3, $P<.001$) 2 weeks after completion of treatment,[31] an index of acute treatment toxicity. At 12 months, the TORS group had returned to baseline swallowing status, whereas diet and FOIS remained impaired in the CRT group. In their report of 45 patients, Moore and coworkers[27] found that only 5 of 22 patients who had gastrostomy tubes required their use beyond 20 days and all had their feeding tubes removed within 4 months.[27] Dean and coworkers[24] compared feeding tube dependence in patients undergoing TORS with those who had open surgery for post-CRT oropharyngeal SCC failures and found that although 43% of the open resection group were G-tube-dependent at 6 months, none of the TORS patients required feeding tube supplementation. Such comparisons are affected by case selection, and randomized trials will be required to ascertain whether patients experience differences in outcome when treated with either best current surgical or nonsurgical approaches. Such studies are currently underway.

Although much attention has been devoted to improved outcomes of oropharyngeal SCC in the HPV era, there remains a significant portion of patients at risk for local relapse and other causes of limited survival. This cohort is primarily represented by those with a significant smoking history (>10 pack-years) whose tumors are not caused by HPV.[10] Surgical resection is one potential means of augmenting current CRT with a potential to improve local control and OS. Interestingly, a SEER (Surveillance, Epidemiology, and End Results) analysis of early stage tonsillar patients treated with a nononcologic tonsillectomy in addition to standard therapy suggested improved survival even when controlling for age and decade of treatment.[32] Perhaps surgical reduction of tumor volume, even with a nononcologic resection, improved patient outcomes. This finding supports a hypothesis that surgical resection could potentially benefit high-risk cohorts. Although traditional surgical approaches have been associated with significant morbidity, TORS offers an opportunity to intensify local therapy, delivering an oncologic procedure in combination with well-established adjuncts, including CRT. Efforts to establish the proposition through prospective trials have been frustrated by poor accrual.

Radiation Therapy

Definitive RT schedules for SCCHN were studied extensively before the acceptance of combined modality regimens.[33–35] Altered fractionation regimens relied on manipulating treatment time to exploit radiobiological principles such as reassortment of cells into the sensitive phase of the cell cycle (hours), repair of normal tissues (hours), reoxygenation (hours to days), and repopulation of tumor cells (weeks). In general, conventional dose and fractionation consist of 2.0 Gy per day to a total dose of 70.0 Gy. Pure hyperfractionation is delivery of the same total dose in the same overall treatment time but with more fractions (eg, 2 fractions per day). Total dose must be increased to account for the lower dose per fraction to achieve equivalent local control. When hyperfractionation is applied clinically, typically 2 fractions are delivered per day (with a 6-hour interfraction interval to allow for normal tissue repair). A common "hyperfractionation" schedule is 81.6 Gy delivered in 1.2-Gy fractions over about 7 weeks. This schedule allows for a higher total dose with a minimal increase in late toxicity because of the lower dose per fraction. Another approach, acceleration with concomitant boost, delivers conventional fractionation during the first portion of treatment, while the final 12 treatments are delivered twice per day. This approach effectively shortens the overall time to deliver a curative dose, a treatment strategy designed specifically to address tumor repopulation. Other approaches have been developed to accelerate the treatment course and address repopulation, including a 6 fraction per week strategy used in DAHANCA 7.[35] Clinical trials reveal that hyperfractionation and accelerated fractionation regimens have improved LRC and, in some trials, also survival. In a meta-analysis of 15 phase III trials with more than 6000 patients, altered fraction RT was associated with a 3.4% absolute benefit in 5-year OS when compared with conventional fractionation.[33] Although altered fractionation in combination with chemotherapy increases toxicity without a statistically significant improvement in clinical outcomes in comparison with standard fractionation,[10] definitive RT-alone regimens (including altered fractionation) are again being proposed as a deintensification strategy.

In addition to the improved understanding of the radiobiology of SCCHN, there have been technological improvements in the delivery of RT. The most widely used technique for improving the therapeutic ratio of RT is intensity-modulated radiation therapy (IMRT).[36] IMRT uses fundamentally different means of radiation planning and delivery when compared with conventional head and neck RT. Specifically, conventional RT combines 3 or 4 large fields in which the RT dose to most normal structures (eg, parotid glands, pharyngeal walls) is the same as the dose to the target volumes of the tumor and regional lymphatics. IMRT combines numerous small and irregularly shaped radiation beams of variable intensities to achieve a radiation dose distribution that is highly conformal to the target volumes. In addition, accelerated hyperfractionation, which was previously accomplished by delivered 2 fractions per day for the last 12 treatments, is now possible using a one fraction per day approach with IMRT. Here, the dose delivered is varied based on disease burden using a concept described as a simultaneous integrated boost (SIB). In the case of an SIB, the radiation dose per fraction varies throughout the disease risk areas from 1.6 to 2.2 Gy per fraction. Completing the definitive treatment course in 30 total fractions in comparison with the more common 35 fractions accelerates the treatment.

Although IMRT improves the dosimetry of RT, its effects on clinical outcomes are still being investigated. Small randomized trials of IMRT versus standard RT for nasopharynx cancer did not show a significant QoL benefit (despite showing significantly increased parotid gland flow with IMRT).[37] In the UK PARSPORT trial, conventional RT was compared prospectively with that of IMRT in regards to parotid sparring and subsequent reduction of xerostomia in patients with pharyngeal carcinoma.[38] The findings from this study at 12 and 24 months revealed that grade 2 or worse xerostomia was significantly lower in the IMRT group than in the conventional RT group. These findings were attributed to benefits in recovery of saliva secretion with IMRT compared with conventional treatment.

Systemic Therapy

The identification of HPV as a prognostic factor in oropharyngeal malignancies has promoted efforts to stratify patients into various risk categories; this has the potential to influence treatment. There may be patients that would benefit from deintensification to ameliorate toxicity (without a decline in survivorship), whereas others have a more guarded prognosis. In addition to its prognostic significance, HPV positivity predicts response to chemotherapy. As noted earlier, in ECOG 2399, patients with HPV+ cancers had higher response rates after induction chemotherapy (82% vs 55%, $P = .01$). OS at 2 years was significantly better in patients with HPV+ cancers compared with patients with HPV− cancers (95% vs 62%; $P = .005$). In ECOG 1308, complete clinical response at the primary site was used as a dynamic response biomarker; complete responders were treated with a 20% reduction in radiation dose (54.0 Gy vs 69.3 Gy). These findings support investigation of induction therapy as a means of selecting HPV+ patients that may benefit from dose-reduced IMRT.

The development of clinical risk classification for oropharyngeal SCC, integrating HPV and tobacco status, has also framed investigational priorities for high-risk disease. Deintensification strategies are being tested in patients with good risk HPV+ SCCHN (ECOG 1308; RTOG 1016; ECOG 3311); intensification approaches represent the major unmet need for HPV− disease, where survivorship has not improved despite increasingly aggressive application of CRT in a variety of means.[39,40] In addition, most head and neck oncologists argue that intermediate-risk HPV+ disease demonstrates PFS unacceptable for deintensification (2-year PFS 60%–70%, based on RTGO 0129). The intermediate group identified in RTOG 0129 consists of those with HPV+ disease, greater than 10 pack-years of smoking along with N2b-N3 disease. In addition, those with HPV− disease along with a less than or equal to 10 pack-year history of smoking and T2–3 disease comprised this intermediate subset. Recent data also indicate intermediate PFS in patients with HPV+ disease and T3–4 tumors or N3 nodal disease, irrespective of smoking status. These subgroups are also viewed as suboptimal for deintensification.[41,42]

The unexpected result of RTOG 0522, where the addition of cetuximab to cisplatin-RT did not improve PFS or OS in locally advanced HPV+ or HPV − SCCHN, prompted experiments in radiobiology to identify non-cross-resistant agents that may successfully increase response, and not simply toxicity. In preclinical models of SCCHN, cetuximab enhances the activity of docetaxel-RT but is less effective at enhancing platinum-RT. Perhaps cetuximab and cisplatin radiosensitize through a similar mechanism (specifically the repair of DNA double-strand breaks through nonhomologous end-joining), whereas docetaxel (a taxane microtubule inhibitor) radiosensitizes through a different mechanism.[43] In the adjuvant high-risk setting, this did not inform design of the RTOG 0234 randomized phase II trial of cisplatin-cetuximab-RT or docetaxel-cetuximab-RT.[44] The primary endpoint of that phase II trial, comparing DFS with the historical control of the RTOG 9501 trial's cisplatin-RT arm, was significantly improved only for the cetuximab-docetaxel arm (hazard ratio [HR] 0.69, $P = .012$). As a result, it is important to ascertain whether the improved DFS is attributed to the taxane alone, or to its combination with cetuximab. In the high-risk adjuvant setting, a randomized phase II/III study of cisplatin-RT versus docetaxel-RT versus docetaxel-cetuximab-RT is being conducted (RTOG 1216).

Additional evidence supporting the use of cetuximab in SCCHN is derived from the recurrent/metastatic setting. In platinum-refractory recurrent/metastatic SCCHN, cetuximab monotherapy has a response rate of approximately 11%,[45] providing evidence that cetuximab exerts its effects via pathways distinct from DNA damaging agents such as cisplatin or RT. In first-line therapy for recurrent/metastatic SCCHN, the addition of cetuximab to fluorouracil (5-FU)/platinum significantly improved OS in the EXTREME study.[46] This study was the first randomized study to demonstrate a benefit in OS (10.1 vs 7.4 months, HR = 0.797, $P = .036$) with a molecular-targeted therapy added to the classical platinum plus 5-FU combination in the first-line treatment of recurrent or metastatic SCCHN.

Targeted Therapy and Immunotherapy

In addition to multidrug regimens for high-risk patients, there is heightened interest in immunotherapy. SCCHN is an immunosuppressive disease; patients demonstrate lower absolute lymphocyte counts than healthy subjects,[47] impaired activity of natural killer cells (the major effector cell of innate immunity),[48,49] poor antigen-presenting function by dendritic cells,[50,51] and impaired function of tumor infiltrating T lymphocytes (the major effector cell of adaptive immunity) with a strong impact on clinical outcome.[52] With progressive insight into the genetics of SCCHN, novel targets likely to be of interest in the definitive management of oropharyngeal SCC[53,54] are increasingly recognized. The PI3-Kinase/Akt/mTOR signaling pathway is the most commonly mutated oncogenic pathway in SCCHN, and patients with HPV+ cancers are disproportionately affected.[55,56]

In addition, a new therapeutic approach for p53-deficient cancers, a nearly universal phenotype in SCCHN on the basis of *TP53* mutation (a typical result of tobacco abuse) or viral degradation of p53 protein, is under development. This synthetic-lethal stratagem pairs a DNA-damaging agent, such as cisplatin or RT, with a cell cycle checkpoint inhibitor (Wee1 or Chk1) to precipitate mitotic catastrophe.[57–59] Epidermal growth factor receptor (EGFR)-independent activation of intracellular proliferative signaling also suggests novel targets for drug development, including accessory receptor tyrosine kinases (alternate HER family members, cMet, insulin growth factor receptor, fibroblast growth factor receptor, or vascular endothelial growth factor receptor), downstream EGFR signaling nodes (RAS, PI3-Kinase, STAT3, SRC), or cell cycle promoters (aurora kinase, CDK4/6).[60] These potentially promising approaches warrant active investigation.

SUMMARY

The increased understanding of molecular and immunologic features of SCCHN heralds the development of novel approaches that can be integrated with advanced radiotherapy and surgical techniques. This understanding may permit rational deintensification in good-risk, HPV+ oropharyngeal cancer or intensification in high- or intermediate-risk disease. Understanding the anatomy and adjacent structures of the oropharynx is crucial to designing oncologically effective treatments that retain functional capabilities of this region, which is crucially important for swallowing.

REFERENCES

1. Siegel R, Naishadham D, Jemal A. Cancer statistics, 2013. CA Cancer J Clin 2013;63:11–30.
2. Pignon JP, le Maître A, Maillard E, et al. Meta-analysis of chemotherapy in head and neck cancer (MACH-NC): An update on 93 randomised trials and 17,346 patients. Radiother Oncol 2009;92:4–14.
3. Gillison ML. Oropharyngeal cancer: a potential consequence of concomitant HPV and HIV infection. Curr Opin Oncol 2009;21:439–44.
4. D'Souza G, Kreimer AR, Viscidi R, et al. Case-control study of human papillomavirus and oropharyngeal cancer. N Engl J Med 2007;356:1944–56.
5. Chaturvedi AK, Engels EA, Anderson WF, et al. Incidence trends for human papillomavirus-related and -unrelated oral squamous cell carcinomas in the United States. J Clin Oncol 2008;26:612–9.
6. Ragin CC, Taioli E. Survival of squamous cell carcinoma of the head and neck in relation to human papillomavirus infection: review and meta-analysis. Int J Cancer 2007;121:1813–20.

7. Fakhry C, Westra WH, Li S, et al. Improved survival of patients with human papillomavirus-positive head and neck squamous cell carcinoma in a prospective clinical trial. J Natl Cancer Inst 2008;100:261–9.
8. Fakhry C, Westra WH, Li S, et al. Improved survival of patients with human papillomavirus-positive head and neck squamous cell carcinoma in a prospective clinical trial. J Natl Cancer Inst 2008;100:261–9.
9. Lassen P, Eriksen JG, Hamilton-Dutoit S, et al. Effect of HPV-associated p16INK4A expression on response to radiotherapy and survival in squamous cell carcinoma of the head and neck. J Clin Oncol 2009;27:1992–8.
10. Ang KK, Harris J, Wheeler R, et al. Human papillomavirus and survival of patients with oropharyngeal cancer. N Engl J Med 2010;363:24–35.
11. Mehta V, Yu GP, Schantz SP. Population-based analysis of oral and oropharyngeal carcinoma: changing trends of histopathologic differentiation, survival and patient demographics. Laryngoscope 2010;120:2203–12.
12. Walvekar RR, Li RJ, Gooding WE, et al. Role of surgery in limited (T1-2, N0-1) cancers of the oropharynx. Laryngoscope 2008;118:2129–34.
13. Steiner W, Fierek O, Ambrosch P, et al. Transoral laser microsurgery for squamous cell carcinoma of the base of the tongue. Arch Otolaryngol Head Neck Surg 2003;129:36–43.
14. Gapany M. Transoral Laser microsurgery as primary treatment for advanced-stage oropharyngeal cancer: a United States Multicenter Study. Yearb. Otolaryngol Neck Surg 2012;2012:32–3.
15. Huang K, Xia P, Chuang C, et al. Intensity-modulated chemoradiation for treatment of stage III and IV oropharyngeal carcinoma: the University of California-San Francisco experience. Cancer 2008;113:497–507.
16. Grant DG, Hinni ML, Salassa JR, et al. Oropharyngeal cancer: a case for single modality treatment with transoral laser microsurgery. Arch Otolaryngol Head Neck Surg 2009;135:1225–30.
17. Hockstein NG, Nolan JP, O'Malley BW, et al. Robot-assisted pharyngeal and laryngeal microsurgery: results of robotic cadaver dissections. Laryngoscope 2005;115:1003–8.
18. Weinstein GS, O'malley BW, Hockstein NG. Transoral robotic surgery: supraglottic laryngectomy in a canine model. Laryngoscope 2005;115:1315–9.
19. Hockstein NG, Weinstein GS, O'malley BW Jr. Maintenance of hemostasis in transoral robotic surgery. ORL J Otorhinolaryngol Relat Spec 2005;67:220–4.
20. O'Malley BW, Weinstein GS, Snyder W, et al. Transoral robotic surgery (TORS) for base of tongue neoplasms. Laryngoscope 2006;116:1465–72.
21. Weinstein GS, O'Malley BW, Snyder W, et al. Transoral robotic surgery: radical tonsillectomy. Arch Otolaryngol Head Neck Surg 2007;133:1220–6.
22. Genden EM, Desai S, Sung CK. Transoral robotic surgery for the management of head and neck cancer: a preliminary experience. Head Neck 2009;31:283–9.
23. Boudreaux BA, Rosenthal EL, Magnuson JS, et al. Robot-assisted surgery for upper aerodigestive tract neoplasms. Arch Otolaryngol Head Neck Surg 2009;135:397–401.
24. Dean NR, Rosenthal EL, Carroll WR, et al. Robotic-assisted surgery for primary or recurrent oropharyngeal carcinoma. Arch Otolaryngol Head Neck Surg 2010;136:380–4.
25. Hurtuk A, Agrawal A, Old M, et al. Outcomes of transoral robotic surgery: a preliminary clinical experience. Otolaryngol Head Neck Surg 2011;145:248–53.
26. Weinstein GS, O'Malley BW, Cohen MA, et al. Transoral robotic surgery for advanced oropharyngeal carcinoma. Arch Otolaryngol Head Neck Surg 2010;136:1079–85.

27. Moore EJ, Olsen KD, Kasperbauer JL. Transoral robotic surgery for oropharyngeal squamous cell carcinoma: a prospective study of feasibility and functional outcomes. Laryngoscope 2009;119:2156–64.

28. Weinstein GS, Quon H, O'Malley BW, et al. Selective neck dissection and deintensified postoperative radiation and chemotherapy for oropharyngeal cancer: a subset analysis of the University of Pennsylvania transoral robotic surgery trial. Laryngoscope 2010;120:1749–55.

29. Leonhardt FD, Quon H, Abrahão M, et al. Transoral robotic surgery for oropharyngeal carcinoma and its impact on patient-reported quality of life and function. Head Neck 2012;34:146–54.

30. Sinclair CF, McColloch NL, Carroll WR, et al. Patient-perceived and objective functional outcomes following transoral robotic surgery for early oropharyngeal carcinoma. Arch Otolaryngol Head Neck Surg 2011;137:1112–6.

31. Genden EM, Park R, Smith C, et al. The role of reconstruction for transoral robotic pharyngectomy and concomitant neck dissection. Arch Otolaryngol Head Neck Surg 2011;137:151–6.

32. Holliday MA, Tavaluc R, Zhuang T, et al. Oncologic benefit of tonsillectomy in stage I and II tonsil cancer: a surveillance epidemiology and end results database review. JAMA Otolaryngol Head Neck Surg 2013;139:362–6.

33. Bourhis J, Overgaard J, Audry H, et al. Hyperfractionated or accelerated radiotherapy in head and neck cancer: a meta-analysis. Lancet 2006;368:843–54.

34. Fu KK, Pajak TF, Trotti A, et al. A Radiation Therapy Oncology Group (RTOG) phase III randomized study to compare hyperfractionation and two variants of accelerated fractionation to standard fractionation radiotherapy for head and neck squamous cell carcinomas: first report of RTOG 9003. Int J Radiat Oncol Biol Phys 2000;48:7–16.

35. Overgaard J, Hansen HS, Specht L, et al. Five compared with six fractions per week of conventional radiotherapy of squamous-cell carcinoma of head and neck: DAHANCA 6 and 7 randomised controlled trial. Lancet 2003;362:933–40.

36. Beadle BM, Liao KP, Elting LS, et al. Improved survival using intensity-modulated radiation therapy in head and neck cancers: A SEER-Medicare analysis. Cancer 2014;120:702–10.

37. Kam MK, Leung SF, Zee B, et al. Prospective randomized study of intensity-modulated radiotherapy on salivary gland function in early-stage nasopharyngeal carcinoma patients. J Clin Oncol 2007;25:4873–9.

38. Nutting CM, Morden JP, Harrington KJ, et al. Parotid-sparing intensity modulated versus conventional radiotherapy in head and neck cancer (PARSPORT): a phase 3 multicentre randomised controlled trial. Lancet Oncol 2011;12:127–36.

39. Ang K, Pajak T, Wheeler R, et al. A phase III trial to test accelerated versus standard fractionation in combination with concurrent cisplatin for head and neck carcinomas (RTOG 0129): report of efficacy and toxicity. Int J Radiat Oncol Biol Phys 2010;77:1–2.

40. Loo SW, Geropantas K, Roques TW. DeCIDE and PARADIGM: nails in the coffin of induction chemotherapy in head and neck squamous cell carcinoma? Clin Transl Oncol 2013;15:248–51.

41. O'Sullivan B, Huang SH, Perez-Ordonez B, et al. Outcomes of HPV-related oropharyngeal cancer patients treated by radiotherapy alone using altered fractionation. Radiother Oncol 2012;103:49–56.

42. Marur S, Li S, Cmelak A, et al. E 1308: a phase II trial of induction chemotherapy followed by cetuximab with low dose versus standard dose IMRT in patients with

human papilloma virus-associated resectable squamous cell carcinoma of the oropharynx. J Clin Oncol 2013;31(Suppl 15):6005.

43. Dittmann K, Mayer C, Rodemann HP. Inhibition of radiation-induced EGFR nuclear import by C225 (Cetuximab) suppresses DNA-PK activity. Radiother Oncol 2005;76:157–61.

44. Kies MS, Harris J, Rotman MZ, et al. Phase II randomized trial of postoperative chemoradiation plus cetuximab for high-risk squamous cell carcinoma of the head and neck (RTOG 0234). Int J Radiat Oncol Biol Phys 2009;75:S14–5.

45. Vermorken JB, Trigo J, Hitt R, et al. Open-label, uncontrolled, multicenter phase II study to evaluate the efficacy and toxicity of cetuximab as a single agent in patients with recurrent and/or metastatic squamous cell carcinoma of the head and neck who failed to respond to platinum-based the. J Clin Oncol 2007;25:2171–7.

46. Vermorken JB, Mesia R, Rivera F, et al. Platinum-based chemotherapy plus cetuximab in head and neck cancer. N Engl J Med 2008;359:1116–27.

47. Kuss I, Hathaway B, Ferris RL, et al. Decreased absolute counts of T lymphocyte subsets and their relation to disease in squamous cell carcinoma of the head and neck. Clin Cancer Res 2004;10:3755–62.

48. Dasgupta S, Bhattacharya-Chatterjee M, O'Malley BW, et al. Inhibition of NK cell activity through TGF-beta 1 by down-regulation of NKG2D in a murine model of head and neck cancer. J Immunol 2005;175:5541–50.

49. Bauernhofer T, Kuss I, Henderson B, et al. Preferential apoptosis of CD56dim natural killer cell subset in patients with cancer. Eur J Immunol 2003;33:119–24.

50. Ferris RL, Whiteside TL, Ferrone S. Immune escape associated with functional defects in antigen-processing machinery in head and neck cancer. Clin Cancer Res 2006;12:3890–5.

51. López-Albaitero A, Nayak JV, Ogino T, et al. Role of antigen-processing machinery in the in vitro resistance of squamous cell carcinoma of the head and neck cells to recognition by CTL. J Immunol 2006;176:3402–9.

52. Galon J, Costes A, Sanchez-Cabo F, et al. Type, density, and location of immune cells within human colorectal tumors predict clinical outcome. Science 2006;313:1960–4.

53. Agrawal N, Frederick MJ, Pickering CR, et al. Exome sequencing of head and neck squamous cell carcinoma reveals inactivating mutations in NOTCH1. Science 2011;333:1154–7.

54. Stransky N, Egloff AM, Tward AD, et al. The mutational landscape of head and neck squamous cell carcinoma. Science 2011;333:1157–60.

55. Lui VW, Hedberg ML, Li H, et al. Frequent mutation of the PI3K pathway in head and neck cancer defines predictive biomarkers. Cancer Discov 2013;3:761–9.

56. Chiosea SI, Grandis JR, Lui VW, et al. PIK3CA, HRAS and PTEN in human papillomavirus positive oropharyngeal squamous cell carcinoma. BMC Cancer 2013; 13:602.

57. Hirai H, Iwasawa Y, Okada M, et al. Small-molecule inhibition of Wee1 kinase by MK-1775 selectively sensitizes p53-deficient tumor cells to DNA-damaging agents. Mol Cancer Ther 2009;8:2992–3000.

58. Gadhikar MA, Sciuto MR, Alves MV, et al. Chk1/2 inhibition overcomes the cisplatin resistance of head and neck cancer cells secondary to the loss of functional p53. Mol Cancer Ther 2013;12:1860–73.

59. Bridges KA, Hirai H, Buser CA, et al. MK-1775, a novel Wee1 kinase inhibitor, radiosensitizes p53-defective human tumor cells. Clin Cancer Res 2011;17:5638–48.

60. Burtness B, Bauman JE, Galloway T. Novel targets in HPV-negative head and neck cancer: overcoming resistance to EGFR inhibition. Lancet Oncol 2013;14:e302–9.

Treatment/Comparative Therapeutics
Cancer of the Larynx and Hypopharynx

Caitlin P. McMullen, MD, Richard V. Smith, MD*

KEYWORDS

- Laryngeal cancer • Hypopharynx cancer • Head and neck cancer treatment
- Transoral laser microsurgery • Conservation surgery • Radiation

KEY POINTS

- Multidisciplinary management, including surgery, radiation, and medical oncology, with speech and swallow therapy, is essential for optimal outcomes in laryngeal and hypopharyngeal cancers.
- Transoral surgical techniques provide equal or better oncologic and functional outcomes compared with open surgical techniques and definitive radiation for appropriate candidates.
- Multimodality therapy is essential to achieve control in advanced disease.
- Organ preservation protocols using concurrent chemoradiation result in similar oncologic outcomes while maintaining laryngeal preservation for select tumors compared with initial total laryngectomy.
- Long-term surveillance allows for early detection of second primary tumors and management of the sequelae of therapy.

INTRODUCTION

A multidisciplinary approach to patients with squamous cell carcinoma of the larynx and hypopharynx is essential. These tumors and their treatment affect a patient's ability to communicate, swallow, and function in society. When managing patients with these diseases, the physician should be mindful of the importance of maintaining quality of life, in addition to the importance of a definitive cure. Long-term survivorship, a primary goal, should be balanced with the known sequelae of therapy.

The authors have nothing to disclose.
Department of Otorhinolaryngology–Head and Neck Surgery, Montefiore Medical Center, Albert Einstein College of Medicine, 3400 Bainbridge Avenue, Bronx, NY 10467, USA
* Corresponding author.
E-mail address: rsmith@montefiore.org

Surg Oncol Clin N Am 24 (2015) 521–545
http://dx.doi.org/10.1016/j.soc.2015.03.013   surgonc.theclinics.com

PATIENT EVALUATION OVERVIEW

A thorough pretreatment assessment is essential for a patient with potential laryngeal or hypopharyngeal cancer. Smoking and alcohol history should be elicited and addressed. Severe malnourishment should be addressed immediately with enteral feeding tube placement, because nutritional status affects treatment outcomes.[1,2] Physical examination should include inspection for second primary lesions, palpation and inspection of the neck, and flexible or indirect nasopharyngolaryngoscopy. Early tracheotomy may be needed for airway protection or management, and dental evaluation, with necessary dental work, should be performed before radiation.

Additional diagnostic tests are also important in the workup of patients with laryngopharyngeal cancers. Patients with limited early stage glottic cancers, without involvement of the anterior commissure, may be spared imaging, however. Hypopharyngeal, supraglottic, and subglottic tumors have a high risk of nodal disease or early local extension due to anatomic factors and therefore should undergo imaging of the neck with computed tomography (CT) with intravenous iodinated contrast or MRI in equivocal cases. PET-CT is useful for diseases of unknown primary, equivocal nodal disease, and advanced cases where distant or nodal metastases are suspected.[3,4] Laryngeal swallowing function and possible aspiration should be evaluated with a modified barium swallow study before initiation of treatment. For early stage laryngeal cancer without nodal disease, chest radiography is adequate to evaluate for second primary tumors. For hypopharynx cancer, chest CT or PET-CT may be necessary for a complete evaluation. Panendoscopy should be performed to assess the dimensions and extent of the lesion, to assess for second primary disease, and to perform a biopsy for pathologic analysis (**Fig. 1**).

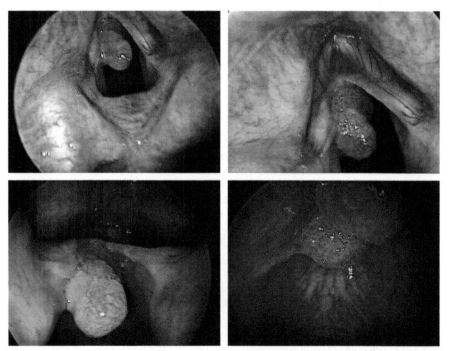

Fig. 1. Endoscopic assessment of a T1a left glottic carcinoma and anterior glottic web with a 0°, 30°, 120°, and 70° telescope (clockwise from upper left).

GENERAL PRINCIPLES OF THERAPY

Laryngeal and hypopharyngeal cancers are defined by their subsites, which portend patterns of spread and outcome (**Table 1**). Larynx and hypopharynx cancers are staged according to American Joint Committee on Cancer criteria.[5] Early stage cancers are initially managed with single-modality therapy such as radiation or surgical resection for accessible lesions. Advanced cases are usually treated with multiple modalities. Organ-preservation protocols involve radiation and chemotherapy, reserving total laryngectomy (TL) for salvage therapy.

RADIATION THERAPY IN EARLY STAGE DISEASE
Principles of Radiotherapy in Head and Neck Cancer

Radiotherapy (RT) is a cornerstone of therapy for head and neck cancer. RT is frequently curative as a single-modality treatment in early stage laryngeal and hypopharyngeal cancers and may be used in combination with surgery or chemotherapy in advanced cases.

External Beam Radiotherapy

External beam RT is the most common form of radiation in the treatment of head and neck tumors. Typical radiation doses for definitive therapy are 66 to 70 Gy. Intensity-modulated radiation therapy is a form of external beam radiation that is intended to minimize radiation doses to uninvolved, critical structures. Various fractionation and dosing schedules exist for the delivery of radiation in head and neck cancers. Hyperfractionated radiation can deliver higher total doses of radiation over the same time course as standard radiation. Accelerated radiation delivers the same dose as standard RT but in a shorter time frame. Hyperfractionated dosing may improve long-term oncologic outcomes.[6,7]

Proton delivery is an emerging and promising external beam radiation technique that improves dose distribution. Proton therapy may decrease radiation dose to normal tissues while maintaining or improving the dose to targeted tissues, potentially reducing xerostomia and swallowing dysfunction.[8,9] Unfortunately, particle accelerators required for proton therapy are not widely available, and the applications of proton therapy in head and neck cancers are still experimental.

Radiotherapy for Early Stage Glottic Tumors

Radiation alone is the most common treatment for early stage glottic cancers. Oncologic outcomes and preservation of function are excellent. Large retrospective reviews have demonstrated high local control and laryngeal preservation rates at 5 years in patients with early glottic laryngeal cancers treated with definitive RT.[10–13] A review of outcomes for early glottis cancers treated with definitive radiation or transoral laser microsurgery (TLM) is provided (**Table 2**). Expectant management of the neck is

Table 1 Laryngeal and hypopharyngeal anatomic subsites			
Laryngeal Subsites			
Supraglottis	**Glottis**	**Subglottis**	**Hypopharyngeal Subsites**
Epiglottis	True vocal folds		Pyriform sinus
Suprahyoid	Anterior commissure		Posterior and lateral
Infrahyoid	Posterior commissure		Postcricoid space
Aryepiglottic folds			
Arytenoids			
False vocal folds			
Laryngeal ventricle			

Table 2
Outcomes for glottic cancers

Author, Year	N	Treatment	OS (%)	DFS (%)	LC (%)	Recurrence (N)
Early Glottic Cancer						
Tis						
Smee et al,[130] 2010	24	RT		87.5	75	2
Garcia-Serra et al,[131] 2002	30	RT		100	88	3
Spayne et al,[132] 2001	67	RT		100	98	1
Peretti et al,[79] 2010	71	TLM		100	93	16
Roedel et al,[133] 2009	35	TLM		100	93	4
Damm et al,[134] 2000	29	TLM		100	87	4
T1						
Stoeckli et al,[78] 2003		RT	88	93	85	
Sjogren et al,[135] 2008	108	RT	80	92	75	34
Smee et al,[130] 2010	356	RT		95	83	61
Cellai et al,[75] 2005	831	RT	77	95	84	121
Franchin et al,[136] 2003	232	RT	66	90	91	27
Peretti et al,[79] 2010	404	TLM		99	95	54
Motta et al,[71] 2005	432	TLM	85	97	96	58
Stoeckli et al,[78] 2003		TLM	85	96	86	
Sjogren et al,[135] 2008	70	TLM	84	99	89	7
T2						
Stoeckli et al,[78] 2003		RT	78	88	67	
Smee et al,[130] 2010	142	RT		85	72	40
Frata et al,[137] 2005	256	RT	59	86	73	62
Garden et al,[138] 2003	230	RT	73	92	72	67
Peretti et al,[79] 2010	109	TLM		98	87	24
Motta et al,[71] 2005	236	TLM	77	86	87	84
Grant et al,[80] 2007	21	TLM	93	93	93	1
Stoeckli et al,[78] 2003		TLM	83	83	89	
T3						
Mendenhall et al,[139] 1997	75	RT	51	78 (DSS)	63	25
Johansen et al,[140] 2002	128	RT	43	63 (DSS)	63	62
Canis et al,[141] 2014	122	TLM	59	84 (DSS)	58	21
Vilaseca et al,[142] 2010	51	TLM	73	86 (DSS)	88	27
Motta et al,[71] 2005	51	TLM	64	72 (DSS)	70	21
Grant et al,[80] 2007	10	TLM	64	40 (DSS)	45	6

Abbreviations: DFS, disease-free survival; DSS, disease-specific survival; LC, local control; OS, overall survival.

indicated in N0 early glottic cancers. Primary early stage glottic cancers have a very low rate of nodal metastases, observed to be 0% to 5% in T1 and T2 tumors confined to the glottis.[14,15] The following factors are associated with worse outcomes after definitive RT for early stage glottic cancers:

- Involvement of the anterior commissure[16–19]
- Treatment interruptions and a protracted treatment course[20]

- Impaired vocal fold mobility[21]
- Larger tumor size and higher histologic grade[11]
- Smoking during treatment[22,23]
- Pretreatment hemoglobin less than or equal to 13 g/dL.[24]

Radiotherapy for Early Stage Supraglottic Tumors

RT as a single-modality treatment is feasible and effective for early and moderately advanced supraglottic cancers. Bulky lesions with pretreatment airway compromise may not be appropriate for initial definitive RT. Tumor volume greater than 6 cubic centimeters on pretreatment CT is a poor prognostic indicator.[25] Because of the high risk of lymphatic spread in supraglottic cancers, nodal basins in the neck, at minimum levels of II to IV, should be included in the radiation field.[26] A review of outcomes for T1 and T2 supraglottic tumors is provided (**Table 3**). Five-year local control with definitive RT for T1–T2 supraglottic tumors ranges between approximately 40% and 95%, but significantly higher ultimate control rates can be achieved when including salvage surgery.[27–30] Voice preservation with RT has been reported to be 96% to 100% in T1 and 80% to 86% in T2 lesions.[28,29]

Radiotherapy for Early Stage Subglottic and Hypopharyngeal Carcinoma

Subglottic and hypopharyngeal tumors frequently present at an advanced stage because of anatomic features that encourage early spread of disease. Treatment typically involves multiple modalities, and lesions are rarely treated with RT alone. Primary carcinoma of the subglottis has a 50% overall survival and 63.2% disease-free survival with RT alone for early stage disease.[31] Elective management of the neck is indicated in clinically N0 cases, including the central neck and upper mediastinum in subglottic cancer and level V and retropharyngeal nodes in hypopharyngeal cancer. Large tumor volume and extension to the pyriform apex in hypopharynx cancers are poor predictors of outcome.[32–35] Ultimately, the risks of recurrence, second malignancy, and distant metastases are high, and multimodality therapy is the norm in subglottic and hypopharyngeal cancers.

Complications of RT include edema, chondritis, chondronecrosis, laryngeal scarring and stenosis, and stenosis of the cervical esophagus. Rarely, persistent edema of the larynx and supraglottic structures may delay diagnosis of persistent or recurrent disease. Edema may become obstructive and result in the necessity of a tracheotomy or feeding tube.

COMBINATION THERAPIES

Chemoradiotherapy (CRT) protocols were developed with the aim of laryngeal preservation in appropriate patients. Patients who are not candidates may be elderly or have a poor performance status, whereby straightforward surgical management with TL may provide more rapid return to swallowing function.

Chemoradiotherapy for Advanced Laryngeal and Hypopharyngeal Cancers

Two landmark articles guide the standard management of advanced laryngeal cancers: the Veteran's Affairs (VA) study and the Radiation Therapy Oncology Group (RTOG) 91-11. The VA study, published in 1991, randomized 332 patients with stage III and IV laryngeal cancers to either TL and adjuvant RT (TL + postoperative radiotherapy [PORT]) or induction chemotherapy followed by radiation (ICRT). The 2-year survival rates were similar between the TL + PORT group and the ICRT group (68%), but there was a 64% rate of laryngeal preservation in the ICRT.[36] Of note,

Table 3
Outcomes for supraglottic cancers

Author, Year	N	Treatment	OS (%)	DFS (%)	LC (%)	Recurrence (N)
			Supraglottic Cancer			
T1						
Johansen et al,[143] 2002	154	RT	55	71	67	56
Daugaard et al,[30] 1998	220	RT			50	
Nakfoor et al,[28] 1998	23	RT		78	96	
Carl et al,[27] 1996	161	RT			58	
Hinerman et al,[29] 2002	18	RT			100	0
Grant et al,[144] 2007	8	TLM	100	80	100	1.0
Motta et al,[87] 2004	45	TLM	91	97	98	12
Iro et al,[145] 1998	39	TLM		86		8
Ambrosch et al,[88] 1998	12	TLM			100	0
Zeitels et al,[146] 1994	13	TLM			100	0
T2						
Johansen et al,[143] 2002	86	RT	52	74	73	32
Daugaard et al,[30] 1998	134	RT			41	
Nakfoor et al,[28] 1998	73	RT		82	86	
Hinerman et al,[29] 2002	109	RT			85	12
Grant et al,[144] 2007	14	TLM	74	91	100	1
Motta et al,[87] 2004	61	TLM	88	94	90	21
Iro et al,[145] 1998	54	TLM		75		7
Ambrosch et al,[88] 1998	34	TLM			89	4
Zeitels et al,[146] 1994	6	TLM			100	0
T3						
Johansen et al,[143] 2002	87	RT	45	52	43	44
Daugaard et al,[30] 1998	147	RT			30	
Nakfoor et al,[28] 1998	51	RT		64	76	
Hinerman et al,[29] 2002	87	RT			62	
Grant et al,[144] 2007	8	TLM	67	73	100	0
Motta et al,[87] 2004	18	TLM	81	81	90	7
Vilaseca et al,[142] 2010	96	TLM	46	62	70	29

Abbreviations: DFS, disease-free survival; LC, local control; OS, overall survival.

the rate of locoregional recurrence was higher in the ICRT group than the surgery group (12% vs 2%). The conclusion was that induction chemotherapy results in higher laryngeal preservation rates without compromising patient survival.

The RTOG 91-11 study randomized 547 patients with advanced laryngeal cancers to ICRT, concurrent chemoradiotherapy (CCRT), or RT alone. Failures received salvage TL. The 5-year survival rates were similar among the 3 arms, but CCRT resulted in the highest laryngeal preservation rate (84%) and local control (78%). Although acute toxic effects were much higher in the chemotherapy arms, late toxic effects were comparable in all 3 groups.[37] The study concluded that CCRT may result in superior outcomes than ICRT or RT alone. At 10-year follow-up, CCRT maintained higher laryngeal preservation and locoregional control rates but had worse overall survival and more seemingly unrelated deaths when compared with ICRT (30.8% vs

20.8%). This finding may be a random occurrence or related to older RT techniques administered in this 2-decade-old study, but it is unclear whether these deaths may in fact be due to late effects of concurrent therapy.[38]

Despite this evidence, caution should be used when generalizing the results to all patients. Patients were accrued for those studied 20 to 30 years ago, before advances in RT and surgical techniques. Long-term results demonstrating increased rates of unexplained deaths in CCRT is of significant concern. As CRT-based organ preservation protocols have been increasingly used, the overall survival for laryngeal cancer has actually declined during this same time period, especially for T3N0M0 glottic cancers.[39] Recent evidence suggests that there may in fact be a survival advantage with initial surgical therapy.[40] Despite this suggestion, organ preservation with CCRT is recommended as the initial treatment of T3 and T4 laryngeal and hypopharyngeal cancers without significant cartilage invasion, base of tongue involvement, or extension into the neck soft tissues.

Since the publication of these studies, there seemed to be a reduced role for open surgery in all laryngeal cancers.[41] Recently, however, the pendulum seems to be swinging back toward the importance of initial surgical management for T4 tumors.[40] Cost-effectiveness may also become a consideration. TL with PORT is nearly $3000 less than organ preservation protocols for chemoradiation in advanced laryngeal cancers.[42]

Postoperative Radiotherapy and Chemoradiotherapy

Postoperative adjuvant therapy is indicated when there is an increased risk of locoregional or distant recurrence of disease after resection. Adjuvant therapy can be considered in patients who have undergone conservation surgery or TL for advanced disease with the following high-risk features[43–46]:

- T3 or T4 disease
- Perineural invasion
- Lymphoid or vascular invasion
- N2 disease or greater
- Positive (or close, <5 mm) resection margins
- Extracapsular extension of nodal disease (ECS)

PORT significantly improves overall survival, locoregional control, and disease-specific survival in patients with high-risk features compared with surgery alone.[47–50] PORT is adequate for patients with moderately increased risk, but those with highest-risk features (positive, or close, margins, and ECS) should receive postoperative CCRT.

Postoperative CCRT has been demonstrated to improve outcomes in multiple large, randomized studies. In 2004, the European Organisation for Research and Treatment of Cancer (EORTC) (22931) and RTOG (9501) simultaneously published randomized trials comparing postoperative CCRT to PORT alone in high-risk patients. The addition of chemotherapy significantly improved locoregional control compared with PORT alone (82% vs 69% in the EORTC trial; 82% vs 72% in the RTOG trial).[51,52] Of note, a significant increase in acute toxicities was noted with the addition of chemotherapy. The RTOG trial cited a 77% incidence of acute adverse effects of grade 3 or greater acute adverse effects in the CCRT group, compared with 34% incidence in the PORT group (P<.001), with 4 deaths directly associated with CCRT.[51] When the data from these 2 studies were pooled, extracapsular extension and positive surgical margins were the only factors that significantly benefitted from the addition of postoperative CCRT.[53] The 10-year follow-up of the RTOG 9501 trial also reported that only patients with positive margins and ECS significantly benefitted from the addition of chemotherapy.[54]

Monoclonal antibodies such as cetuximab (Erbitux, developed by Merck, under license from ImClone) may be used as a single agent or in combination with other modalities in advanced, recurrent, or metastatic head and neck cancers. Cetuximab produces modest improvements in the duration of locoregional control and overall survival.[55,56] However, recent studies suggest that the addition of cetuximab to standard CCRT is of questionable benefit with significant toxicity and should not be used routinely.[57]

SURGICAL TREATMENT OPTIONS

Surgical techniques used in the management of laryngeal and hypopharyngeal tumors have evolved over the last 3 decades with the increasing application of transoral surgery. Open partial procedures are now rarely indicated. Transoral CO_2 laser microsurgery is the most common endoscopic technique, but transoral robotic surgery (TORS) has also been used for glottic and supraglottic lesions.[58–60] Transoral conservation surgery is useful for T1, T2, and highly select T3 and T4 tumors.

Transoral techniques have many benefits over open conservative laryngeal procedures and RT.[41] TLM significantly reduces the need for tracheotomy, feeding tube placement, length of hospital stay, and the rate of postoperative pharyngocutaneous fistulae compared with open resection.[41,61–63] TLM is usually an ambulatory procedure; RT requires daily or twice-daily therapy for several weeks. From a cost-effectiveness perspective, TLM greatly outweighs definitive RT.[64,65] Poor candidates for TLM include the following:

- Tumors with cartilage invasion
- Large tumors that would require extensive removal resulting in aspiration
- Bilateral arytenoid involvement
- Poor intraoperative visualization of the tumor
- Direct extension into the neck soft tissues
- Significant extension into the base of tongue, hypopharynx, or subglottis
- Patients with poor pulmonary function

Preoperative assessment of pulmonary status by the ability to walk up 2 flights of stairs, rather than pulmonary function tests, is adequate to determine if the patient will be able to tolerate some degree of inevitable postoperative aspiration.[66]

Endoscopic Surgery for Early Glottic Tumors

A classification system for endoscopic cordectomies based on extent of resection was initially proposed[67] in 2000 by the European Laryngological Society and then revised[68] in 2007 to include lesions involving the anterior commissure (**Table 4**).

Transoral surgery for early laryngeal tumors has excellent oncologic and functional results (**Figs. 2** and **3**). Evidence increasingly demonstrates that, in experienced hands, the oncologic and functional outcomes are comparable to RT and may in fact be superior, with the added benefit of the ability to reserve RT for locoregionally recurrent disease. For Tis, T1, and T2 glottic cancers, several studies have reported excellent oncologic outcomes with both transoral resection and RT (see **Table 1**).

Vocal quality after laser resection in glottic cancers has been shown to be no different than those for RT.[69] Ultimate laryngeal preservation rates are higher with TLM: 94% to 100% of patients,[64,68,70–74] compared with 90% to 98% for T1 and 75% to 87% for T2 with RT alone.[75–77] Oncologic outcomes with TLM are excellent,

Table 4
Classification of cordectomies for transoral laser resection of glottic carcinoma according to the European Laryngological Society

Type	Procedure	Cordectomy for Glottic Carcinoma Details
I	Subepithelial cordectomy	Resection of the vocal fold epithelium, through the superficial layer of the lamina propria
II	Subligamental cordectomy	Resection of the epithelium, Reinke space, and vocal ligament
III	Transmuscular cordectomy	Resection of the epithelium, lamina propria, and part of the vocalis muscle
IV	Total or complete cordectomy	Resection from the vocal process to the anterior commissure, to the internal perichondrium of the thyroid ala ± perichondrium
Va	Extended cordectomy encompassing the contralateral vocal fold	Type IV + a segment of the entire contralateral vocal fold, along the cartilage at the height of the anterior commissure, removing Broyle ligament
Vb	Extended cordectomy encompassing the arytenoid	In cases where the lesion is involving the vocal process but sparing the arytenoid, resection can include the cartilage up to the posterior arytenoid mucosa
Vc	Extended cordectomy encompassing the ventricular fold	For superiorly spreading lesions involving the ventricle or transglottic cancers, resection includes Type IV, the ventricular fold and Morgagnis ventricle, down to the inferior extent of the vocal fold
Vd	Extended cordectomy encompassing the subglottis	Resection is continued 1 cm under the glottis with exposure of the cricoid cartilage
VI	Anterior bilateral cordectomy and commissurectomy	Includes removal of Broyle ligament

Modified from Remacle M, Eckel HE, Antonelli A, et al. Endoscopic cordectomy. A proposal for a classification by the Working Committee, European Laryngological Society. Eur Arch Otorhinolaryngol 2000;257:227–31.

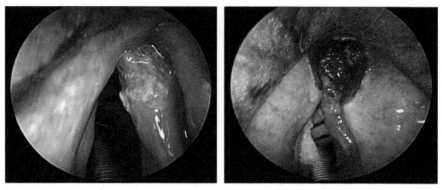

Fig. 2. Assessment of a T1 glottic squamous cell carcinoma, and subsequent transoral vestibulotomy for additional exposure.

with 5-year local control rates of 83% to 99% for T1–T2 tumors.[71,78–80] Involvement of the anterior commissure may imply worse oncologic outcomes, especially local control, regardless of the treatment modality.[17,81] Despite worse oncologic outcomes, involvement of the anterior commissure does not preclude the use of TLM therapy.

Endoscopic Surgery for Early Supraglottic Tumors

The European Laryngological Society also introduced a classification system for endoscopic supraglottic laryngectomy procedures based on location and extent of resection (**Table 5**).[82] Bilateral necks, at minimum levels of II, III, and IV, should also be electively treated due to the high risk of occult nodal disease, which has been reported to be up to 25% in T1 and T2 supraglottic tumors.[83,84] Adjuvant PORT to the primary site and neck can be combined with transoral surgical resection for initial treatment of supraglottic cancers, but one should try to avoid that. Compared with primary RT and open surgery, oncologic outcomes and laryngeal preservation rates may be higher with TLM (**Fig. 4**) for supraglottic cancers.[85,86] Five-year local control has been reported as 98% to 100% for T1 and 89% to 100% for T2 disease with TLM,[87,88] compared with lower rates with RT alone.[28,89,90]

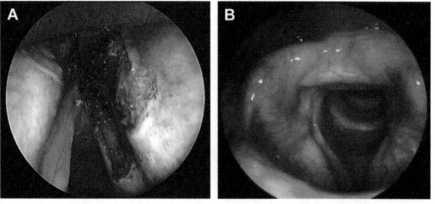

Fig. 3. (A) Final resection and (B) appearance at 1 year postoperatively of the T1a tumor demonstrated in **Fig. 2.**

Table 5
Classification of transoral procedures for supraglottic carcinoma according to the European Laryngological Society

Type	Procedure	Transoral Laser Surgery for Supraglottic Carcinoma	
		Details
I	Limited excision	For small superficial lesions
II	Resection of the pre-epiglottic space	Resection of half of the suprahyoid epiglottis (IIa) or total epiglottectomy (IIb) for lesions on the laryngeal surface of the epiglottis
III	Medial SGL with resection of the pre-epiglottic space	The epiglottis and entire pre-epiglottic space are removed along the inner thyroid lamina (IIIa). For tumors of the infrahyoid epiglottis, the tissue up to the ventricular folds is included (IIIb)
IV	Lateral SGL	The AE fold, the pharyngo-epiglottic fold, free edge of the epiglottis, and ventricular fold are resected, with (IVb) or without (IVa) the arytenoid

Abbreviation: SGL, supraglottic laryngectomy.
Modified from Remacle M, Hantzakos A, Eckel H, et al. Endoscopic supraglottic laryngectomy: a proposal for a classification by the working committee on nomenclature, European Laryngological Society. Eur Arch Otorhinolaryngol 2009;266:993–8.

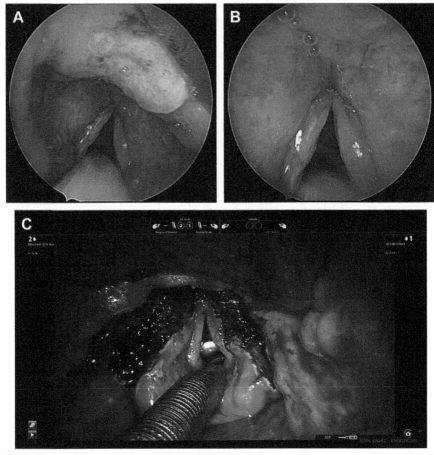

Fig. 4. Tumor endoscopy and excision defect of a T2N0M0 supraglottic squamous cell carcinoma (SCCA). (*A*) Laryngeal surface epiglottic tumor. (*B*) Involvement of the right false vocal fold and bilateral true vocal fold leukoplakia. (*C*) Defect following a transoral robotic resection using the CO_2 laser.

Endoscopic Surgery for Early Hypopharynx Tumors

Similar transoral techniques have been applied to select hypopharynx tumors with acceptable oncologic and functional results. Limited lesions of the pyriform sinus and of the pharyngeal walls are particularly amenable to TLM or TORS. Conservation procedures should not be performed for lesions involving the deep pyriform sinus apex or invading the postcricoid space. Five-year overall survival is approximately 70% for early disease and 40% to 50% for late stage disease.[91–94] TLM is feasible for limited hypopharynx cancers, but the majority present in later stages and are treated with nonsurgical organ conservation protocols.

Open Laryngeal Conservation Surgery

As mentioned previously, open conservation surgery for laryngeal hypopharyngeal tumors has largely been replaced by transoral techniques. A temporary tracheotomy and a feeding tube are almost always required for these procedures. Indications and contraindications for open laryngeal conservation surgeries parallel those for endo-scopic conservation techniques. Open partial procedures may be carefully considered an alternative to RT or TL in select glottic or supraglottic cancers. Organ-preserving open procedures are also feasible for certain hypopharynx cancers via a suprahyoid pharyngotomy approach, partial lateral pharyngotomy, or extended supraglottic partial laryngectomy.

Glottic lesions can be resected through simple laryngofissure with cordectomy or vertical partial laryngectomy, where the endolarynx is approached through a vertical midline incision at the anterior commissure. Reconstruction of the resulting defect with local muscle flaps, epiglottic laryngoplasty, or even free tissue reconstruction may be necessary.[95] Five-year disease-free survival is 93% to 98% for T1 and T2 lesions, with ultimate laryngeal preservation rates of 95% to 100%.[61,96,97]

For supraglottic lesions, horizontal partial laryngectomy procedures access the endolarynx through a horizontal incision in the thyroid cartilage and allow for partial removal of the supraglottic structures (**Fig. 5**). If the tumor has significant inferior extension, supracricoid laryngectomy is required. The supracricoid laryngectomy with crico-hyoido-epiglottopexy (SCL-CHEP) is indicated in more extensive supraglot-tic and transglottic tumors. SCL-CHEP involves resection of the entire thyroid cartilage and its contents, the epiglottis, one arytenoid complex, paraglottic space, and pree-piglottic space, leaving the cricoid, hyoid, and one arytenoid complex intact. The hyoid bone is aligned with and sutured to the cricoid cartilage for reconstruction. Laccour-reye and colleagues[98] reported a 71% 3-year overall survival rate with no local failures in 68 patients. Chevalier and Piquet[99] reported a 79% 5-year survival rate and a 3.3% local failure rate for 61 patients with T1–4 supraglottic cancers.

Complications of open partial laryngeal procedures include bleeding, infection, pharyngocutaneous fistula formation, severe dysphonia, tracheostomy dependence, and chronic aspiration. Severe dysphagia and aspiration occur in many patients.[100] Late stenosis and granulation can be managed endoscopically with serial debride-ment or dilation, with or without steroid injection. Complications are more likely to occur in salvage cases.[101] Open partial procedures for laryngeal and hypopharyngeal cancers have a great deal more adverse effects compared with TLM, and subse-quently, their use has widely fallen out of favor.

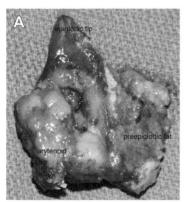 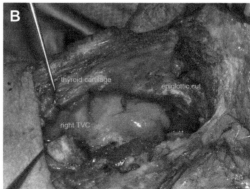

Fig. 5. A combination of a left supraglottic horizontal partial laryngectomy with a left ante-rolateral vertical partial laryngectomy for SCCA involving the false vocal folds, arytenoids, and true vocal fold. (*A*) Labeled medial aspect of the resection specimen. (*B*) Surgical defect showing right-sided structures left intact.

Total Laryngectomy

TL remains the mainstay of therapy for advanced laryngeal and hypopharyngeal tumors. After TL, most patients will still require adjuvant therapy. TL is appropriate for patients with severe aspiration, airway compromise, thyroid cartilage destruction, extralaryngeal spread, posterior commissure involvement, bilateral arytenoid complex involvement, and significant extension superiorly or inferiorly involving the base of tongue, subglottis, or cricoid cartilage. These patients are unlikely to maintain organ function with organ-sparing CRT protocols. TL is also indicated for treatment failures, recurrence, intractable aspiration, or chondronecrosis after organ-sparing treatments. Total laryngopharyngectomy is necessary for extensive hypopharyngeal tumors involving the pyriform sinuses, postcricoid tissues, with extension into the esophageal inlet or extensive involvement of the posterior pharyngeal wall.

For vocal rehabilitation, tracheoesophageal puncture (TEP) for tracheoesophageal speech can be performed at the time of primary surgery or as a secondary procedure. Primary placement of the TEP avoids the morbidity of a second procedure and may have better vocal rehabilitation outcomes.[102,103] A primary TEP can even be placed when free tissue is used for reconstruction.[104] Postoperatively, oral feeding typically begins at 1 week in nonirradiated patients and about 10 to 14 days in radiated patients. Some suggest oral feeding earlier, at 48 hours postoperatively, for nonradiated patients who did not undergo partial pharyngectomy.[105] Patients usually maintain good quality of life, including speech, swallow, and minimal social disruption.[106,107]

Oncologic outcomes after primary TL are acceptable. The VA trial in 1991 reported a 2-year overall survival of 68% after TL, with significantly fewer local recurrences than with organ preservation therapy (2% vs 12%, respectively, $P = .001$).[36] Woodard and colleagues[106] reviewed outcomes for 143 patients who underwent primary or salvage TL. Median survival time was 21 months for T4 disease and 58 months for T3 disease. Hypopharyngeal primary tumors had significantly worse median survival than laryngeal primary tumors: 16 months versus 42 months, respectively ($P = .005$). Multiple comorbidities, cardiovascular comorbidities, and N2 or higher disease were predictive of worse survival.

Complications of Total Laryngectomy

Complications following TL are either early or late in onset. Early complications after TL include infection, bleeding, hematoma, and wound breakdown. Paratracheal node dissection and thyroidectomy may result in chyle leak or temporary or permanent hypocalcemia. Hypocalcemia can be managed with postoperative monitoring of calcium levels and supplementation. Thyroid hormone placement should be initiated if total thyroidectomy is performed to prevent hypothyroidism and subsequent wound-healing issues. The approximate long-term prevalence of hypothyroidism is notable, with clinical hypothyroidism in 25% and subclinical hypothyroidism in 27%. Intraoperative hemithyroidectomy and combined therapy with RT appear to be significant prognostic factors of hypothyroidism.[108]

Pharyngocutaneous fistula is a common complication after TL, especially in salvage cases.[109] Development of a fistula typically occurs between 5 and 10 days postoperatively and prolongs rehabilitation and hospitalization.[110] The fistula rate is approximately 20% to 30% in salvage cases, although augmentation with a vascularized flap may potentially decrease the rate or severity of fistula.[111-113] Early signs of fistula formation include fever, swelling, increased pain, elevated white blood cell count, and murky material in the drains. Operative management of fistulae with placement of a salivary bypass tube or with tissue reconstruction is necessary when conservative management fails or great vessels are at risk. Persistent or recurrent cancers should be ruled out in the case of late fistula formation. Stomal stenosis is a potential late complication of TL, which can be managed conservatively by placement of a laryngectomy tube or surgically with stomal dilation via stomaplasty. Stenosis of the esophagus and neopharynx may also occur long term and require esophageal dilation and gastrostomy tube feeding.

Management of the Neck

All clinically positive nodal disease should be addressed. Selective neck dissection is usually feasible, even in N2–3 cases, but modified radical dissection with resection of any involved structures may be necessary. In N0 disease, the neck should be treated when the risk of occult metastases is greater than 20%. For tumors treated endoscopically, neck management principles are the same according to tumor site and stage.

Early glottic primary disease has an extremely low rate of occult nodal metastases, approaching 0%.[14,15] Therefore, initial observation of the neck is appropriate in T1N0 and T2N0 glottic cancers. T3 and T4 glottic carcinomas in clinically N0 cases have up to a 30% risk of occult nodal disease, and therefore, elective neck dissection should be performed.[114] Transglottic spread and extralaryngeal extension are important predictors of occult nodal metastases, arguably more than T stage, and this feature should be considered when determining the management of the neck.[114] In limited glottic tumors, unilateral neck dissection may be acceptable; however, bilateral dissection should be performed in large tumors with significant soft tissue extension, extension into adjacent subsites, and lesions approaching the midline. RT alone to the neck is an alternative treatment of endoscopically managed primary tumors with N0 or N1 disease. Consolidation to a single treatment modality in these situations should be the goal, however.

Supraglottic, subglottic, and hypopharyngeal cancers have rich bilateral lymphatic drainage and a high likelihood of occult nodal disease, even in T1 and T2 cases. Because the contralateral neck is a common site for failure, bilateral selective neck dissection is routine in supraglottic cancer and improves outcomes for select T1 and all T2–T4 cases.[115–117] Subglottic carcinoma requires dissection of bilateral levels II–IV, total thyroidectomy, and paratracheal node dissection. Although level V and retropharyngeal nodes may be involved in hypopharyngeal primaries, surgical dissection may not improve overall survival.[118] Selective nodal dissection of levels II–IV is usually sufficient for N0 disease in hypopharynx cancer.

TREATMENT RESISTANCE AND RECURRENCE

Response to therapy should be assessed 3 months after treatment with imaging. If there is no clinical response to definitive RT or CRT at 6 weeks after therapy, workup and surgical salvage can be initiated sooner. Stomal recurrences have a particularly dismal prognosis, and salvage surgical management may require heroic measures. Appropriately selected candidates, such as those with early stage recurrences, may have acceptable outcomes with salvage treatment. Poor prognostic factors include previous chemotherapy or CRT, advanced stage at recurrence presentation, short time to recurrence, and nonlaryngeal recurrence sites.[119–121]

Surgical Salvage

Salvage TL is indicated for patients who fail initial therapy with RT, CRT, or conservation laryngeal surgery. The RTOG 91-11 trial in 2003, described previously, analyzed outcomes after salvage TL following ICRT, CCRT, or RT alone. Overall, 129 of 517 patients underwent TL. The incidence of TL in each group was 28%, 15%, and 31% for ICRT, CCRT, and RT, respectively. Locoregional control was achieved in 90% of RT-alone patients and 74% in ICRT and CCRT patients, with no significant difference in overall survival among the 3 arms (69%–76%).[111] In a comprehensive meta-analysis, 5-year survival after salvage surgery for recurrent glottic carcinoma with either TL or salvage conservation surgery was 83% and 36% for early and late stage disease, respectively.[120] Five-year survival after surgical salvage for recurrent supraglottic cancers after initial RT is lower, at 29%.[122] Outcomes for recurrent hypopharyngeal cancers, despite salvage surgery, are especially poor. Minimally invasive, partial laryngectomy salvage procedures are indicated for highly selected patients with well-defined glottic and supraglottic tumors. Unlike open partial laryngectomy, extensive disease found during an endoscopic procedure does not require immediate TL, therefore extending the initial indications of such an approach.

Management of the neck at the time of surgical salvage after initial RT should be guided by the presalvage imaging.[123] The general management principles are similar to those for primary therapy. Persistent nodal disease after definitive treatment with RT or CRT that is PET-CT and biopsy-positive for squamous cell carcinoma should be managed with neck dissection, if resectable. Even in clinically N0 necks after initial nonsurgical therapy, there is a significant risk of occult nodal disease, especially with recurrent transglottic and supraglottic primary tumors. Therefore, standard selective neck dissection is suggested in these cases.[124]

Reirradiation

Reirradiation for locoregionally recurrent disease may be feasible for patients who are not candidates for salvage surgery or who have high-risk pathologic features on surgical salvage. Two-year survival rates after reirradiation for recurrent head and neck cancers are approximately 20% to 40%, but most studies include disease from all sites and vary significantly in terms of patient selection.[125–127]

Reirradiation doses are significant and the potential adverse effects are as well. Potential adverse effects include pseudoaneurysm, osteoradionecrosis of the vertebrae and facial skeleton, severe mucositis, and spinal cord and brainstem injury. Free or regional tissue transfer may be necessary before reirradiation to prevent carotid rupture. The RTOG group examined outcomes after reirradiation combined with CCRT for unresectable head and neck cancers (RTOG 9610). The incidence of grade 5 toxicities was 7.6%, and estimated 2- and 5-year survival rates were 15.3% and 3.8%, respectively.[128] In the RTOG 99-11 study, a high incidence of grade 5 toxicities was observed with reirradiation and chemotherapy (8%), with a 2-year overall survival rate of only 26%.[129] These combination salvage therapies should be reserved for experimental protocols and used with caution because of the high risk and limited reward. Proton therapy may prove to be a significant benefit in the salvage reirradiation patient, but the data are not yet available.

EVALUATION OF OUTCOME AND LONG-TERM RECOMMENDATIONS

Patients with head and neck cancer are at significant risk of recurrence, second primaries, and adverse effects of therapy. Patients should be evaluated on a monthly basis for the first year, progressing to every 2 to 4 months in the second and third years. Five years after treatment, patients can be seen annually. Patients who had RT to the neck should have thyroid-stimulating hormone levels measured every 6 to 12 months. Imaging with PET-CT is recommended 3 months after completion of therapy or sooner if recurrent or persistent disease is suspected. False positives may occur, but a negative PET-CT scan is satisfactory to exclude recurrent disease. Suspicious lesions on imaging should undergo fine-needle aspiration. It is common practice to perform a PET/CT at a year following completion of therapy as well. Residual or recurrent disease in the neck should be treated with neck dissection. Local disease recurrence or persistence will likely necessitate salvage surgical therapy with TL or a partial procedure if appropriate.

Continued surveillance for distant metastases and second primary tumors is also an essential component of long-term patient follow-up. Patients at high risk for lung cancer, including those with greater than 20 pack-years smoking history, should undergo annual chest CT. The physician should routinely provide counseling for tobacco and alcohol cessation and screen for depression when appropriate.

SUMMARY/DISCUSSION

Many advances have been made over the past 2 decades that greatly improve the care of patients with laryngeal and hypopharyngeal cancer. The development and refinement of transoral surgery have significantly reduced the morbidities that patients experience when treated surgically. Not all patients are candidates for TLM, however, and organ-sparing therapy with CCRT is the favored management strategy for most advanced cases. Unfortunately, oncologic outcomes have remained relatively stagnant despite these apparent advances in therapy. TL is the definitive procedure for advanced cases with nonfunctioning larynges and salvage cases. Long-term surveillance for second primary disease in these smoking-related cancers is a critical component of follow-up.

REFERENCES

1. Goodwin WJ Jr, Byers PM. Nutritional management of the head and neck cancer patient. Med Clin North Am 1993;77:597–610.
2. Capuano G, Gentile PC, Bianciardi F, et al. Prevalence and influence of malnutrition on quality of life and performance status in patients with locally advanced head and neck cancer before treatment. Support Care Cancer 2010;18:433–7.
3. Agarwal V, Branstetter BF 4th, Johnson JT. Indications for PET/CT in the head and neck. Otolaryngol Clin North Am 2008;41:23–49, v.
4. Schoder H, Yeung HW, Gonen M, et al. Head and neck cancer: clinical usefulness and accuracy of PET/CT image fusion. Radiology 2004;231:65–72.
5. Edge SB, Byrd DR, Compton CC, et al. AJCC cancer staging manual. New York: Springer; 2010.
6. Fu KK, Pajak TF, Trotti A, et al. A Radiation Therapy Oncology Group (RTOG) phase III randomized study to compare hyperfractionation and two variants of accelerated fractionation to standard fractionation radiotherapy for head and neck squamous cell carcinomas: first report of RTOG 9003. Int J Radiat Oncol Biol Phys 2000;48:7–16.
7. Beitler JJ, Zhang Q, Fu KK, et al. Final results of local-regional control and late toxicity of RTOG 9003: a randomized trial of altered fractionation radiation for locally advanced head and neck cancer. Int J Radiat Oncol Biol Phys 2014; 89:13–20.
8. van de Water TA, Bijl HP, Schilstra C, et al. The potential benefit of radiotherapy with protons in head and neck cancer with respect to normal tissue sparing: a systematic review of literature. Oncologist 2011;16:366–77.
9. van der Laan HP, van de Water TA, van Herpt HE, et al. The potential of intensity-modulated proton radiotherapy to reduce swallowing dysfunction in the

treatment of head and neck cancer: a planning comparative study. Acta Oncol 2013;52:561–9.

10. Chera BS, Amdur RJ, Morris CG, et al. T1N0 to T2N0 squamous cell carcinoma of the glottic larynx treated with definitive radiotherapy. Int J Radiat Oncol Biol Phys 2010;78:461–6.

11. Mendenhall WM, Amdur RJ, Morris CG, et al. T1-T2N0 squamous cell carcinoma of the glottic larynx treated with radiation therapy. J Clin Oncol 2001;19: 4029–36.

12. Marshak G, Brenner B, Shvero J, et al. Prognostic factors for local control of early glottic cancer: the Rabin Medical Center retrospective study on 207 patients. Int J Radiat Oncol Biol Phys 1999;43:1009–13.

13. Burke LS, Greven KM, McGuirt WT, et al. Definitive radiotherapy for early glottic carcinoma: prognostic factors and implications for treatment. Int J Radiat Oncol Biol Phys 1997;38:37–42.

14. Yang CY, Andersen PE, Everts EC, et al. Nodal disease in purely glottic carcinoma: is elective neck treatment worthwhile? Laryngoscope 1998;108:1006–8.

15. Johnson JT, Myers EN, Hao SP, et al. Outcome of open surgical therapy for glottic carcinoma. Ann Otol Rhinol Laryngol 1993;102:752–5.

16. Maheshwar AA, Gaffney CC. Radiotherapy for T1 glottic carcinoma: impact of anterior commissure involvement. J Laryngol Otol 2001;115:298–301.

17. Rodel RM, Steiner W, Muller RM, et al. Endoscopic laser surgery of early glottic cancer: involvement of the anterior commissure. Head Neck 2009;31:583–92.

18. Mlynarek A, Kost K, Gesser R. Radiotherapy versus surgery for early T1-T2 glottic carcinoma. J Otolaryngol 2006;35:413–9.

19. Hirota S, Soejima T, Obayashi K, et al. Radiotherapy of T1 and T2 glottic cancer: analysis of anterior commissure involvement. Radiat Med 1996;14:297–302.

20. Groome PA, O'Sullivan B, Mackillop WJ, et al. Compromised local control due to treatment interruptions and late treatment breaks in early glottic cancer: population-based outcomes study supporting need for intensified treatment schedules. Int J Radiat Oncol Biol Phys 2006;64:1002–12.

21. McCoul ED, Har-El G. Meta-analysis of impaired vocal cord mobility as a prognostic factor in T2 glottic carcinoma. Arch Otolaryngol Head Neck Surg 2009; 135:479–86.

22. Browman GP, Mohide EA, Willan A, et al. Association between smoking during radiotherapy and prognosis in head and neck cancer: a follow-up study. Head Neck 2002;24:1031–7.

23. Browman GP, Wong G, Hodson I, et al. Influence of cigarette smoking on the efficacy of radiation therapy in head and neck cancer. N Engl J Med 1993;328: 159–63.

24. Fein DA, Lee WR, Hanlon AL, et al. Pretreatment hemoglobin level influences local control and survival of T1-T2 squamous cell carcinomas of the glottic larynx. J Clin Oncol 1995;13:2077–83.

25. Freeman DE, Mancuso AA, Parsons JT, et al. Irradiation alone for supraglottic larynx carcinoma: can CT findings predict treatment results? Int J Radiat Oncol Biol Phys 1990;19:485–90.

26. Levendag P, Vikram B. The problem of neck relapse in early stage supraglottic cancer–results of different treatment modalities for the clinically negative neck. Int J Radiat Oncol Biol Phys 1987;13:1621–4.

27. Carl J, Andersen LJ, Pedersen M, et al. Prognostic factors of local control after radiotherapy in T1 glottic and supraglottic carcinoma of the larynx. Radiother Oncol 1996;39:229–33.

28. Nakfoor BM, Spiro IJ, Wang CC, et al. Results of accelerated radiotherapy for supraglottic carcinoma: a Massachusetts General Hospital and Massachusetts Eye and Ear Infirmary experience. Head Neck 1998;20:379–84.
29. Hinerman RW, Mendenhall WM, Amdur RJ, et al. Carcinoma of the supraglottic larynx: treatment results with radiotherapy alone or with planned neck dissection. Head Neck 2002;24:456–67.
30. Daugaard BJ, Sand HH. Primary radiotherapy of carcinoma of the supraglottic larynx–a multivariate analysis of prognostic factors. Int J Radiat Oncol Biol Phys 1998;41:355–60.
31. Dahm JD, Sessions DG, Paniello RC, et al. Primary subglottic cancer. Laryngoscope 1998;108:741–6.
32. Chen SW, Yang SN, Liang JA, et al. Value of computed tomography-based tumor volume as a predictor of outcomes in hypopharyngeal cancer after treatment with definitive radiotherapy. Laryngoscope 2006;116:2012–7.
33. Pameijer FA, Mancuso AA, Mendenhall WM, et al. Evaluation of pretreatment computed tomography as a predictor of local control in T1/T2 pyriform sinus carcinoma treated with definitive radiotherapy. Head Neck 1998;20:159–68.
34. Rabbani A, Amdur RJ, Mancuso AA, et al. Definitive radiotherapy for T1-T2 squamous cell carcinoma of pyriform sinus. Int J Radiat Oncol Biol Phys 2008;72:351–5.
35. Amdur RJ, Mendenhall WM, Stringer SP, et al. Organ preservation with radiotherapy for T1-T2 carcinoma of the pyriform sinus. Head Neck 2001;23:353–62.
36. Induction chemotherapy plus radiation compared with surgery plus radiation in patients with advanced laryngeal cancer. The Department of Veterans Affairs Laryngeal Cancer Study Group. N Engl J Med 1991;324:1685–90.
37. Forastiere AA, Goepfert H, Maor M, et al. Concurrent chemotherapy and radiotherapy for organ preservation in advanced laryngeal cancer. N Engl J Med 2003;349:2091–8.
38. Vokes EE. Competing roads to larynx preservation. J Clin Oncol 2013;31:833–5.
39. Hoffman HT, Porter K, Karnell LH, et al. Laryngeal cancer in the United States: changes in demographics, patterns of care, and survival. Laryngoscope 2006;116:1–13.
40. Gourin CG, Conger BT, Sheils WC, et al. The effect of treatment on survival in patients with advanced laryngeal carcinoma. Laryngoscope 2009;119:1312–7.
41. Silver CE, Beitler JJ, Shaha AR, et al. Current trends in initial management of laryngeal cancer: the declining use of open surgery. Eur Arch Otorhinolaryngol 2009;266:1333–52.
42. Davis GE, Schwartz SR, Veenstra DL, et al. Cost comparison of surgery vs organ preservation for laryngeal cancer. Arch Otolaryngol Head Neck Surg 2005;131:21–6.
43. Olsen KD, Caruso M, Foote RL, et al. Primary head and neck cancer. Histopathologic predictors of recurrence after neck dissection in patients with lymph node involvement. Arch Otolaryngol Head Neck Surg 1994;120:1370–4.
44. Jacobs JR, Ahmad K, Casiano R, et al. Implications of positive surgical margins. Laryngoscope 1993;103:64–8.
45. Snyderman NL, Johnson JT, Schramm VL Jr, et al. Extracapsular spread of carcinoma in cervical lymph nodes. Impact upon survival in patients with carcinoma of the supraglottic larynx. Cancer 1985;56:1597–9.
46. Fagan JJ, Collins B, Barnes L, et al. Perineural invasion in squamous cell carcinoma of the head and neck. Arch Otolaryngol Head Neck Surg 1998;124:637–40.

47. Kokal WA, Neifeld JP, Eisert D, et al. Postoperative radiation as adjuvant treatment for carcinoma of the oral cavity, larynx, and pharynx: preliminary report of a prospective randomized trial. J Surg Oncol 1988;38:71–6.

48. Huang DT, Johnson CR, Schmidt-Ullrich R, et al. Postoperative radiotherapy in head and neck carcinoma with extracapsular lymph node extension and/or positive resection margins: a comparative study. Int J Radiat Oncol Biol Phys 1992; 23:737–42.

49. Lundahl RE, Foote RL, Bonner JA, et al. Combined neck dissection and postoperative radiation therapy in the management of the high-risk neck: a matched-pair analysis. Int J Radiat Oncol Biol Phys 1998;40:529–34.

50. Lavaf A, Genden EM, Cesaretti JA, et al. Adjuvant radiotherapy improves overall survival for patients with lymph node-positive head and neck squamous cell carcinoma. Cancer 2008;112:535–43.

51. Cooper JS, Pajak TF, Forastiere AA, et al. Postoperative concurrent radiotherapy and chemotherapy for high-risk squamous-cell carcinoma of the head and neck. N Engl J Med 2004;350:1937–44.

52. Bernier J, Domenge C, Ozsahin M, et al. Postoperative irradiation with or without concomitant chemotherapy for locally advanced head and neck cancer. N Engl J Med 2004;350:1945–52.

53. Bernier J, Cooper JS, Pajak TF, et al. Defining risk levels in locally advanced head and neck cancers: a comparative analysis of concurrent postoperative radiation plus chemotherapy trials of the EORTC (#22931) and RTOG (#9501). Head Neck 2005;27:843–50.

54. Cooper JS, Zhang Q, Pajak TF, et al. Long-term follow-up of the RTOG 9501/intergroup phase III trial: postoperative concurrent radiation therapy and chemotherapy in high-risk squamous cell carcinoma of the head and neck. Int J Radiat Oncol Biol Phys 2012;84:1198–205.

55. Bonner JA, Harari PM, Giralt J, et al. Radiotherapy plus cetuximab for squamous-cell carcinoma of the head and neck. N Engl J Med 2006;354:567–78.

56. Burtness B, Goldwasser MA, Flood W, et al, Eastern Cooperative Oncology Group. Phase III randomized trial of cisplatin plus placebo compared with cisplatin plus cetuximab in metastatic/recurrent head and neck cancer: an Eastern Cooperative Oncology Group study. J Clin Oncol 2005;23:8646–54.

57. Ang KK, Zhang Q, Rosenthal DI, et al. Randomized phase III trial of concurrent accelerated radiation plus cisplatin with or without cetuximab for stage III to IV head and neck carcinoma: RTOG 0522. J Clin Oncol 2014;32(27):2940–50.

58. Mendelsohn AH, Remacle M, Van Der Vorst S, et al. Outcomes following transoral robotic surgery: supraglottic laryngectomy. Laryngoscope 2013;123:208–14.

59. Lallemant B, Chambon G, Garrel R, et al. Transoral robotic surgery for the treatment of T1-T2 carcinoma of the larynx: preliminary study. Laryngoscope 2013; 123:2485–90.

60. Kayhan FT, Kaya KH, Sayin I. Transoral robotic cordectomy for early glottic carcinoma. Ann Otol Rhinol Laryngol 2012;121:497–502.

61. Mantsopoulos K, Psychogios G, Koch M, et al. Comparison of different surgical approaches in T2 glottic cancer. Head Neck 2012;34:73–7.

62. Cabanillas R, Rodrigo JP, Llorente JL, et al. Functional outcomes of transoral laser surgery of supraglottic carcinoma compared with a transcervical approach. Head Neck 2004;26:653–9.

63. Peretti G, Piazza C, Cattaneo A, et al. Comparison of functional outcomes after endoscopic versus open-neck supraglottic laryngectomies. Ann Otol Rhinol Laryngol 2006;115:827–32.

64. Gallo A, de Vincentiis M, Manciocco V, et al. CO2 laser cordectomy for early-stage glottic carcinoma: a long-term follow-up of 156 cases. Laryngoscope 2002;112:370–4.

65. Smith JC, Johnson JT, Cognetti DM, et al. Quality of life, functional outcome, and costs of early glottic cancer. Laryngoscope 2003;113:68–76.

66. Chow JM, Block RM, Friedman M. Preoperative evaluation for partial laryngectomy. Head Neck Surg 1988;10:319–23.

67. Remacle M, Eckel HE, Antonelli A, et al. Endoscopic cordectomy. A proposal for a classification by the Working Committee, European Laryngological Society. Eur Arch Otorhinolaryngol 2000;257:227–31.

68. Remacle M, Van Haverbeke C, Eckel H, et al. Proposal for revision of the European Laryngological Society classification of endoscopic cordectomies. Eur Arch Otorhinolaryngol 2007;264:499–504.

69. Delsupehe KG, Zink I, Lejaegere M, et al. Voice quality after narrow-margin laser cordectomy compared with laryngeal irradiation. Otolaryngol Head Neck Surg 1999;121:528–33.

70. Schrijvers ML, van Riel EL, Langendijk JA, et al. Higher laryngeal preservation rate after CO2 laser surgery compared with radiotherapy in T1a glottic laryngeal carcinoma. Head Neck 2009;31:759–64.

71. Motta G, Esposito E, Motta S, et al. CO2 laser surgery in the treatment of glottic cancer. Head Neck 2005;27:733.

72. Eckel HE, Thumfart W, Jungehulsing M, et al. Transoral laser surgery for early glottic carcinoma. Eur Arch Otorhinolaryngol 2000;257:221–6.

73. Ledda GP, Puxeddu R. Carbon dioxide laser microsurgery for early glottic carcinoma. Otolaryngol Head Neck Surg 2006;134:911–5.

74. Mortuaire G, Francois J, Wiel E, et al. Local recurrence after CO2 laser cordectomy for early glottic carcinoma. Laryngoscope 2006;116:101–5.

75. Cellai E, Frata P, Magrini SM, et al. Radical radiotherapy for early glottic cancer: results in a series of 1087 patients from two Italian radiation oncology centers. I. The case of T1N0 disease. Int J Radiat Oncol Biol Phys 2005;63:1378–86.

76. Jorgensen K, Godballe C, Hansen O, et al. Cancer of the larynx–treatment results after primary radiotherapy with salvage surgery in a series of 1005 patients. Acta Oncol 2002;41:69–76.

77. Fein DA, Mendenhall WM, Parsons JT, et al. T1-T2 squamous cell carcinoma of the glottic larynx treated with radiotherapy: a multivariate analysis of variables potentially influencing local control. Int J Radiat Oncol Biol Phys 1993;25:605–11.

78. Stoeckli SJ, Schnieper I, Huguenin P, et al. Early glottic carcinoma: treatment according patient's preference? Head Neck 2003;25:1051–6.

79. Peretti G, Piazza C, Cocco D, et al. Transoral CO2 laser treatment for Tis-T3 glottic cancer: the University of Brescia experience on 595 patients. Head Neck 2010;32:977–83.

80. Grant DG, Salassa JR, Hinni ML, et al. Transoral laser microsurgery for untreated glottic carcinoma. Otolaryngol Head Neck Surg 2007;137:482–6.

81. Steiner W, Ambrosch P, Rodel RM, et al. Impact of anterior commissure involvement on local control of early glottic carcinoma treated by laser microresection. Laryngoscope 2004;114:1485–91.

82. Remacle M, Hantzakos A, Eckel H, et al. Endoscopic supraglottic laryngectomy: a proposal for a classification by the working committee on nomenclature, European Laryngological Society. Eur Arch Otorhinolaryngol 2009;266:993–8.

83. Cummings CW. Incidence of nodal metastases in T2 supraglottic carcinoma. Arch Otolaryngol 1974;99:268–9.
84. Till JE, Bruce WR, Elwan A, et al. A preliminary analysis of end results for cancer of the larynx. Laryngoscope 1975;85:259–75.
85. Cabanillas R, Rodrigo JP, Llorente JL, et al. Oncologic outcomes of transoral laser surgery of supraglottic carcinoma compared with a transcervical approach. Head Neck 2008;30:750–5.
86. Ambrosch P. The role of laser microsurgery in the treatment of laryngeal cancer. Curr Opin Otolaryngol Head Neck Surg 2007;15:82–8.
87. Motta G, Esposito E, Testa D, et al. CO2 laser treatment of supraglottic cancer. Head Neck 2004;26:442–6.
88. Ambrosch P, Kron M, Steiner W. Carbon dioxide laser microsurgery for early supraglottic carcinoma. Ann Otol Rhinol Laryngol 1998;107:680–8.
89. Mendenhall WM, Parsons JT, Mancuso AA, et al. Radiotherapy for squamous cell carcinoma of the supraglottic larynx: an alternative to surgery. Head Neck 1996;18:24–35.
90. Sykes AJ, Slevin NJ, Gupta NK, et al. 331 cases of clinically node-negative supraglottic carcinoma of the larynx: a study of a modest size fixed field radiotherapy approach. Int J Radiat Oncol Biol Phys 2000;46:1109–15.
91. Steiner W, Ambrosch P, Hess CF, et al. Organ preservation by transoral laser microsurgery in piriform sinus carcinoma. Otolaryngol Head Neck Surg 2001; 124:58–67.
92. Rudert HH, Hoft S. Transoral carbon-dioxide laser resection of hypopharyngeal carcinoma. Eur Arch Otorhinolaryngol 2003;260:198–206.
93. Vilaseca I, Blanch JL, Bernal-Sprekelsen M, et al. CO2 laser surgery: a larynx preservation alternative for selected hypopharyngeal carcinomas. Head Neck 2004;26:953–9.
94. Martin A, Jackel MC, Christiansen H, et al. Organ preserving transoral laser microsurgery for cancer of the hypopharynx. Laryngoscope 2008;118:398–402.
95. Gilbert RW, Goldstein DP, Guillemaud JP, et al. Vertical partial laryngectomy with temporoparietal free flap reconstruction for recurrent laryngeal squamous cell carcinoma: technique and long-term outcomes. Arch Otolaryngol Head Neck Surg 2012;138:484–91.
96. Thomas JV, Olsen KD, Neel HB 3rd, et al. Early glottic carcinoma treated with open laryngeal procedures. Arch Otolaryngol Head Neck Surg 1994;120:264–8.
97. Laccourreye O, Muscatello L, Laccourreye L, et al. Supracricoid partial laryngectomy with cricohyoidoepiglottopexy for "early" glottic carcinoma classified as T1-T2N0 invading the anterior commissure. Am J Otolaryngol 1997;18: 385–90.
98. Laccourreye H, Laccourreye O, Weinstein G, et al. Supracricoid laryngectomy with cricohyoidopexy: a partial laryngeal procedure for selected supraglottic and transglottic carcinomas. Laryngoscope 1990;100:735–41.
99. Chevalier D, Piquet JJ. Subtotal laryngectomy with cricohyoidopexy for supraglottic carcinoma: review of 61 cases. Am J Surg 1994;168:472–3.
100. Lewin JS, Hutcheson KA, Barringer DA, et al. Functional analysis of swallowing outcomes after supracricoid partial laryngectomy. Head Neck 2008;30:559–66.
101. Ganly I, Patel SG, Matsuo J, et al. Analysis of postoperative complications of open partial laryngectomy. Head Neck 2009;31:338–45.
102. Cheng E, Ho M, Ganz C, et al. Outcomes of primary and secondary tracheoesophageal puncture: a 16-year retrospective analysis. Ear Nose Throat J 2006; 85(262):264–7.

103. Chone CT, Gripp FM, Spina AL, et al. Primary versus secondary tracheoesophageal puncture for speech rehabilitation in total laryngectomy: long-term results with indwelling voice prosthesis. Otolaryngol Head Neck Surg 2005;133:89–93.

104. Divi V, Lin DT, Emerick K, et al. Primary TEP placement in patients with laryngopharyngeal free tissue reconstruction and salivary bypass tube placement. Otolaryngol Head Neck Surg 2011;144:474–6.

105. Medina JE, Khafif A. Early oral feeding following total laryngectomy. Laryngoscope 2001;111:368–72.

106. Woodard TD, Oplatek A, Petruzzelli GJ. Life after total laryngectomy: a measure of long-term survival, function, and quality of life. Arch Otolaryngol Head Neck Surg 2007;133:526–32.

107. Vilaseca I, Chen AY, Backscheider AG. Long-term quality of life after total laryngectomy. Head Neck 2006;28:313–20.

108. Leon X, Gras JR, Perez A, et al. Hypothyroidism in patients treated with total laryngectomy. A multivariate study. Eur Arch Otorhinolaryngol 2002;259:193–6.

109. Ganly I, Patel S, Matsuo J, et al. Postoperative complications of salvage total laryngectomy. Cancer 2005;103:2073–81.

110. Papazoglou G, Doundoulakis G, Terzakis G, et al. Pharyngocutaneous fistula after total laryngectomy: incidence, cause, and treatment. Ann Otol Rhinol Laryngol 1994;103:801–5.

111. Weber RS, Berkey BA, Forastiere A, et al. Outcome of salvage total laryngectomy following organ preservation therapy: the Radiation Therapy Oncology Group trial 91-11. Arch Otolaryngol Head Neck Surg 2003;129:44–9.

112. Withrow KP, Rosenthal EL, Gourin CG, et al. Free tissue transfer to manage salvage laryngectomy defects after organ preservation failure. Laryngoscope 2007;117:781–4.

113. Fung K, Teknos TN, Vandenberg CD, et al. Prevention of wound complications following salvage laryngectomy using free vascularized tissue. Head Neck 2007;29:425–30.

114. Kligerman J, Olivatto LO, Lima RA, et al. Elective neck dissection in the treatment of T3/T4 N0 squamous cell carcinoma of the larynx. Am J Surg 1995;170:436–9.

115. Lutz CK, Johnson JT, Wagner RL, et al. Supraglottic carcinoma: patterns of recurrence. Ann Otol Rhinol Laryngol 1990;99:12–7.

116. Redaelli de Zinis LO, Nicolai P, Tomenzoli D, et al. The distribution of lymph node metastases in supraglottic squamous cell carcinoma: therapeutic implications. Head Neck 2002;24:913–20.

117. Chiu RJ, Myers EN, Johnson JT. Efficacy of routine bilateral neck dissection in the management of supraglottic cancer. Otolaryngol Head Neck Surg 2004;131:485–8.

118. Amatsu M, Mohri M, Kinishi M. Significance of retropharyngeal node dissection at radical surgery for carcinoma of the hypopharynx and cervical esophagus. Laryngoscope 2001;111:1099–103.

119. Ho AS, Kraus DH, Ganly I, et al. Decision making in the management of recurrent head and neck cancer. Head Neck 2014;36:144–51.

120. Goodwin WJ Jr. Salvage surgery for patients with recurrent squamous cell carcinoma of the upper aerodigestive tract: when do the ends justify the means? Laryngoscope 2000;110:1–18.

121. Choe KS, Haraf DJ, Solanki A, et al. Prior chemoradiotherapy adversely impacts outcomes of recurrent and second primary head and neck cancer treated with concurrent chemotherapy and reirradiation. Cancer 2011;117:4671–8.

122. Parsons JT, Mendenhall WM, Stringer SP, et al. Salvage surgery following radiation failure in squamous cell carcinoma of the supraglottic larynx. Int J Radiat Oncol Biol Phys 1995;32:605–9.
123. Farrag TY, Lin FR, Cummings CW, et al. Neck management in patients undergoing postradiotherapy salvage laryngeal surgery for recurrent/persistent laryngeal cancer. Laryngoscope 2006;116:1864–6.
124. Koss SL, Russell MD, Leem TH, et al. Occult nodal disease in patients with failed laryngeal preservation undergoing surgical salvage. Laryngoscope 2014;124:421–8.
125. Stevens KR Jr, Britsch A, Moss WT. High-dose reirradiation of head and neck cancer with curative intent. Int J Radiat Oncol Biol Phys 1994;29:687–98.
126. Dawson LA, Myers LL, Bradford CR, et al. Conformal re-irradiation of recurrent and new primary head-and-neck cancer. Int J Radiat Oncol Biol Phys 2001;50:377–85.
127. Goldstein DP, Karnell LH, Yao M, et al. Outcomes following reirradiation of patients with head and neck cancer. Head Neck 2008;30:765–70.
128. Spencer SA, Harris J, Wheeler RH, et al. Final report of RTOG 9610, a multiinstitutional trial of reirradiation and chemotherapy for unresectable recurrent squamous cell carcinoma of the head and neck. Head Neck 2008;30:281–8.
129. Langer CJ, Harris J, Horwitz EM, et al. Phase II study of low-dose paclitaxel and cisplatin in combination with split-course concomitant twice-daily reirradiation in recurrent squamous cell carcinoma of the head and neck: results of Radiation Therapy Oncology Group Protocol 9911. J Clin Oncol 2007;25:4800–5.
130. Smee RI, Meagher NS, Williams JR, et al. Role of radiotherapy in early glottic carcinoma. Head Neck 2010;32:850–9.
131. Garcia-Serra A, Hinerman RW, Amdur RJ, et al. Radiotherapy for carcinoma in situ of the true vocal cords. Head Neck 2002;24:390–4.
132. Spayne JA, Warde P, O'Sullivan B, et al. Carcinoma-in-situ of the glottic larynx: results of treatment with radiation therapy. Int J Radiat Oncol Biol Phys 2001;49:1235–8.
133. Roedel RM, Christiansen H, Mueller RM, et al. Transoral laser microsurgery for carcinoma in situ of the glottic larynx. A retrospective follow-up study. ORL J Otorhinolaryngol Relat Spec 2009;71:45–9.
134. Damm M, Sittel C, Streppel M, et al. Transoral CO2 laser for surgical management of glottic carcinoma in situ. Laryngoscope 2000;110:1215–21.
135. Sjogren EV, Langeveld TP, Baatenburg de Jong RJ. Clinical outcome of T1 glottic carcinoma since the introduction of endoscopic CO2 laser surgery as treatment option. Head Neck 2008;30:1167–74.
136. Franchin G, Minatel E, Gobitti C, et al. Radiotherapy for patients with early-stage glottic carcinoma: univariate and multivariate analyses in a group of consecutive, unselected patients. Cancer 2003;98:765–72.
137. Frata P, Cellai E, Magrini SM, et al. Radical radiotherapy for early glottic cancer: results in a series of 1087 patients from two Italian radiation oncology centers. II. The case of T2N0 disease. Int J Radiat Oncol Biol Phys 2005;63:1387–94.
138. Garden AS, Forster K, Wong PF, et al. Results of radiotherapy for T2N0 glottic carcinoma: does the "2" stand for twice-daily treatment? Int J Radiat Oncol Biol Phys 2003;55:322–8.
139. Mendenhall WM, Parsons JT, Mancuso AA, et al. Definitive radiotherapy for T3 squamous cell carcinoma of the glottic larynx. J Clin Oncol 1997;15:2394–402.
140. Johansen LV, Grau C, Overgaard J. Glottic carcinoma–patterns of failure and salvage treatment after curative radiotherapy in 861 consecutive patients. Radiother Oncol 2002;63:257–67.

141. Canis M, Martin A, Ihler F, et al. Transoral laser microsurgery in treatment of pT2 and pT3 glottic laryngeal squamous cell carcinoma - results of 391 patients. Head Neck 2014;36:859–66.

142. Vilaseca I, Bernal-Sprekelsen M, Luis Blanch J. Transoral laser microsurgery for T3 laryngeal tumors: prognostic factors. Head Neck 2010;32:929–38.

143. Johansen LV, Grau C, Overgaard J. Supraglottic carcinoma: patterns of failure and salvage treatment after curatively intended radiotherapy in 410 consecutive patients. Int J Radiat Oncol Biol Phys 2002;53:948–58.

144. Grant DG, Salassa JR, Hinni ML, et al. Transoral laser microsurgery for carcinoma of the supraglottic larynx. Otolaryngol Head Neck Surg 2007;136:900–6.

145. Iro H, Waldfahrer F, Altendorf-Hofmann A, et al. Transoral laser surgery of supraglottic cancer: follow-up of 141 patients. Arch Otolaryngol Head Neck Surg 1998;124:1245–50.

146. Zeitels SM, Koufman JA, Davis RK, et al. Endoscopic treatment of supraglottic and hypopharynx cancer. Laryngoscope 1994;104:71–8.

Nasopharyngeal Carcinoma

Sophia C. Kamran, MD[a], Nadeem Riaz, MD[b], Nancy Lee, MD[b],*

KEYWORDS

- Head and neck cancer • Epstein-Barr virus • Nasopharyngeal carcinoma
- EBV molecular biology

KEY POINTS

- Nasopharyngeal carcinoma (NPC) is uncommon in the United States, with only 0.2 to 0.5 cases per 100,000 people; this is in contrast to southern China and Hong Kong, where the incidence is 25 to 50 per 100,000 people.
- There is a potential link between Epstein-Barr virus (EBV) and the development of NPC.
- Radiotherapy alone as a single modality leads to similar 10-year survival rates in the United States, Denmark, and Hong Kong (34%, 37%, and 43%, respectively). Multiple studies have shown an advantage to concurrent chemoradiation in the treatment of advanced disease.
- Radiation therapy remains the mainstay of salvage therapy, and modern techniques have allowed clinicians to achieve adequate local control without excessive toxicity.

INTRODUCTION
Epidemiology

Nasopharyngeal is an uncommon disease in the United States. The incidence is approximately 0.2 to 0.5 cases per 100,000 people.[1] In Southeast Asia, North Africa, and parts of the Mediterranean basin, however, approximately 80 cases per 100,000 of the population are reported.[2] Among the Inuit who reside in Alaska and Greenland, the incidence is also high (15 to 20 cases per 100,000 people). Several etiologic factors have been implicated. Dr John Ho's observations in the 1970s on boat people in southern China with a high incidence of NPC led him in the search and identification of salted fish as a carcinogen.[3] Cantonese salted fish is now identified as a group 1 human carcinogen according to the International Agency for Research on Cancer (http://monographs.iarc.fr/ENG/Monographs/vol100E/mono100E-12.pdf). Other etiologic risk factors include alcohol consumption, cigarette smoking, and exposure to

The authors have nothing to disclose.
[a] Harvard Radiation Oncology Program, Brigham and Women's Hospital, 75 Francis Street, Boston, MA 02115, USA; [b] Department of Radiation Oncology, Memorial Sloan Kettering Cancer Center, 1275 York Avenue, New York, NY 10065, USA
* Corresponding author.
E-mail address: leen2@mskcc.org

Surg Oncol Clin N Am 24 (2015) 547–561
http://dx.doi.org/10.1016/j.soc.2015.03.008

dust, fumes, and formaldehyde.[4,5] The role of alcohol and cigarette smoking has been controversial, because prior studies have suggested no association.[6–8] A case-control study conducted in 1992, however, showed that both cigarette smoking and alcohol consumption were risk factors for NPC. NPC risk was increased 3-fold with heavy smoking (adjusted for alcohol consumption), and an excess risk of 80% was demonstrated for heavy alcohol consumption (adjusted for cigarette usage).[5] The possibility that environmental factors are important in the pathogenesis of NPC is supported by the finding that incidence rates decrease for successive generations of people who emigrated from southern China to California.[8] Socioeconomic development in Hong Kong, along with dramatic lifestyle changes (including the marked decrease in consumption of salted fish and tobacco), as well as increased consumption of fresh vegetables, has led to a to a decrease in the age-standardized incidence rate of NPC in Hong Kong by more than 50% over 30 years.[3]

In endemic areas, EBV has been tightly associated with the development of NPC. EBV infection is found in 90% to 100% of NPC cases in endemic regions.[9] EBV is typically associated with mononucleosis or malignancies, such as Burkitt lymphoma and Hodgkin disease, in Western countries whereas in Asia it is closely linked to NPC. This association was described more than 30 years ago. Molecular biology advances have furthered understanding of the association. EBV infection is ubiquitous; this and other evidence suggests that that NPC has a multifactorial etiology.

Pathology

The tumor arises from epithelial cells on the surface of the nasopharynx. There are 3 different histologic subtypes according to the World Health Organization (WHO): keratinizing squamous cell carcinoma (WHO type I), nonkeratinizing differentiated carcinoma (WHO type II), and nonkeratinizing undifferentiated carcinoma (WHO type III). Nonkeratinized undifferentiated carcinoma comprise 90% to 95% of cases in endemic regions, such as southern China. EBV is more tightly associated with NPC in endemic regions. In contrast, keratinizing squamous cell carcinomas are most commonly found in Western countries. EBV DNA is detected less frequently in patients with keratinizing squamous cell carcinomas. The prognosis for keratinizing squamous cell carcinomas has been poorer as compared to nonkeratinizing histologic subtypes. However, a recent study of 2436 new cases in the United States demonstrated that Chinese keratinizing squamous cell carcinoma NPC patients had statistically improved survival as compared to keratinizing squamous cell carcinoma NPC patients from other ethnicities, suggesting that ethnicity plays a role in NPC pathogenesis.[10]

Molecular Biology

The causal link between EBV and the development of NPC remains to be elucidated, despite advances in molecular biology confirming the association. EBV-encoded proteins are expressed from the EBV genome on entry into host cells, such as latent membrane proteins (LMPs) 1, 2A, and 2B; 6 EBV nuclear antigens (EBNAs) 1, 2, 3A to C, and LP; and 2 small noncoding nuclear RNAs (EBERs).[11–13] EBV has been shown to immortalize and transform B cells into lymphoblastoid cells. Infection of epithelial cells by EBV is inefficient, however, and how EBV infects epithelium and transforms the cells is unknown. Perhaps EBV infection of the nasopharyngeal epithelium is an early event, with further processes leading to malignant transformation. Recent studies have suggested that a transcription factor, signal transducer and activator of transcription 3 (STAT3), may be the mechanism for NPC pathogenesis. STAT3 overexpression has been demonstrated in greater than 75% of NPCs in endemic regions.[14,15] EBV infection can induce the activation of STAT3, a well-characterized oncogenic transcription factor.[14,16,17]

EBV DNA levels in pretreatment and postradiotherapy plasma samples from patients in Hong Kong correlated with outcome,[18] which could be useful in risk stratification and therapeutic interventions.

High levels of EBNA-1 DNA after treatment of NPC in plasma predicted a high risk of distant metastases and low risk of survival. The DNA was measured by real-time polymerase chain reaction (qPCR) techniques. The median follow-up time during this study was 30 months, suggesting a promising biomarker to predict those patients at risk for metastasis or even relapse and potentially allowing high-risk patients to receive more intensive treatment.[18]

Recently, mutational analysis of NPC using single nucleotide polymorphism arrays revealed 9 significantly mutated genes, many of which were novel. Several cellular processes and pathways were involved, including chromatin modifications, autophagy, and ERBB-PI3K signaling. This study identified new pathways and genes that are novel and potential targets for drug treatment (druggable). The work affords new insights into the pathogenesis of NPC.[19]

PATIENT EVALUATION OVERVIEW
Prevention and Detection

Nasopharynx cancer often is not detected until a tumor has grown large enough to invade a critical structure. The association of EBV and NPC might play a role in screening for tumors. A study from China of 338,868 patients who underwent serologic screening for EBV titer revealed that of nearly 10,000 patients who had antibodies to EBV, NPC was detected in 113 (approximately 1.2%). Most (>85%) were early-stage cancers.[20]

qPCR techniques may be helpful in detecting early nasopharyngeal cancer. Screening for LMP1 in nasopharyngeal swabs was shown to be a promising screening tool in high-risk populations, with a sensitivity of 87% and a specificity of 98%.[21] Technological advances and other genetic or environmental markers proving useful in the detection of early NPC may lead to the identification of populations benefitting from rigorous screening or chemoprevention.

Clinical Manifestations

Nasopharyngeal cancer is rare in the Western countries and therefore seldom suspected when patients present with early symptoms. In a Texas series analyzing 378 patients,[22] presenting symptoms included a neck mass in 41%; ear complaints (including hearing loss and drainage) in 27%; nasal bleeding/obstruction in 21%; cranial nerve deficits in 8%; and other nonspecific symptoms in 8%. Level VA lymph nodes were most commonly enlarged (54% of patients), followed by the level II nodes (49% of patients). The level III and lower-level VA/upper-level VB groups were involved in 24% and 22% of patients, respectively. Level IV, lower-level VB, and supraclavicular lymph nodes were less commonly involved (approximately 10%–13%). Cranial nerve VI was the nerve most frequently affected.

Detection/Patient Evaluation

All patients who have a diagnosis of NPC must undergo a history and physical examination. Documentation of the clinically involved lymph nodes in the neck is helpful, especially when a radiotherapy boost is considered. All patients should have nasopharyngoscopy to determine involvement of mucosal surfaces. This is also useful for a biopsy of the primary lesion.

CT and MRI of the head and neck are valuable in the evaluation of the tumor and associated lymphadenopathy. MRI may be more useful in delineating soft tissue invasion outside the nasopharynx, which is required for T staging, and extent of retropharyngeal lymph node involvement[23]; hence, MRI is necessary for evaluating nasopharyngeal tumors. MRI is also superior to CT for assessing clival involvement and perineural invasion. Positron emission tomography (PET)/CT evaluation for distant metastases completes the staging/work-up. It may be useful after treatment, when persistent anatomic changes limits the ability of other modalities to detect local recurrence.

Blood tests as well as a preradiation therapy dental assessment and audiology evaluation should be undertaken.

Staging

Clinical staging has been a matter of controversy. The most common staging systems used in North America and Europe include those of the American Joint Committee on Cancer (AJCC)[24,25] and the International Union Against Cancer (Union Internationale Contre le Cancer [UICC]).[26] In Asia, the Ho classification system, developed in Hong Kong, is widely used.[27] In China, specifically, physicians adopted an independent classification, similar to the Ho system (**Table 1**).[28] The AJCC/UICC staging is most commonly used in the English literature.

The Ho system uses lymph node location in N-stage assignment, and it allows a more even distribution of nodal disease in stage grouping. It takes into account supraclavicular nodal involvement, which carries a worse prognosis, assigning it stage IV. Modifications have been implemented in the AJCC system to incorporate lymph node location in N-category assignment, include involvement of the supraclavicular nodes, and provide a more even stage distribution.[25]

T1 and T2 lesions are segregated by invasion into the soft tissues. Parapharyngeal soft tissue involvement carries prognostic value; hence the updated edition of the AJCC system now groups lesions with parapharyngeal involvement into T2, whereas all other soft tissue involvement falls into T1.[31–33] Cranial nerve involvement has a worse prognosis than base-of-skull involvement[29,34–37]; hence, the most recent edition of the AJCC has reclassified base-of-skull involvement to T3.

The current AJCC edition considers disease that has spread to the retropharyngeal lymph nodes as N1. These nodes are involved in 83% of patients with NPC compared with 74% involvement of the level II or IV nodes.[38]

Improved imaging modalities have allowed for precise evaluation of tumor invasion and lymph node involvement, permitting more accurate staging.

PRIMARY THERAPY
Single Modality Therapy

The nasopharynx has not been easy to approach surgically due to the complicated anatomy. Primary surgical intervention fell out of favor in the 1950s, and most treatment consists of concurrent chemoradiation.

Radiation alone has been previously shown to have 10-year survival rates of 34%, 37%, and 43%, from studies from the United States, Denmark, and Hong Kong, respectively.[22,39,40] The Hong Kong trial has the highest 10-year survival rate, although this series had many patients with early-stage disease (node-negative in 39%) and few patients with the poor-prognosis keratinizing histology (0.3%). The United States and European groups had a higher percentage of patients with keratinizing histology.

In the study out of the United States, researchers found that advanced T stage, squamous cell histology, and cranial nerve deficits predict poor prognosis using radiation alone.[22] Good tumor control can be achieved through radiation alone with earlystage lesions, but combined modality treatments, such as chemoradiation, are necessary for advanced cancers. Significant improvements in the treatment of advanced stage disease were made with combined chemoradiation and evolving radiotherapy techniques, however the use of intensity-modulated radiation therapy (IMRT) has allowed for higher doses of radiation to the tumor as well as reduced significant radiation-associated toxicities, thus making IMRT the radiation modality of choice in both early stage and advanced stage lesions.[41,42]

COMBINATION THERAPIES
Radiation Plus Chemotherapy

Several groups have conducted phase III trials specific to nasopharyngeal primary tumors comparing chemotherapy plus radiation to radiation alone (**Table 2**).

Intergroup study 0099 showed a dramatic improvement in survival rates with combined modality treatment.[43] Patients were randomized to receive either chemoradiotherapy or radiotherapy alone. Patients received standard radiation to 70 Gy to the gross disease in daily fractions of 1.8 to 2 Gy. The addition of chemotherapy was 100 mg/m^2 of cisplatin on days 1, 22, and 43 of radiation, and cisplatin (80 mg/m^2) and 5-fluorouracil (5-FU) (1000 mg/m^2) every 3 weeks for 3 cycles after radiation ended. As shown in **Table 3**, there was a statistically significant improvement in both disease-free survival (DFS) and overall survival (OS) in the combined modality arm; the 5-year OS for patients with the keratinizing squamous cell carcinoma histologic type (WHO type I) was 37%; the differentiated nonkeratinizing histologic type (WHO type II), 55%; and the undifferentiated nonkeratinizing histologic type (WHO type III), 60%. The trial was criticized on several grounds. It was a US-based study and performed in a nonendemic population. Studies in Chinese patients[57] have demonstrated either severe toxicities or high rates of distant metastases outside of the radiated field.[58] Other analyses have suggested that the radiotherapy-only group did poorly as a result of radiation techniques.[59] Nevertheless, the results of this trial changed the standard of care for nasopharynx cancers. Indeed, the dramatic improvement in outcomes with combined modality therapy has limited the use of single modality radiation to patients with T1 disease.

Trials conducted in endemic areas, including Taiwan, Hong Kong, and Singapore, confirmed the advantage of a cisplatin-based chemoradiation plan.[46–48] A meta-analysis of 7 endemic-region phase III trials of concurrent chemoradiation versus radiotherapy alone, including 1608 patients, demonstrated an OS advantage of the concurrent regimen, with a relative risk of 0.74 at 5 years.[60] This survival advantage is less than that seen in trials from nonendemic regions.

LOCAL RECURRENCE/RESISTANCE
Surgery

Recurrent or resistant lymph node disease in NPC is often resected with neck dissection. Primary site recurrence, however, generates the same difficulties frustrating surgery as does initial treatment. The choice of a salvage surgical approach depends on the size and location of the recurrent cancer. Recent series suggest locoregional control and OS of 40% to 72% and 30% to 54%, respectively, when addressing recurrence.[61–64]

Radiation

Reirradiation is a cornerstone of treatment of recurrent nasopharyngeal cancer. Earlier stage at recurrence and longer time to recurrence are associated with improved

Table 1
A comparison of staging systems

Classification	American Joint Committee on Cancer[24]	2002/1997 American Joint Committee on Cancer[29,30]	Ho[27]	2008 Chinese[28]
T1	Confined to nasopharynx, or extends to oropharynx and/or nasal cavity	Confined to nasopharynx	Confined to nasopharynx	Confined to nasopharynx
T2	With parapharyngeal extension	Soft tissue invasion a. Without parapharyngeal extension b. With parapharyngeal extension	Nasal fossa, oropharynx, muscle, or nerves below base of skull	Nasal cavity, oropharynx, parapharyngeal extension
T3	Bony or paranasal sinus extension	Bony or paranasal sinus extension	a. Bone involvement below base of skull b. Involves base of skull c. Cranial nerves d. Orbits, laryngopharynx, or infratemporal fossa[a]	Skull base or medial pterygoid extension
T4	Intracranial extension, or cranial nerve or infratemporal fossa,[a] hypopharynx, or orbital involvement	Intracranial extension, or cranial nerve or infratemporal fossa,[a] hypopharynx, or orbital involvement	—	Cranial nerves, paranasal sinuses, masticator space[a] (excluding medial pterygoid muscles), intracranial (cavernous sinus, dural meninges) extension
N1	Unilateral, ≤6 cm and/or unilateral or bilateral retropharyngeal ≤6 cm	Unilateral, ≤6 cm	Upper neck above thyroid notch	a. Retropharyngeal b. Unilateral level Ib, II, III, and Va or ≤3 cm

N2	Bilateral, ≤6 cm	Bilateral, ≤6 cm	Below thyroid notch above line joining end of clavicle and superior margin of trapezius muscle	Bilateral level Ib, II, III, and Va or >3 cm or with extranodal spread
N3	a. >6 cm node b. Supraclavicular involvement	a. >6 cm node b. Supraclavicular involvement	Supraclavicular fossa[b] or skin involvement	Level IV or Vb involvement
M1	—	Metastases	Metastases	Metastases
Stage I	T1N0M0	T1N0M0	T1N0	T1N0M0
Stage II	T1N1 T2N0 T2N1	a. T2aN0M0 b. T1-2aN1M0 or T2bN0M0	T2 and/or N1	T1N1a-1bM0 or T2N0-1bM0
Stage III	T1N2M0 T2N2M0 T3N0-2M0	T1-2bN2M0 T3N0-2M0	T3 and/or N2	T1-2N2M0 or T3N0-2M0
Stage IV	a. T4N0-2M0 b. Any TN3M0 c. Any T any NM1	a. T4N0-2M0 b. Any TN3M0 c. Any T any NM1	N3 (any T)	a. T1-3N3M0 or T4N0-3M0 b. Any T any NM1
Stage V	—	—	M1	—

[a] Masticator space is defined as infratemporal fossa.
[b] Supraclavicular fossa as described by Ho is a triangular space defined by 3 points: (1) the superior margin of the sternal end of the clavicle, (2) the superior margin of the lateral end of the clavicle, and (3) the point where the neck meets the shoulder. This includes the caudal portion of levels IV and Vb lymph nodes.

Table 2
A comparison of the major concurrent chemoradiotherapy randomized trials

Study	No. Patients	Stage	Randomization	Disease-free Survival (%), 5 y	P Value	Overall Survival (%), 5 y	P Value
Intergroup study 0099,[43] 1998	150	AJCC 1992 stage III: T3N0; T1-3N1M0 AJCC 1992 stage IV: T4N0-1; any TN2-3M0	70 Gy/7-8 wk 70 Gy/7-8 wk with cisplatin, followed by 3 cycles of cisplatin/5-FU	29 58	<.001	37 67	.005
Chan et al,[44] 2002; Chan et al,[45] 2005	350	Ho system N2-3 or any nodes ≥4 cm	66 Gy/6.5 wk ± 10-20 Gy boost 66 Gy/6.5 wk ± 10-20 Gy boost with cisplatin	52 60	NS	59 70	.065
Lin et al,[46] 2003	284	AJCC 1992: III-IV (M0)	70-74 Gy/6-7 wk 70-74 Gy/6-7 wk with infusional cisplatin/ 5-FU × 2	53 72	.0012	54 72	.0022
Wee et al,[47] 2005	221	AJCC 1997: stage III or IV; WHO type 2 or 3	70 Gy/7 wk 70 Gy/7 wk with infusional cisplatin, followed by 3 cycles of cisplatin/5-FU	53 (3 y) 72 (3 y)	.01	65 (3 y) 80 (3 y)	.01
Lee et al,[48] 2005	348	AJCC 1997: T1-4N2-3M0; WHO type 2 or 3	>66 Gy/7-8 wk >66 Gy/7-8 wk with cisplatin, followed by 3 cycles of cisplatin/5-FU	62 72	.027	78 78	.97

Abbreviation: NS, not significant.

Table 3
Nasopharyngeal carcinoma reirradiation studies

Study	No. Patients	T3/T4 (%)	Median Follow-up (mo)	5-y Local Control (%)	5-y Overall Survival (%)	Major Complications (%)	Patients Retreated with Chemotherapy (%)
Conventional or 3-D Conformal EBRT Techniques Alone or in Combination with Radiosurgery or Brachytherapy							
Lee et al,[49] 1997	654	48[a]	17	23	16	26	Unknown
Chua et al,[50] 1998	97	70	18	—	36	34 (neurologic)	18
Hwang et al,[51] 1998	74	66[a]	20	—	37	33	30
Teo et al,[52] 1998	103	56	20	15	8	20 (neurologic)	16
Leung et al,[53] 2000	91	44	27–55	38	30	57	19
IMRT Alone or in Combination with Radiosurgery or Brachytherapy							
Lu et al,[54] 2004	49	73	9	100 (9 mo)	—	N/A	6
Chua et al,[55] 2005	31	74	11	65 (1 y)	63	70, Grade ≥3	68
Koutcher et al,[56] 2010	29	48	45	52	69	31, Grade ≥3	93

Abbreviation: N/A, not applicable.
[a] Eighty-three percent of the patients were treated with IMRT.

outcomes.[49,52,65] Higher doses are also more effective, which can be accomplished with intensity-modulated radiation therapy (IMRT). After radiation therapy for the primary tumor, however, it can be difficult to distinguish true recurrence from postradiation effects. Biopsy is considered the gold standard. The interval between primary treatment and retreatment of persistence remains a controversial topic. Some investigators advocate early treatment to prevent further progression, whereas others recommend waiting at least 10 weeks because late histologic regressions may continue. In a study[66] of 803 patients, serial post-treatment biopsies were performed to examine the histology. After treatment, 77% of biopsies were negative whereas 23% remained positive. Of the 23% positive biopsies, 4% normalized within 5 weeks, and 12% did so between weeks 5 and 10. Thus, 70% (12% + 4% = 16%/23% = 70%) of post-treatment positive biopsies converted to normal within 12 weeks. No additional treatment was given at the time.

Brachytherapy has been used to treat nasopharyngeal cancer recurrence since the 1920s. Intracavitary brachytherapy is an excellent modality for patients with recurrent tumors confined to the mucosal or submucosal nasopharynx. Stereotactic radiation is a promising approach as well and can be used in combination with external beam radiation therapy (EBRT). It is typically reserved for smaller lesions, and studies have shown that it can provide good control with an improved toxicity profile.[61] EBRT and IMRT allow for higher doses ($\geq$60 Gy) with decreased toxicity. In a New York series, 29 patients were treated with radiation for recurrence between 1996 and 2008: 16 received EBRT alone and 13 received EBRT to 45 Gy followed by intracavitary brachytherapy to 20 Gy; 24 patients were treated with IMRT; and 93% of patients received chemotherapy. Five-year local control and OS rates were 52% and 60%, respectively. There was no significant difference between the combined brachytherapy/EBRT and EBRT groups but the combined radiation therapy approach resulted in fewer late complications.[56] A Hong Kong study reported on 103 patients treated with EBRT reirradiation techniques. With a median follow-up time of 20 months, the 5-year local control and OS rates were 15% and 8%, respectively. Major complications occurred in 20% of patients; these were mainly neurologic.[52] Unfortunately, residual or recurrent disease is most common in regions where sophisticated techniques are not available; hence, these treatment options may not be available to most patients. **Table 3** compares studies using the different modalities.

Chemotherapy

Chemotherapy for locally recurrent or resistant disease is typically reserved for lesions that cannot be easily treated with surgery or radiation alone. NPC is sensitive to cisplatin regimens, and response rate in patients with recurrent disease is 50% to 80%.[67–69] The combination of chemoradiation is thought superior to chemotherapy alone, similar to the initial treatment of the disease, and many salvage irradiation studies have included cisplatin-based chemotherapy.

EVALUATION OF OUTCOME AND LONG-TERM RECOMMENDATIONS

Patients typically should be followed closely after treatment of NPC with CT and/or PET. PET has been shown to be useful in patients treated with radiation. Xie and coworkers[70] studied the association of maximal standardized uptake value (SUVmax) on fludeoxyglucose F 18–PET/CT and the outcome of 62 patients treated with radiation. Patients with a lower SUVmax (<8) of tumor had a higher 5-year OS and DFS than those with a higher SUVmax. In a separate study examining 75 patients submitted to radiation therapy, Liu and coworkers[71] found that patients with a lower SUVmax ($\leq$5) had a better 5-year local failure-free survival and DFS than those with a higher SUV-max (>5).

The rate of distant metastasis remains high in NPC. Hence, the advent of EBV as a potential biomarker for treatment response is promising. EBV-specific antibodies are increased in sera of most NPC patients.[72] Genomic DNA of EBV is elevated in peripheral blood and body fluids of NPC patients. In a Thai study, serum/plasma EBV DNA disappeared in 92% of patients (12/13) during early treatment, and EBV DNA could not be detected in 100% of patients (32/32) who achieved complete remission. EBV DNA was detectable in 60% of cases (3/5) with recurrence or partial response.[73] In the recent prospective study by Lin & coworkers, EBV DNA proved a useful biomarker to predict relapse and metastatic disease. OS and relapse-free survival was significantly lower among patients with elevated EBV DNA prior to treatment (>1500 copies/mL compared with <1000 copies/mL). The elevation of plasma EBV DNA in patients with relapse occurred 6 months before clinical detection of relapse in 8 of 16 patients.[18]

SUMMARY

Nasopharyngeal cancer is a complex disease, but progress has been achieved through breakthroughs in molecular biology and radiation treatment. Surgery has fallen out of favor as a primary therapy. Early-stage disease can respond to radiation with good local control. For stage greater than or equal to T2, or greater than or equal to N1 disease, concurrent chemoradiation is preferred. Development of better therapeutic (as opposed to radiosensitizing) chemotherapy is important in treating nasopharyngeal cancer, because many patients still have a high rate of distant metastasis. Novel techniques, such as the use of post-treatment circulating EBV DNA or EBV-associated antigens for treatment planning, may help clinicians identify patients who would benefit most from more intensive treatments. Investigations to identify and screen high-risk patients using molecular techniques may also help detect nasopharyngeal cancer at an earlier stage.

REFERENCES

1. Yu MC. Nasopharyngeal carcinoma: epidemiology and dietary factors. IARC Sci Publ 1991;39–47.
2. Caponigro F, Longo F, Ionna F, et al. Treatment approaches to nasopharyngeal carcinoma: a review. Anticancer Drugs 2010;21(5):471–7.
3. Lee AW, Ng WT, Chan YH, et al. The battle against nasopharyngeal cancer. Radiother Oncol 2012;104(3):272–8.
4. Henderson BE, Louie E, SooHoo Jing J, et al. Risk factors associated with nasopharyngeal carcinoma. N Engl J Med 1976;295(20):1101–6.
5. Nam JM, McLaughlin JK, Blot WJ. Cigarette smoking, alcohol, and nasopharyngeal carcinoma: a case-control study among U.S. whites. J Natl Cancer Inst 1992;84(8):619–22.
6. Henle G, Henle W. Epstein-barr virus-specific IgA serum antibodies as an outstanding feature of nasopharyngeal carcinoma. Int J Cancer 1976;17(1):1–7.
7. Neel HB 3rd, Pearson GR, Taylor WF. Antibodies to epstein-barr virus in patients with nasopharyngeal carcinoma and in comparison groups. Ann Otol Rhinol Laryngol 1984;93(5 Pt 1):477–82.
8. Buell P. The effect of migration on the risk of nasopharyngeal cancer among chinese. Cancer Res 1974;34(5):1189–91.
9. Ho Y, Tsao SW, Zeng M, et al. STAT3 as a therapeutic target for epstein-barr virus (EBV): associated nasopharyngeal carcinoma. Cancer Lett 2013;330(2):141–9.

10. Ou SH, Zell JA, Ziogas A, et al. Epidemiology of nasopharyngeal carcinoma in the united states: improved survival of chinese patients within the keratinizing squamous cell carcinoma histology. Ann Oncol 2007;18(1):29–35.
11. Raab-Traub N. Epstein-barr virus in the pathogenesis of NPC. Semin Cancer Biol 2002;12(6):431–41.
12. Thompson MP, Kurzrock R. Epstein-barr virus and cancer. Clin Cancer Res 2004; 10(3):803–21.
13. Young LS, Murray PG. Epstein-barr virus and oncogenesis: from latent genes to tumours. Oncogene 2003;22(33):5108–21.
14. Lo AK, Lo KW, Tsao SW, et al. Epstein-barr virus infection alters cellular signal cascades in human nasopharyngeal epithelial cells. Neoplasia 2006;8(3): 173–80.
15. Liu YP, Tan YN, Wang ZL, et al. Phosphorylation and nuclear translocation of STAT3 regulated by the epstein-barr virus latent membrane protein 1 in nasopharyngeal carcinoma. Int J Mol Med 2008;21(2):153–62.
16. Lui VW, Wong EY, Ho Y, et al. STAT3 activation contributes directly to epstein-barr virus-mediated invasiveness of nasopharyngeal cancer cells in vitro. Int J Cancer 2009;125(8):1884–93.
17. Lui VW, Yau DM, Wong EY, et al. Cucurbitacin I elicits anoikis sensitization, inhibits cellular invasion and in vivo tumor formation ability of nasopharyngeal carcinoma cells. Carcinogenesis 2009;30(12):2085–94.
18. Lin JC, Wang WY, Chen KY, et al. Quantification of plasma epstein-barr virus DNA in patients with advanced nasopharyngeal carcinoma. N Engl J Med 2004; 350(24):2461–70.
19. Lin DC, Meng X, Hazawa M, et al. The genomic landscape of nasopharyngeal carcinoma. Nat Genet 2014;46(8):866–71.
20. Deng H, Zeng Y, Lei Y, et al. Serological survey of nasopharyngeal carcinoma in 21 cities of south china. Chin Med J (Engl) 1995;108(4):300–3.
21. Hao SP, Tsang NM, Chang KP. Screening nasopharyngeal carcinoma by detection of the latent membrane protein 1 (LMP-1) gene with nasopharyngeal swabs. Cancer 2003;97(8):1909–13.
22. Sanguineti G, Geara FB, Garden AS, et al. Carcinoma of the nasopharynx treated by radiotherapy alone: determinants of local and regional control. Int J Radiat Oncol Biol Phys 1997;37(5):985–96.
23. Poon PY, Tsang VH, Munk PL. Tumour extent and T stage of nasopharyngeal carcinoma: a comparison of magnetic resonance imaging and computed tomographic findings. Can Assoc Radiol J 2000;51(5):287–95 [quiz: 286].
24. Edge SB, Byrd DR, Compton CC, et al, editors. AJCC Cancer Staging Manual. 7th edition. New York (NY): Springer; 2010. p. 41–56.
25. Beahrs OH, Henson DE, Hutter RVP, et al, editors. Manual for Staging of Cancer. 4th edition. Philadelphia: J.B.Lippincott; 1992. p. 33–8.
26. Pharynx. In: Union internationale contre le cancer: TNM atlas. 2nd edition. Berlin: Springer-Verlag; 1992.
27. Teo PM, Leung SF, Yu P, et al. A comparison of Ho's, International Union Against Cancer, and American Joint Committee Stage Classifications for Nasopharyngeal Carcinoma. Cancer 1991;67(2):434–9.
28. Committee of Chinese Clinical Staging of Nasopharyngeal Carcinoma. Report on the revision of nasopharyngeal carcinoma '92 staging. Chinese Journal of Radiation Oncology 2009;18:2–6.
29. Huang SC. Nasopharyngeal cancer: a review of 1605 patients treated radically with cobalt 60. Int J Radiat Oncol Biol Phys 1980;6(4):401–7.

30. Greene FL, Page DL, Fleming ID, et al. Pharynx. In: AJCC cancer staging manual. 6th edition. New York: Springer-Verlag; 2002.
31. Xiao GL, Gao L, Xu GZ. Prognostic influence of parapharyngeal space involvement in nasopharyngeal carcinoma. Int J Radiat Oncol Biol Phys 2002;52(4):957–63.
32. Mao YP, Xie FY, Liu LZ, et al. Re-evaluation of 6th edition of AJCC staging system for nasopharyngeal carcinoma and proposed improvement based on magnetic resonance imaging. Int J Radiat Oncol Biol Phys 2009;73(5):1326–34.
33. Ho HC, Lee MS, Hsiao SH, et al. Prognostic influence of parapharyngeal extension in nasopharyngeal carcinoma. Acta Otolaryngol 2008;128(7):790–8.
34. Sham JS, Cheung YK, Choy D, et al. Cranial nerve involvement and base of the skull erosion in nasopharyngeal carcinoma. Cancer 1991;68(2):422–6.
35. Perez CA, Devineni VR, Marcial-Vega V, et al. Carcinoma of the nasopharynx: factors affecting prognosis. Int J Radiat Oncol Biol Phys 1992;23(2):271–80.
36. Teo P, Shiu W, Leung SF, et al. Prognostic factors in nasopharyngeal carcinoma investigated by computer tomography–an analysis of 659 patients. Radiother Oncol 1992;23(2):79–93.
37. Roh JL, Sung MW, Kim KH, et al. Nasopharyngeal carcinoma with skull base invasion: a necessity of staging subdivision. Am J Otolaryngol 2004;25(1):26–32.
38. King AD, Ahuja AT, Leung SF, et al. Neck node metastases from nasopharyngeal carcinoma: MR imaging of patterns of disease. Head Neck 2000;22(3):275–81.
39. Johansen LV, Mestre M, Overgaard J. Carcinoma of the nasopharynx: analysis of treatment results in 167 consecutively admitted patients. Head Neck 1992;14(3):200–7.
40. Lee AW, Poon YF, Foo W, et al. Retrospective analysis of 5037 patients with nasopharyngeal carcinoma treated during 1976-1985: overall survival and patterns of failure. Int J Radiat Oncol Biol Phys 1992;23(2):261–70.
41. Lee N, Xia P, Quivey JM, et al. Intensity-modulated radiotherapy in the treatment of nasopharyngeal carcinoma: an update of the UCSF experience. Int J Radiat Oncol Biol Phys 2002;53:12–22.
42. Pow EH, Kwong DL, McMillan AS, et al. Xerostomia and quality of life after intensity-modulated radiotherapy vs. conventional radiotherapy for early-stage nasopharyngeal carcinoma: initial report on a randomized controlled clinical trial. Int J Radiat Oncol Biol Phys 2006;66:981–91.
43. Al-Sarraf M, LeBlanc M, Giri PG, et al. Chemoradiotherapy versus radiotherapy in patients with advanced nasopharyngeal cancer: phase III randomized intergroup study 0099. J Clin Oncol 1998;16(4):1310–7.
44. Chan AT, Teo PM, Ngan RK, et al. Concurrent chemotherapy-radiotherapy compared with radiotherapy alone in locoregionally advanced nasopharyngeal carcinoma: progression-free survival analysis of a phase III randomized trial. J Clin Oncol 2002;20(8):2038–44.
45. Chan AT, Leung SF, Ngan RK, et al. Overall survival after concurrent cisplatin-radiotherapy compared with radiotherapy alone in locoregionally advanced nasopharyngeal carcinoma. J Natl Cancer Inst 2005;97(7):536–9.
46. Lin JC, Jan JS, Hsu CY, et al. Phase III study of concurrent chemoradiotherapy versus radiotherapy alone for advanced nasopharyngeal carcinoma: positive effect on overall and progression-free survival. J Clin Oncol 2003;21(4):631–7.
47. Wee J, Tan EH, Tai BC, et al. Randomized trial of radiotherapy versus concurrent chemoradiotherapy followed by adjuvant chemotherapy in patients with american joint committee on Cancer/International union against cancer stage III and IV nasopharyngeal cancer of the endemic variety. J Clin Oncol 2005;23(27):6730–8.

48. Lee AW, Lau WH, Tung SY, et al. Preliminary results of a randomized study on therapeutic gain by concurrent chemotherapy for regionally-advanced nasopharyngeal carcinoma: NPC-9901 trial by the hong kong nasopharyngeal cancer study group. J Clin Oncol 2005;23(28):6966–75.

49. Lee AW, Foo W, Law SC, et al. Reirradiation for recurrent nasopharyngeal carcinoma: factors affecting the therapeutic ratio and ways for improvement. Int J Radiat Oncol Biol Phys 1997;38(1):43–52.

50. Chua DT, Sham JS, Kwong DL, et al. Locally recurrent nasopharyngeal carcinoma: treatment results for patients with computed tomography assessment. Int J Radiat Oncol Biol Phys 1998;41(2):379–86.

51. Hwang JM, Fu KK, Phillips TL. Results and prognostic factors in the retreatment of locally recurrent nasopharyngeal carcinoma. Int J Radiat Oncol Biol Phys 1998; 41(5):1099–111.

52. Teo PM, Kwan WH, Chan AT, et al. How successful is high-dose (> or = 60 gy) reirradiation using mainly external beams in salvaging local failures of nasopharyngeal carcinoma? Int J Radiat Oncol Biol Phys 1998;40(4):897–913.

53. Leung TW, Tung SY, Sze WK, et al. Salvage radiation therapy for locally recurrent nasopharyngeal carcinoma. Int J Radiat Oncol Biol Phys 2000;48(5):1331–8.

54. Lu TX, Mai WY, Teh BS, et al. Initial experience using intensity-modulated radiotherapy for recurrent nasopharyngeal carcinoma. Int J Radiat Oncol Biol Phys 2004;58(3):682–7.

55. Chua DT, Sham JS, Leung LH, et al. Re-irradiation of nasopharyngeal carcinoma with intensity-modulated radiotherapy. Radiother Oncol 2005;77(3):290–4.

56. Koutcher L, Lee N, Zelefsky M, et al. Reirradiation of locally recurrent nasopharynx cancer with external beam radiotherapy with or without brachytherapy. Int J Radiat Oncol Biol Phys 2010;76(1):130–7.

57. Chua DT, Sham JS, Au GK, et al. Concomitant chemoirradiation for stage III-IV nasopharyngeal carcinoma in chinese patients: results of a matched cohort analysis. Int J Radiat Oncol Biol Phys 2002;53(2):334–43.

58. Baron-Hay S, Clifford A, Jackson M, et al. Life threatening laryngeal toxicity following treatment with combined chemoradiotherapy for nasopharyngeal cancer: a case report with review of the literature. Ann Oncol 1999;10(9):1109–12.

59. Chow E, Payne D, O'Sullivan B, et al. Radiotherapy alone in patients with advanced nasopharyngeal cancer: comparison with an intergroup study is combined modality treatment really necessary? Radiother Oncol 2002;63(3):269–74.

60. Zhang L, Zhao C, Ghimire B, et al. The role of concurrent chemoradiotherapy in the treatment of locoregionally advanced nasopharyngeal carcinoma among endemic population: a meta-analysis of the phase III randomized trials. BMC Cancer 2010;10:558.

61. Chang KP, Hao SP, Tsang NM, et al. Salvage surgery for locally recurrent nasopharyngeal carcinoma-A 10-year experience. Otolaryngol Head Neck Surg 2004;131(4):497–502.

62. Hao SP, Tsang NM, Chang KP, et al. Nasopharyngectomy for recurrent nasopharyngeal carcinoma: a review of 53 patients and prognostic factors. Acta Otolaryngol 2008;128(4):473–81.

63. Danesi G, Zanoletti E, Mazzoni A. Salvage surgery for recurrent nasopharyngeal carcinoma. Skull Base 2007;17(3):173–80.

64. Wei WI. Cancer of the nasopharynx: functional surgical salvage. World J Surg 2003;27(7):844–8.

65. Wang CC. Re-irradiation of recurrent nasopharyngeal carcinoma–treatment techniques and results. Int J Radiat Oncol Biol Phys 1987;13(7):953–6.

66. Kwong DL, Nicholls J, Wei WI, et al. The time course of histologic remission after treatment of patients with nasopharyngeal carcinoma. Cancer 1999;85(7): 1446–53.

67. Boussen H, Cvitkovic E, Wendling JL, et al. Chemotherapy of metastatic and/or recurrent undifferentiated nasopharyngeal carcinoma with cisplatin, bleomycin, and fluorouracil. J Clin Oncol 1991;9(9):1675–81.

68. Taamma A, Fandi A, Azli N, et al. Phase II trial of chemotherapy with 5-fluorouracil, bleomycin, epirubicin, and cisplatin for patients with locally advanced, metastatic, or recurrent undifferentiated carcinoma of the nasopharyngeal type. Cancer 1999;86(7):1101–8.

69. Ngan RK, Yiu HH, Lau WH, et al. Combination gemcitabine and cisplatin chemotherapy for metastatic or recurrent nasopharyngeal carcinoma: report of a phase II study. Ann Oncol 2002;13(8):1252–8.

70. Xie P, Yue JB, Fu Z, et al. Prognostic value of 18F-FDG PET/CT before and after radiotherapy for locally advanced nasopharyngeal carcinoma. Ann Oncol 2010; 21(5):1078–82.

71. Liu WS, Wu MF, Tseng HC, et al. The role of pretreatment FDG-PET in nasopharyngeal carcinoma treated with intensity-modulated radiotherapy. Int J Radiat Oncol Biol Phys 2012;82(2):561–6.

72. Shimakage M, Ikegami N, Chatani M, et al. Serological follow-up study on the antibody levels to epstein-barr virus-determined nuclear antigen (EBNA) patients with nasopharyngeal carcinoma (NPC) after radiation therapy. Biken J 1987; 30(2):45–51.

73. de-Vathaire F, Sancho-Garnier H, de-The H, et al. Prognostic value of EBV markers in the clinical management of nasopharyngeal carcinoma (NPC): a multicenter follow-up study. Int J Cancer 1988;42(2):176–81.

Cancers of the Nose, Sinus, and Skull Base

Victoria Banuchi, MD, MPH[a], Jonathan Mallen, BA[b], Dennis Kraus, MD[c,d,]*

KEYWORDS

- Skull base cancers • Sinonasal carcinoma • Nasal carcinoma
- Sinonasal malignancies

KEY POINTS

- The most common malignancies of the nose, sinus and skull base are squamous cell carcinoma and adenocarcinoma.
- The most common sites of origin are the nasal cavity and the maxillary sinuses.
- Advanced presentation is common and usually involves important structures such as the orbit and the skull base.
- Advances in surgical resection and delivery of radiation have substantially improved outcomes in the last few decades.

INTRODUCTION

Malignancies of the nose, sinus, and skull base are rare, comprising approximately 3% to 5% of cancers of the head and neck[1] with an incidence of 0.556 cases per 100,000 in the United States.[2,3] The most common histologies are squamous cell carcinoma (SCC) (52%) and adenocarcinoma (13%), whereas the most common primary sites are the nasal cavity (44%) and maxillary sinus (36%). Cancers arising in the frontal and sphenoid sinuses are very rare.[4,5]

Management of these tumors is technically challenging because they often present in advanced stages. Nasal cavity tumors have improved survival outcomes compared with sinonasal and skull base tumors. Overall 5-year survivals reported range from 22% to 67%.[6] Tumors that are superior or posterior to Ohngren line are associated with a worse prognosis due to increased incidence of skull base invasion and perineural spread.[7] In the last few decades, advances in surgical resection techniques, as well

The authors have nothing to disclose.

[a] Department of Otolaryngology, Weill Cornell Medical College, 1320 York Avenue, New York, NY 10021, USA; [b] Hofstra North Shore-LIJ School of Medicine, 500 Hofstra University, Hempstead, NY 11549, USA; [c] The Center for Head & Neck Oncology, New York Head & Neck Institute, North Shore-LIJ Cancer Institute, 130 East 77th Street, Black Hall 10th Floor, New York, NY 10075, USA; [d] The Center for Thyroid & Parathyroid Surgery, New York Head and Neck Institute, New York, NY, USA

* Corresponding author. 130 East 77th Street, 10th Floor, New York, NY 10075.

E-mail address: DKraus@NSHS.edu

surgonc.theclinics.com

as improved strategies to deliver adjuvant radiation (minimizing morbidity) have substantially improved the outcomes in patients with malignancies of the sinonasal tract and skull base.

RISK FACTORS

Risk factors associated with sinonasal SCC include occupational exposure to nickel, soft wood dust, radium, mustard gas, and asbestos.[8–10] Adenocarcinomas are associated with exposure to hardwood dust, chrome pigment, textile dust, and leather work. Occupational exposure to formaldehyde is associated with an increased risk of acquiring both sinonasal adenocarcinomas and SCC. Radiation is a significant risk factor in the development of head and neck sarcomas, including sinonasal sarcomas.[11] Significant risk factors, such as alcohol and tobacco use, have not been associated with other less common histologies in malignant sinonasal and skull base tumors.

ANATOMY OF THE NOSE AND SINUS

The nasal cavity is bounded by the cribriform plate and the ethmoid bone superiorly and by the hard palate inferiorly. Anteriorly, it is bounded by the bony pyriform aperture and the external framework of the nose. Posteriorly, the choanae communicate with the nasopharynx. The nasal septum, which divides the 2 sides of the nasal cavity, is formed by cartilaginous and bony components. The cartilage of the septum is quadrangular in shape. Anteriorly, it connects with the nasal bones and is continuous with the anterior margins of the lateral cartilages. Inferiorly it is connected to the medial crura of the alar cartilages by fibrous tissue. It connects posteriorly to the perpendicular plate of the ethmoid and inferiorly to the vomer bone and palatine process of the maxilla. The inferior, middle, and superior turbinates are 3 bony projections from the lateral wall of the nose that help humidify as well as regulate the temperature of inhaled air. The bulla ethmoidalis is the most prominent anterior ethmoid cell.

The roof of the nasal cavity slopes downward at about a 30-degree angle from anterior to posterior. The cribriform plate forms the roof of the nasal cavity medial to the superior attachment of the middle turbinate and transmits the olfactory nerve. Lateral to the middle turbinate, the roof of the ethmoid sinuses is formed by the fovea ethmoidalis. The relationship of the cribriform plate to the fovea ethmoidalis is described by the Keros classification. Keros type I refers to the cribriform plate being in a slightly lower horizontal plane (1–3 mm) than the fovea ethmoidalis. Keros type II refers to the cribriform being moderately lower (3–7 mm) than the fovea ethmoidalis. Keros type III refers to the cribriform plate being significantly lower (8–16 mm) than the fovea ethmoidalis.[12] These are important distinctions during surgical planning for management of tumors involving the nose and sinuses.

The paranasal sinuses are hollows in bones surrounding the nose. The bones in which they lie define the names of the sinuses. They are lined with pseudostratified ciliated columnar epithelium continuous with the mucous membranes of the nasal cavity. Cilia in the mucosa carry secretions from the sinuses into the nasal cavity. The frontal sinus drains into the anterior part of the hiatus semilunaris via the infundibulum. The hiatus semilunaris also receives secretions from the maxillary sinus and the anterior ethmoids. The posterior ethmoids drain into the superior meatus. The sphenoid sinus drains into the sphenoethmoidal recess, a space above the superior concha. The inferior meatus contains the opening of the nasolacrimal ducts, carrying tears into the nasal cavity.

Sensory innervation of the nose is provided by the trigeminal nerve. The ophthalmic division (V1) provides ethmoidal branches to the anterior part of the nose, the floor of the nose, and the sphenoid and ethmoid sinuses. V1 also provides innervation to the frontal sinus via the supraorbital branch. The maxillary division (V2) of the trigeminal nerve innervates the lateral wall of the nose and the maxillary sinus via its infraorbital branch.

The nasal cavity and paranasal sinuses have a rich blood supply, primarily from the sphenopalatine branch of the internal maxillary artery. The internal maxillary artery enters the nose from the pterygopalatine fossa, posterior to the maxillary sinus. The facial artery perfuses the vestibule of the nose through the superior labial branch and the ophthalmic branch of the internal carotid artery supplies the roof of the nose and the nasal septum through the anterior and posterior ethmoidal arteries.

ANATOMY OF THE ANTERIOR SKULL BASE

The anterior skull base is often invaded in cases of sinonasal carcinoma. It is defined as the bony partition between the frontal lobes of the brain in the anterior cranial fossa and the midline and paramedian facial structures, including nasal cavity and orbits.

The gyri of the frontal lobes overlie most of the anterior cranial fossa; the ocular gyri and gyrus rectus lie lateral to the midline. The floor of the anterior cranial fossa is composed of ethmoid, sphenoid, and frontal bones. Anteriorly, it forms the crista galli and cribriform plate of the ethmoid bone covering the upper nasal cavity. The crista galli defines the midline of the anterior skull base. Posteriorly, it forms the planum sphenoidale. Laterally, the frontal bone and lesser wing of the sphenoid form the roof or the orbit and the optic canal; they blend medially into the anterior clinoid process. The cribriform plate is the thinnest portion of the ethmoid bone and transmits the first cranial nerve to the olfactory fossa through multiple foramina.

Tumor of the sinonasal region readily invades the infratemporal fossa, situated inferiorly to the temporal fossa. The temporalis muscle is located in the temporal fossa and inserts into the coronoid process and the mandibular ramus. Distally, the temporalis muscle traverses deep to the zygomatic arch and forms the lateral wall of the infratemporal fossa. The roof of the infratemporal fossa is the floor of the middle cranial fossa. The boundaries of the infratemporal fossa include the maxillary sinus anteriorly, the parotid gland posterolaterally, the ascending ramus of the mandible and the temporalis muscle laterally, the zygomatic arch and the greater wing of the sphenoid posteriorly, as well as the pterygoid fascia. It includes the parapharyngeal space (containing the internal carotid artery, internal jugular vein, cranial nerves VI to XII) and the masticator space, which contains the maxillary and mandibular branches of the trigeminal nerve, the internal maxillary artery, the pterygoid venous plexus, and the pterygoid muscles. The infratemporal fossa is connected to the middle cranial fossa via multiple foramina (eg, carotid canal, jugular foramen, foramen spinosum, foramen ovale, foramen lacerum).

SINONASAL CARCINOMAS

Jackson and colleagues[13] originally described the signs and symptoms of sinonasal tumors, with or without involvement of the skull base, in a retrospective study of 115 subjects. These results were validated by a separate study from Memorial Sloan-Kettering.[14] Their prevalence, in descending order, are nasal obstruction (61%), localized pain (43%), epistaxis (40%), swelling (29%), nasal discharge (26%), epiphora (19%), palate lesion (10%), diplopia (8%), cheek numbness (8%), decreased vision (8%), neck mass (4%), proptosis (3%), and trismus (2%). These manifestations can be used to assess extent of the tumor. The presence of palpable neck masses, trismus, and hearing loss indicate metastatic adenopathy, pterygoid invasion, and eustachian tube invasion, all of which portend a worse prognosis.

SCC is by far the most common of the paranasal sinus tumors. It can arise de novo or in association with inverted papillomas, which account for approximately 10% of the cases.[15,16] Approximately 70% occur in the maxillary sinus, with 12% in the nasal cavity.[17,18] Although most lesions are moderately differentiated on presentation, they are typically aggressive. The 5-year overall survival of sinonasal SCC ranges from 43% to 59%.[19,20] The rate of lymph node metastases of sinonasal SCC is approximately 10%.[21] The verrucous subtype has a fungating appearance and carries a better prognosis.[22] In addition, a subset of sinonasal SCC is associated with human papillomavirus (HPV) infection (up to 20% of cases in a recent study). HPV-positive sinonasal SCC seems to have a significantly better prognosis (80% vs 30% 5-year overall survival).[23] SCC is the only epithelial tumor for which TNM staging criteria are established, in view of the rarity of the other subtypes (**Table 1**). Management is typically primary

Table 1 Staging of primary malignant maxillary and ethmoid sinus tumors	
Primary Tumor: Maxillary Sinus	
TX	Cannot be assessed
T0	No evidence of primary tumor
Tis	Carcinoma in situ
T1	Tumor limited to the maxillary sinus mucosa with no erosion or destruction of bone
T2	Tumor causing bone erosion or destruction, including extension into the hard palate and/or middle nasal meatus, except extension to posterior wall of maxillary sinus and pterygoid plates
T3	Tumor invades any of the following: bone of the posterior wall of maxillary sinus, subcutaneous tissues, floor or medial wall of orbit, pterygoid fossa, ethmoid sinuses
T4a	Tumor invades anterior orbital contents, skin of cheek, pterygoid plates, infratemporal fossa, cribriform plate, sphenoid or frontal sinuses
T4b	Tumor invades any of the following: orbital apex, dura, brain, middle cranial fossa, cranial nerves other than maxillary division of trigeminal nerve (V_2), nasopharynx, or clivus
Primary Tumor: Nasal Cavity and Ethmoid Sinus	
TX	Cannot be assessed
T0	No evidence of primary tumor
Tis	Carcinoma in situ
T1	Tumor restricted to any one subsite, with or without bone invasion
T2	Tumor invading 2 subsites in a single region or extending to involve an adjacent region within the nasoethmoidal complex, with or without bone invasion
T3	Tumor extends to invade the medial wall or floor of the orbit, maxillary sinus, palate, or cribriform plate
T4a	Tumor invades any of the following: anterior orbital contents, skin of nose or cheek, minimal extension to anterior cranial fossa, pterygoid plates, sphenoid or frontal sinuses
T4b	Tumor invades any of the following: orbital apex, dura, brain, middle cranial fossa, cranial nerves other than maxillary division of trigeminal nerve (V_2), nasopharynx, or clivus

surgical resection with or without adjuvant radiation. In cases of advanced unresectable disease, primary chemoradiotherapy is used. Either response or stable disease with primary chemoradiotherapy is suggestive of a favorable outcome. Advanced T classification, bone or neural invasion, intracranial extension, dural or brain involvement, or positive margins are indications for adjuvant radiation as part of combined modality treatment. Depending on the histology and stage of disease, induction, as well as postoperative chemotherapy has been used.[24]

Primary intestinal type adenocarcinoma is the second most common sinonasal tumor. It is chiefly found in the ethmoid sinuses. It arises from the epithelial surface of the sinonasal mucosa. This tumor is associated with woodworkers and leather workers.[25] Adenocarcinomas of the sinonasal tract are a diverse group of malignancies that have been classified according to Barnes[26] into papillary, colonic, solid, mucinous, and mixed. According to Kleinsasser and Schroeder,[27] they have also been classified into well differentiated (papillary, tubular, and papillary-tubular type), moderately differentiated (papillary-mucinous and papillary-tubular-mucinous type), and poorly differentiated (mucinous, alveolar goblet cell, signet-ring type). These tumors, when advanced, are treated with surgery followed by adjuvant radiation. Despite aggressive therapy, there is a high recurrence rate (38%). As with most sinonasal carcinomas, cervical metastases are rare. Recurrence and distant metastasis diminish overall survival.[28] Although adjuvant radiation improved local control, it has not been shown to improve survival outcomes.[29]

Adenoid cystic carcinoma is a salivary gland tumor. Although more common in the major salivary glands, it has been shown to grow insidiously in the paranasal sinuses.[30] Such cancers are typically diagnosed in an advanced stage. Their proximity to vital structures (eg, dura, brain, orbit, and central nerves), as well as propensity for perineural invasion, makes resection with clear margins less likely.[31] Adenoid cystic carcinoma in the sinuses, much like its counterpart in salivary glands, has a high propensity for perineural spread and is associated with intracranial extension, positive surgical margins, and poor prognosis.[29]

The sinonasal tumors with neuroendocrine differentiation consist primarily of esthesioneuroblastomas (ENBs), sinonasal undifferentiated carcinoma (SNUC), sinonasal neuroendocrine carcinoma (SNEC), and small cell carcinoma (SmCC), with respective 5-year survival rates of 93%, 62%, 64%, and 28%.[32–34] Although SNEC and SNUC seem to have a similar clinical behavior, SmCC is clearly more aggressive. Their propensity for distant metastasis and poor prognosis warrant consideration of adjuvant systemic therapy that is mindful of the impact of treatment on the quality of remaining life.[35] The rarity of the disease has frustrated development of clinical trials.

ENB is a rare tumor with the incidence estimated at approximately 0.4 per million people per year.[36] ENB is derived from olfactory neuroepithelium and is responsible for approximately 6% of tumors in the nasal cavity and paranasal sinuses.[37] The age distribution is bimodal, occurring most commonly during the second and sixth decades of life. Neck metastases reported in up to 25% of patients, whereas distant metastases are estimated to occur in 17%.[38–40] In general, these tumors are treated with a combination of surgery and adjuvant radiation.[41] The validated Kadish staging system is the most commonly used for ENB (**Table 2**).

SNUCs are derived from schneiderian epithelium and are characterized by fast progression, extensive tissue destruction, and a poor prognosis.[42–45] Their rapid growth and aggressive behavior often results in extensive local invasion into the sinuses, orbit, and brain. Surgical resection followed by adjuvant radiation has historically been the mainstay of treatment; however, the recent emergence of aggressive trimodality

Table 2	
Modified Kadish staging system for esthesioneuroblastoma	
Type	**Extent**
A	Tumor is limited to the nasal cavity
B	Tumor in the nasal cavity and extending to the paranasal sinuses
C	Tumor extends beyond the nasal cavity and paranasal sinuses, involving the cribriform lamina, the skull base, the orbit, or the intracranial cavity
D	Tumor with neck or distant metastases

Adapted from Morita A, Ebersold MJ, Olsen KD, et al. Esthesioneuroblastoma: prognosis and management. Neurosurgery 1993;32:706–15; with permission.

therapy (incorporating surgery followed by postoperative chemoradiotherapy) has improved local-regional control and overall survival.[46]

Sinonasal mucosal melanoma (SMM) is exceedingly rare. It derives from melanocytes in neural crest cells. SMM accounts for 4% to 13% of sinonasal malignant tumors.[47] The 5-year overall survival rate ranges from 17% to 35%.[48] Cervical metastases have been observed in 6% to 22% of patients; distant metastases are relatively uncommon (4%–10%).[49,50] Surgery to achieve clear margins, when feasible, is the mainstay of treatment.[51] Meleti and colleagues[50] found that rates of locoregional recurrence of head and neck mucosal melanoma were higher with surgery alone than with the combination of surgery with postoperative radiotherapy. These results have been confirmed in other studies.[52–54] Elective neck dissection is not routinely recommended.[55] Chemotherapy fails to prolong survival but is often used as palliative treatment of those with advanced disease.[56]

MANAGEMENT

A very high index of suspicion is necessary to diagnose sinonasal or skull base malignancies at an early stage because many of these tumors do not cause symptoms until they reach a critical size and extension. A suspicious lesion should be biopsied and imaged before embarking on surgical planning. Computed tomography (CT) and MRI are complementary and essential in many cases and should be obtained in axial, coronal, and sagittal planes. A fine-cut CT scan has the advantage of detecting bone erosion whereas MRI with gadolinium-based IV-contrast and with fat-suppression software is used to differentiate tumor from adjacent soft tissue. Evaluation for distant metastases should include CT of the chest and abdomen or a PET study.

Complete surgical excision, with or without postoperative radiotherapy, is the treatment of choice for most sinonasal and skull base carcinomas. Surgery is the most effective single-modality treatment of sinonasal cancers.[2] Tumor extension to the cavernous sinus, internal carotid artery, optic chiasm, extensive brain parenchymal involvement, or distant metastasis are relative contraindications to surgical management.[57] Adjuvant radiotherapy with or without chemotherapy is standard in advanced cases to improve local control[58] but early stage lesions of the sinonasal tract show no survival benefit from the addition of adjuvant radiotherapy.[59]

APPROACHES

Surgical approaches to sinonasal cancers can be divided into endoscopic versus open surgery. Lateral rhinotomy with or without Weber-Ferguson incision, transoral-transpalatal approach, facial degloving, and open craniofacial resection may be appropriate.[60] Choosing the proper approach is essential to achieving adequate oncologic resection, minimal brain retraction, integrity of the dura, protection of neurovascular structures, reconstruction of the skull base, and optimal functional and esthetic outcomes.

Endonasal approaches to the skull base became commonplace after they were reintroduced in the 1960s by Guiot and Hardy as alternatives to approaching the ventral midline cranial base.[61,62] With the introduction of the endoscope, this technique has become increasingly popular.[63] Endoscopic resection of the anterior skull base and dura with reconstruction was first described in 2005.[64] Endoscopic resection avoids large transfacial and scalp incisions, permits better vision through magnification and angled scopes, and avoids brain retraction. The 2 largest recent series evaluating oncologic results of endoscopic skull base resection versus open surgery have demonstrated comparable overall survival, concluding that in well-selected patients endoscopic resection results in acceptable oncologic outcomes.[65–67] An endoscopic approach is contraindicated in cases in which there is involvement of skin and subcutaneous tissue, nasolacrimal sac, anterior table of the frontal sinus, carotid artery, extensive lateral dural invasion, or brain parenchymal involvement.[68] Randomized controlled trials comparing open and endoscopic techniques have not been performed and are unlikely in the future due to rarity of the cases and logistical constraints.

Watertight closure of the skull base defect is important and for many years represented the single greatest challenge of endoscopic resection. Initially, extended endonasal approaches to the skull base were plagued with a postoperative cerebrospinal fluid (CSF) leak of 20% to 30%. Use of the Hadad-Bassagasteguy flap (pedicled nasoseptal mucosal flap) reduces the incidence of CSF leak.[69] One of the largest reported series using vascularized flap repairs in endoscopic skull base series showed an overall postoperative CSF leak rate of 3.3% among patients with intraoperative of the dura,[70] demonstrating that the nasoseptal flap is effective in prevention of postoperative CSF leaks. This advance in surgical technique has contributed substantially to decreasing morbidity associated with endoscopic approaches.

Open transfacial approaches remain the most commonly used for resection of locally advanced sinonasal tumors. Although a lateral rhinotomy is the standard incision, it can be extended with a Weber-Ferguson incision, which adds lip-splitting and subciliary incisions, enhancing exposure of the maxillary bone.[71] Midface degloving and sublabial approaches are more common for large benign sinonasal lesions or selected small malignancies. The degloving approach avoids an external incision and exposes both the inferior and medial maxilla bilaterally. This approach can include a complete transfixion incision of the membranous septum that joins intranasally with a bilateral intercartilaginous incision. The extent of resection in these open approaches can vary from a medial maxillectomy, through total maxillectomy, anterior cranial base resection, and infratemporal fossa dissection with or without orbital exenteration, as needed based on tumor extent.

Medial maxillectomy is indicated for tumors of the nasal cavity, lateral nasal wall, and medial maxillary sinus. This technique is most commonly performed endoscopically.[72] The lateral nasal wall is resected beginning with the inferior osteotomy along the nasal floor below the attachment of the inferior turbinate. This is carried to the posterior maxillary wall. The lamina papyracea can be resected if needed. A complete sphenoethmoidectomy is performed. The anterior frontoethmoidal suture is identified and dissection is performed inferior to its level, to avoid injury the of the anterior skull base. Superior cuts are made above the attachment of the middle turbinate. Frozen sections should be judiciously obtained to determine that the margins are tumor-free.[73] If performed through an open transfacial approach, closure should include the repositioning of the medial canthal tendon.

Inferior maxillectomy is commonly used for neoplasms of the alveolar process with minimal extension into the maxillary sinus. It involves a resection of the inferior maxillary sinus below the infraorbital nerve. It requires a combination of sublabial and palatal incisions. This approach is most commonly applicable to palatal malignancies or early sinonasal tumors.

Total maxillectomy is performed by extending a lateral rhinotomy to a lip-splitting incision. By definition, a total maxillectomy includes a resection of all the 6 walls of the maxilla, including the floor of the orbit. In some instances orbital exenteration is required.[74] A gingiva-buccal incision performed, connecting the lip-splitting incision to the first molar laterally, and over the lateral surface of the maxillary tuberosity. A medial or paramedial incision is performed over the hard palate to the junction of the hard and soft palate posteriorly. The lateral rhinotomy can be extended superiorly below the medial brow to avoid the risk of lower lid complications seen with the Weber-Ferguson extension, such as ectropion and edema.[75] The facial flap is elevated in a subperiosteal plane unless the tumor extends into the anterior wall of the maxillary sinus and adjacent soft tissue. Transection of the infraorbital nerve is performed to expose the entire maxillary bone lateral to the zygomatic extension. The periorbita are dissected along the medial, inferior, and lateral orbital walls. Medial osteotomies are performed along the frontal process of the maxilla below the frontoethmoidal suture line. Lateral osteotomies are performed along the frontal and temporal processes of the zygoma. A midline or paramedian sagittal osteotomy is made through the hard palate. Care is taken to identify, ligate, and transect the internal maxillary artery at its entrance through the pterygomaxillary fissure. The specimen is gently cantilevered and the remaining soft tissue attachments are divided. Brisk bleeding is to be anticipated. At this juncture in the procedure, hemostasis is achieved with packing and electrocautery. Frozen sections are obtained to ensure negative margins. In selected cases an orbital exenteration can be performed. After achieving adequate exposure, the periorbita are incised over the superior and lateral orbital rims. Dissection continues along the roof of the orbit and lateral walls until the superior orbital fissure (SOF) and the optic foramen are exposed. Lidocaine is injected around these structures to prevent autonomic-induced cardiac arrhythmias. The neurovascular structures of the SOF are carefully ligated and divided. The optic nerve and ophthalmic artery are also ligated and divided. The extraocular muscles are transected at the orbital apex. The medial and inferior orbital wall should be removed en bloc.[57] Additional resection margins can be achieved when extending this procedure to the infratemporal fossa.

Craniofacial resection involves resection of the anterior cranial base. Ketcham and colleagues[76] first described this approach in 1963. This is required for patients with sinonasal tumors that invade the cribriform plate or fovea ethmoidalis.[77,78] It is necessary in most cases of ENB,[79] as well as in cases of ethmoid and maxillary sinus carcinoma involving the skull base. Historically, it is the standard of care for treatment of malignancies involving the anterior skull base.[80–83] Dural resection may be sufficient in some patients. In patients with malignant tumors that transgress the dural barrier, however, a limited resection of the involved brain may be indicated. Owing to the poor prognosis associated with involved brain parenchyma, this is usually reserved for cases of limited frontal lobe involvement.[84] In craniofacial resection, combined extracranial and intracranial access to the anterior and lateral skull base is created. The extracranial portion may include transfacial, sublabial, or endonasal approaches, as described previously. Intracranial access is performed by a neurosurgeon. A bicoronal flap is raised with preservation of the pericranium. The posterior scalp is then raised to give appropriate length to the pericranial flap. Two parallel incisions are made in the calvarial periosteum on either side of the frontal skull to the origin of the temporalis muscle. Incisions are connected across the vertex posterior to the scalp incision. The flap is elevated down to the supraorbital rims. The pericranial flap is pedicled on the supraorbital and supratrochlear vessels.[85,86] A low, limited, craniotomy is performed as needed to extirpate the intracranial extent of tumor and provide adequate exposure for management of the frontal sinus. Tumors invading dura or brain should be cleared with an adequate margin. The specimen should be delivered en bloc with the intranasal portion of the tumor. After resection, multiple frozen sections are obtained to ensure clearance of margins. Any dural defect is repaired with temporalis fascia, fascia lata, lyophilized dura, or bovine pericardium grafts. The pericranial flap is placed under the dural reconstruction and sutured between the healthy dura and beyond the posterior extremity of the defect and the residual anterior fossa floor at this site. A dacryocystorhinostomy may be performed with placement of a sialastic stent through the lacrimal puncta if the duct has been severed.[87] One of the most common complications of this approach is CSF leak, leading to meningitis. The likelihood of this complication is diminished with vascularized free flap reconstruction of the skull base. Many groups advocate the use of free microvascular flaps for reconstruction of larger defects resulting from extirpation of a significant volume of tissue, including cases of orbital exenteration and for posterior defects.[88–91] The selection of a free flap is based on the size of the defect, the length of the pedicle needed, and the reconstructive surgeon's preference. Reconstruction with rectus abdominis, latissimus dorsi, radial forearm, and fibula free flaps has been described.[92] In a series of 25 subjects with free flap reconstruction who underwent craniofacial resection for malignancies involving the skull base and the infratemporal fossa, none had evidence of a CSF leak.[93] Wound complications observed in other series include wound dehiscence, infection, neurologic impairment, fistula, and free flap failure.[94]

ROLE OF RADIATION

Current data support the use of surgical resection of skull base lesions, followed by adjuvant radiation therapy for high-risk disease, dural invasion, or positive margins on final pathologic testing.[95] Surgery followed by adjuvant radiation shows improved rates of locoregional control and disease free-survival when compared with primary radiation treatment in patients with sinonasal carcinoma.[96] Radiosensitivity depends on histology and growth rate of tumor. Implementation of intensity-modulated radiotherapy (IMRT) allows delivery of higher doses to the target and minimized radiation-induced toxicity without sacrificing survival outcomes. It is considered the standard radiotherapy modality for sinonasal carcinomas.[97] IMRT in patients with sinonasal carcinoma allows for increased dose at target and minimizes morbidity to surrounding structures.[98] Brachytherapy is used at some centers but there are little data supporting its use. A recent series of 35 subjects suggests that interdisciplinary perioperative image-adapted brachytherapy is well tolerated with low toxicity and is associated with excellent locoregional control and survival rates.[99]

ROLE OF CHEMOTHERAPY

The role of primary chemoradiotherapy in sinonasal carcinoma treatment is unclear. There are reports on concurrent chemoradiation in sinonasal carcinomas, albeit limited to advanced SCC and SNUC.[100,101]

SUMMARY

Sinonasal carcinomas are rare and carry significant challenges in terms of management. When presenting at advanced stages, sinonasal carcinomas tend to invade important structures such as the orbit and the skull base. Orbital or intracranial involvement are both associated with poor prognosis and make treating these tumors a challenging, often morbid, endeavor including a significant risk of treatment-associated mortality.

Recent advances, such as endoscopic resection of sinonasal tumors involving the skull base combined with targeted craniotomies in an interdisciplinary setting, have transpired. In addition, advances in imaging and delivery of radiation therapy with the use of IMRT have led to improved survival outcomes and decreased morbidity associated with treatment. When using these techniques, multiple institutions report an average of approximately 50% overall survival at 5 years in complicated sinonasal cases involving the skull base. Although there have been significant improvements in the field, new modalities of therapy for high-risk tumors must still be pursued to improve on these results.

REFERENCES

1. Lund VJ, Stammberger H, Nicolai P, et al. European position paper on endoscopic management of tumours of the nose, paranasal sinuses and skull base. Rhinol Suppl 2010;1:1–143.
2. Turner JH, Reh DD. Incidence and survival in patients with sinonasal cancer: a historical analysis of population-based data. Head Neck 2012;34(6): 877–85.
3. Dulguerov P, Jacobsen MS, Allal AS, et al. Nasal and paranasal sinus carcinoma: are we making progress? A series of 220 patients and a systematic review. Cancer 2001;92:3012–29.
4. Osguthorpe JD, Richardson M. Frontal sinus malignancies. Otolaryngol Clin North Am 2001;34:269–81.
5. DeMonte F, Ginsberg LE, Clayman GL. Primary malignant tumors of the sphenoid sinus. Neurosurgery 2000;46:1084–91.
6. Khademi B, Moradi A, Hoseini S, et al. Malignant neoplasms of the sinonasal tract: report of 71 patients and literature review and analysis. Oral Maxillofac Surg 2009;13:191–9.
7. Ohngren LG. Malignant tumors of the maxilla-ethmoidal region. Clinical study with special reference to treatment with electrocautery and irradiation. Acta Otolaryngol 1933;19(Suppl):1–476.
8. Luce D, Leclerc A, Begin D, et al. Sinonasal cancer and occupational exposures: a pooled data analysis of 12 case-control studies. Cancer Causes Control 2002;13:147–57.
9. Roush GC. Epidemiology of cancer of the nose and paranasal sinuses, current concepts. Head Neck Surg 1979;2:3–11.
10. Lund VJ. Malignancy of the nose and sinuses: epidemiological and aetiological considerations. Rhinology 1991;29:57–68.
11. Patel SG, See AC, Williamson PA, et al. Radiation induced sarcoma of the head and neck. Head Neck 1999;21:346–54.
12. Bolger WE. Anatomy of the paranasal sinuses. In: Kennedy DW, Bolger WE, Zinreich SJ, editors. Diseases of the sinuses: diagnosis and management. Toronto (Canada): BC Decker; 2001. p. 1–12.

13. Jackson RT, Fitz-Hugh GS, Constable WC. Malignant neoplasms of the nasal cavities and paranasal sinuses: (a retrospective study). Laryngoscope 1977; 87:726–36.
14. Sisson GA, Toriumi DM, Atiyah RA. Paranasal sinus malignancy: a comprehensive update. Laryngoscope 1989;99:143–50.
15. Yoskovitch AY, Braverman I, Nachtigal D, et al. Sinonasal schneiderian papilloma. J Otolaryngol 1998;27:122–6.
16. von Buchwald C, Bradley PJ. Risks of malignancy in inverted papilloma of the nose and paranasal sinuses. Curr Opin Otolaryngol Head Neck Surg 2007;15: 95–8.
17. Tiwari R, Hardillo JA, Mehta D, et al. Squamous cell carcinoma of maxillary sinus. Head Neck 2000;22(2):164–9.
18. Lewis JS, Castro EB. Cancer of the nasal cavity and paranasal sinuses. J Laryngol Otol 1972;86:255–62.
19. Ganly I, Patel SG, Singh B, et al. Craniofacial resection for malignant paranasal sinus tumors: Report of an International Collaborative Study. Head Neck 2005; 27:575–84.
20. Lee CH, Hur DG, Roh HJ, et al. Survival rates of sinonasal squamous cell carcinoma with the new AJCC staging system. Arch Otolaryngol Head Neck Surg 2007;133:131–4.
21. Cantù G, Bimbi G, Miceli R, et al. Lymph node metastases in malignant tumors of the paranasal sinuses: prognostic value and treatment. Arch Otolaryngol Head Neck Surg 2008;134:170.
22. Durden FL Jr, Moore CE, Muller S. Verrucous carcinoma of the paranasal sinuses: a case report. Ear Nose Throat J 2010;89(7):E21–3.
23. Alos L, Moyano S, Nadal A, et al. Human papillomaviruses are identified in a subgroup of sinonasal squamous cell carcinomas with favorable outcome. Cancer 2009;115:2701.
24. Kazi M, Awan S, Junaid M, et al. Hassan management of sinonasal tumors: prognostic factors and outcomes: a 10 year experience at a tertiary care hospital. Indian J Otolaryngol Head Neck Surg 2013;65(Suppl 1):155–9.
25. Bornholdt J, Hansen J, Steiniche T, et al. K-ras mutations in sinonasal cancers in relation to wood dust exposure. BMC Cancer 2008;8:53.
26. Barnes L. Intestinal-type adenocarcinoma of the nasal cavity and paranasal sinuses. Am J Surg Pathol 1986;10:192–202.
27. Kleinsasser O, Schroeder HG. Adenocarcinomas of the inner nose after exposure to wood dust. Morphological findings and relationships between histopathology and clinical behavior in 79 cases. Arch Otorhinolaryngol 1988;245:1–15.
28. Camp S, Van Gerven L, Vander Poorten V, et al. Long-term follow-up of 123 patients with adenocarcinoma of the sinonasal tract treated with endoscopic resection and postoperative radiation therapy. Head Neck 2014. [Epub ahead of print].
29. Lupinetti AD, Roberts DB, Williams MD, et al. Sinonasal adenoid cystic carcinoma: the M. D. Anderson Cancer Center experience. Cancer 2007;110(12): 2726–31.
30. Gil Z, Carlson DL, Gupta A, et al. Patterns and incidence of neural invasion in patients with cancers of the paranasal sinuses. Arch Otolaryngol Head Neck Surg 2009;135(2):173–9.
31. Patel SG, Singh B, Polluri A, et al. Craniofacial surgery for malignant skull base tumors: report of an international collaborative study. Cancer 2003;98(6): 1179–87.

32. Hyams VJ, Batsakis JG, Michaels L. Tumors of the upper respiratory tract and ear. In: Armed Forces Institute of Pathology Fascicles, 2nd series. Washington: American Registry of Pathology Press; 1988.

33. Kameya T, Shimosato Y, Adachi I, et al. Neuroendocrine carcinoma of the paranasal sinus: a morphological and endocrinological study. Cancer 1980;45(2): 330–9.

34. Sirsath NT, Babu KG, Das U, et al. Paranasal sinus neuroendocrine carcinoma: a case report and review of the literature. Case Rep Oncol Med 2013;2013: 728479.

35. van der Laan TP, Bij HP, van Hemel BM, et al. The importance of multimodality therapy in the treatment of sinonasal neuroendocrine carcinoma. Eur Arch Otorhinolaryngol 2013;270(9):2565–8.

36. Theilgaard SA, Buchwald C, Ingeholm P, et al. Esthesioneuroblastoma: a Danish demographic study of 40 patients registered between 1978 and 2000. Acta Otolaryngol 2003;123:433–9.

37. Svane-Knudsen V, Jorgensen KE, Hansen O, et al. Cancer of the nasal cavity and paranasal sinuses a series of 115 patients. Rhinology 1998; 36(1):12–4.

38. Rinaldo A, Ferlito A, Shaha AR, et al. Esthesioneuroblastoma and cervical lymph node metastases: clinical and therapeutic implications. Acta Otolaryngol 2002; 122:215–21.

39. Ferlito A, Rinaldo A, Rhys-Evans PH. Contemporary clinical commentary: esthesioneuroblastoma: an update on management of the neck. Laryngoscope 2003; 113:1935–8.

40. Dulguerov P, Allal AS, Calcaterra TC. Esthesioneuroblastoma: a meta-analysis and review. Lancet Oncol 2001;2001(2):683–90.

41. Lund V, Howard D, Wei W, et al. Olfactory neuroblastoma: past, present, and future? Laryngoscope 2003;113:502–7.

42. Frierson HF Jr, Mills SE, Fechner RE, et al. Sinonasal undifferentiated carcinoma. An aggressive neoplasm derived from schneiderian epithelium and distinct from olfactory neuroblastoma. Am J Surg Pathol 1986;10:771–9.

43. Goel R, Ramalingam K, Ramani P, et al. Sino nasal undifferentiated carcinoma: A rare entity. J Nat Sci Biol Med 2012;3:101–4.

44. Levine PA, Frierson HF Jr, Stewart FM, et al. Sinonasal undifferentiated carcinoma: a distinctive and highly aggressive neoplasm. Laryngoscope 1987; 97(8 Pt 1):905–8.

45. Houston GD, Gillies E. Sinonasal undifferentiated carcinoma: a distinctive clinicopathologic entity. Adv Anat Pathol 1999;6:317–23.

46. Yoshida E, Aouad R, Fragoso R, et al. Improved clinical outcomes with multimodality therapy for sinonasal undifferentiated carcinoma of the head and neck. Am J Otolaryngol 2013;34(6):658–63.

47. Gavriel H, McArthur G, Sizeland A, et al. Review: mucosal melanoma of the head and neck. Melanoma Res 2011;21:257–66.

48. Jethanamest D, Vila PM, Sikora AG, et al. Predictors of survival in mucosal melanoma of the head and neck. Ann Surg Oncol 2011;18:2748–56.

49. Bartell HL, Bedikian AY, Papadopoulos NE, et al. Biochemotherapy in patients with advanced head and neck mucosal melanoma. Head Neck 2008;30: 1592–8.

50. Meleti M, Leemans CR, de Bree R, et al. Head and neck mucosal melanoma: experience with 42 patients, with emphasis on the role of postoperative radiotherapy. Head Neck 2008;30:1543–51.

51. Sun CZ, Li QL, Hu ZD, et al. Treatment and prognosis in sinonasal mucosal melanoma: A retrospective analysis of 65 patients from a single cancer center. Head Neck 2014;36(5):675–81.

52. Krengli M, Masini L, Kaanders JH, et al. Radiotherapy in the treatment of mucosal melanoma of the upper aerodigestive tract: analysis of 74 cases. A Rare Cancer Network study. Int J Radiat Oncol Biol Phys 2006;65:751–9.

53. Temam S, Mamelle G, Marandas P, et al. Postoperative radiotherapy for primary mucosal melanoma of the head and neck. Cancer 2005;103:313–9.

54. Owens JM, Roberts DB, Myers JN. The role of postoperative adjuvant radiation therapy in the treatment of mucosal melanomas of the head and neck region. Arch Otolaryngol Head Neck Surg 2003;129:864–8.

55. Moreno MA, Hanna EY. Management of mucosal melanomas of the head and neck: did we make any progress? Curr Opin Otolaryngol Head Neck Surg 2010;18:101–6.

56. Mucke T, Holzle F, Kesting MR, et al. Tumor size and depth in primary malignant melanoma in the oral cavity influences survival. J Oral Maxillofac Surg 2009;67: 1409–15.

57. Hanna EY, DeMonte F. Comprehensive management of skull base tumors. New York: Informa Healthcare USA, Inc; 2008. p. 256–7.

58. Bristol IJ, Ahamad A, Garden AS, et al. Postoperative radiotherapy for maxillary sinus cancer: Long-term outcomes and toxicities of treatment. Int J Radiat Oncol Biol Phys 2007;68(3):719–30.

59. Blanch JL, Ruiz AM, Alos L, et al. Treatment of 125 sinonasal tumors: prognostic factors, outcome, and follow-up. Otolaryngol Head Neck Surg 2004; 131:973–6.

60. Hanna Ey, Westfall CT, Myers EN, et al. Cancer of the nasal cavity, paranasal sinuses and orbit. In: Myers EN, Suen JY, Myers JN, et al, editors. Cancer of the head and neck. Philadelphia: Saunders; 2003. p. 155–206.

61. Frank G, Sciarretta V, Calbucci F, et al. The endoscopic transnasal transsphenoidal approach for the treatment of cranial base chordomas and chondrosarcomas. Neurosurgery 2006;59(Suppl 1):ONS50–7.

62. Frank G, Sciarretta V, Mazzatenta D, et al. Transsphenoidal endoscopic approach in the treatment of Rathke's cleft cyst. Neurosurgery 2005;56:124–9.

63. Ciric I, Mikhael M, Stafford T, et al. Transsphenoidal microsurgery of pituitary macroadenomas with long-term follow-up results. J Neurosurg 1983;59: 395–401.

64. Kassam A, Snyderman CH, Mintz A, et al. Expanded endonasal approach: the rostrocaudal axis. Part I. Crista galli to the sella turcica. Neurosurg Focus 2005; 19:E3.

65. Nicolai P, Battaglia P, Bignami M, et al. Endoscopic surgery for malignant tumors of the sinonasal tract and adjacent skull base: a 10-year experience. Am J Rhinol 2008;22:308–16.

66. Hanna E, DeMonte F, Ibrahim S, et al. Endoscopic resection of sinonasal cancers with and without craniotomy: oncologic results. Arch Otolaryngol Head Neck Surg 2009;135:1219–24.

67. de Almeida JR, Su SY, Koutourousiou M, et al. endonasal endoscopic surgery for squamous cell carcinoma or the sinonasal cavities and skull base: Oncologic outcomes based on treatment strategy and tumor etiology. Head Neck Surg 2014. [Epub ahead of print].

68. Su SY, Kupferman ME, DeMonte F, et al. Endoscopic resection of sinonasal cancers. Curr Oncol Rep 2014;16(2):369.

69. Hadad G, Bassagasteguy L, Carrau RL, et al. A novel reconstructive technique after endoscopic expanded endonasal approaches: vascular pedicle nasoseptal flap. Laryngoscope 2006;116:1882–6.

70. Thorp BD, Sreenath SB, Ebert CS, et al. Endoscopic skull base reconstruction: a review and clinical case series of 152 vascularized flaps used for surgical skull base defects in the setting of intraoperative cerebrospinal fluid leak. Neurosurg Focus 2014;37(4):E4.

71. Fergusson W. Operation on the upper jaw. A system of practical surgery. London (United Kingdom): J Churchill & Co; 1842. p. 484.

72. Sadeghi N, Al-Dhahri S, Manoukian JJ. Transnasal endoscopic medial maxillectomy for inverting papilloma. Laryngoscope 2003;113(4):749–53.

73. Gandour-Edwards RF, Donald PJ, Boggan JE. Intraoperative frozen section diagnosis in skull base surgery. Skull Base Surg 1993;3(3):159–63.

74. Cordeiro PG, Santamaria E, Kraus DH, et al. Reconstruction of total maxillectomy defects with preservation of the orbital contents. Plast Reconstr Surg 1998;102:1874–84 [discussion: 1885–7].

75. Vural E, Hanna E. Extended lateral rhinotomy incision for total maxillectomy. Otolaryngol Head Neck Surg 2000;123(4):512–3.

76. Ketcham AS, Wilkins RH, Vanburen JM, et al. A combined intracranial facial approach to the paranasal sinuses. Am J Surg 1963;106:698–703.

77. Shah JP, Kraus DH, Bilsky MH, et al. Craniofacial resection for malignant tumors involving the anterior skull base. Arch Otolaryngol Head Neck Surg 1997;123:1312–7.

78. Bridger PG, Kwok B, Baldwin M, et al. Craniofacial resection for paranasal sinus cancers. Head Neck 2000;22:772–80.

79. Patel SG, Singh B, Stambuk HE, et al. Craniofacial surgery for esthesioneuroblastoma: report of an international collaborative study. J Neurol Surg B Skull Base 2012;73(3):208–20.

80. Van Buren JM, Ommaya AK, Ketcham AS. Ten years' experience with radical combined craniofacial resection of malignant tumors of the paranasal sinuses. J Neurosurg 1968;28:341–50.

81. Gil Z, Patel SG, Singh B, et al. Analysis of prognostic factors in 146 patients with anterior skull base sarcoma: an international collaborative study. Cancer 2007;110:1033–41.

82. Shah JP, Galicich JH. Craniofacial resection for malignant tumors of ethmoid and anterior skull base. Arch Otolaryngol 1977;103:514–7.

83. Fliss DM, Abergel A, Cavel O, et al. Combined subcranial approaches for excision of complex anterior skull base tumors. Arch Otolaryngol Head Neck Surg 2007;133:888–96.

84. Feiz-Erfran I, Suki D, Hanna E, et al. Prognostic significance of transdural invasion of cranial base malignancies in patients undergoing craniofacial resection. Neurosurgery 2007;61(6):1178–85.

85. Boyle JO, Shah KC, Shah JP. Craniofacial resection for malignant neoplasms of the skull base: an overview. J Surg Oncol 1998;69:275–84.

86. Schramm VL Jr, Myers EN, Maroon JC. Anterior skull base surgery for benign and malignant disease. Laryngoscope 1979;89:1077–91.

87. Andersen PE, Kraus DH, Arbit E, et al. Management of the orbit during anterior fossa craniofacial resection. Arch Otolaryngol Head Neck Surg 1996 Dec;122(12):1305–7.

88. Jones NF, Sekhar LN, Schramm VL. Free rectus abdominis muscle flap reconstruction of the middle and posterior cranial base. Plast Reconstr Surg 1986;78:471.

89. Shestak KC, Jones NF, Ramasastry SS. Microvascular reconstruction of the cranial base. In: Sekhar LN, Jenecka IP, editors. Surgery of cranial base tumors. New York: Raven Press; 1993. p. 427–34.

90. Chang DW, Langstein HN, Gupta A, et al. Reconstructive management of cranial base defects after tumor ablation. Plast Reconstr Surg 2001;107(6): 1346–55 [discussion: 1356–7].

91. Neligan PC, Mulholland S, Irish J, et al. Flap selection in cranial base reconstruction. Plast Reconstr Surg 1996;98(7):1159–66 [discussion: 1167–8].

92. Valentini V, Fabiani F, Nicolai G, et al. Use of microvascular free flaps in the reconstruction of the anterior and middle skull base. J Craniofac Surg 2006; 17(4):790–6.

93. Bilsky MH, Bentz B, Vitaz T, et al. Craniofacial resection for cranial base malignancies involving the infratemporal fossa. Neurosurgery 2005;57(Suppl 4): 339–47 [discussion: 339–47].

94. Richtsmeier WJ, Briggs RJ, Koch WM, et al. Complications and early outcome of anterior craniofacial resection. Arch Otolaryngol Head Neck Surg 1992;118: 913–7.

95. Bentz BG, Bilsky MH, Shah JP, et al. Anterior skull base surgery for malignant tumors: A multivariate analysis of 27 years of experience. Head Neck 2003; 25(7):515–20.

96. Mendenhall WM, Amdur RJ, Morris CG, et al. Carcinoma of the nasal cavity and paranasal sinuses. Laryngoscope 2008;119:899.

97. Duprez F, Madani I, Morbée L, et al. IMRT for sinonasal tumors minimizes severe late ocular toxicity and preserves disease control and survival. Int J Radiat Oncol Biol Phys 2012;83(1):252–9.

98. Bradford S, Hoppe MD, Suzanne L, et al. Postoperative intensity-modulated radiation therapy for cancers of the paranasal sinuses, nasal cavity, and lacrimal glands: Technique, early outcomes, and toxicity. Head Neck 2008;30(7):925–32.

99. Teudt IU, Meyer JE, Ritter M, et al. Perioperative image-adapted brachytherapy for the treatment of paranasal sinus and nasal cavity malignancies. Brachytherapy 2014;13(2):178–86.

100. Nishimura G, Tsukuda M, Mikami Y, et al. The efficacy and safety of concurrent chemoradiotherapy for maxillary sinus squamous cell carcinoma. Auris Nasus Larynx 2009;36:547–54.

101. Enepekides DJ. Sinonasal undifferentiated carcinoma: an update. Curr Opin Otolaryngol Head Neck Surg 2005;13:222–5.

Evaluation and Management of Head and Neck Squamous Cell Carcinoma of Unknown Primary

Jeffrey M. Martin, MD, Thomas J. Galloway, MD*

KEYWORDS

- Unknown primary • Head and neck cancer • Radiation therapy • Surgery
- Squamous cell carcinoma

KEY POINTS

- Enhanced diagnostic techniques have narrowed the population of patients with an unknown primary and should be considered when comparing results to historical literature.
- Application of the general principles of head and neck oncology to squamous cell carcinoma of unknown primary generally results in a gratifying control rate.
- Evolution of the delivery of radiation therapy requires oncologists to give further consideration to which tissues to target and which to spare.

INTRODUCTION

Squamous cell carcinoma of an unknown primary of the head and neck (SCCUP) is defined as metastatic disease in the lymph nodes of the neck without any evidence of a primary tumor of the mucosa[1] after "appropriate investigation."[2] It is a diagnosis of exclusion: what constitutes an appropriate investigation depends on the expertise of the physician assigning the diagnosis and pretreatment diagnostic investigations.

Epidemiology

SCCUP accounts for approximately 1% to 4% of all cancers of the head and neck.[3] Recent series suggest that an increasing proportion of SCCUP is associated with human papilloma virus (HPV),[4] and that the incidence is increasing at a rate similar to that of "known-primary" oropharynx cancer.[5]

The authors have nothing to disclose.
Department of Radiation Oncology, Fox Chase Cancer Center, 333 Cottman Avenue, Philadelphia, PA 19111, USA
* Corresponding author.
E-mail address: Thomas.galloway@fccc.edu

Surg Oncol Clin N Am 24 (2015) 579–591
http://dx.doi.org/10.1016/j.soc.2015.03.007
1055-3207/15/$ – see front matter © 2015 Elsevier Inc. All rights reserved.

surgonc.theclinics.com

Histology

Most cases of unknown primary of the head and neck are SCC.[6,7] Adenocarcinoma represents a minority of unknown primary cases and typically presents in the low neck or supraclavicular fossa.[8] A primary presentation of unknown primary adenocarcinoma in this location is suggestive of a primary site below the clavicles.[9] Thyroid cancer, lymphoma, melanoma, and other diseases occasionally present with a palpable neck metastasis, similar to the presentation of SCCUP. Management of these histologies will not be addressed here.

PATIENT EVALUATION

Mechanisms used to identify a small primary tumor of the head and neck have evolved over the past 70 years. Increasing sophistication of imaging and examination has narrowed the population of patients typically considered as "unknown primary." This is an important consideration when evaluating SCCUP in the literature; a patient with what was once an "unknown primary" in a historical series may now instead prove to have a small primary tumor.

Clinical Presentation and Imaging

The most common presentation of SCCUP is a painless neck mass that is refractory to antibiotics. In the absence of an identifiable primary, most patients with SCCUP deny upper aerodigestive tract symptoms.

Level II is the most commonly involved with SCCUP. Presentation of SCCUP in level III without concurrent involvement of level II suggests a primary in the supraglottic larynx or hypopharynx, because these locations more commonly drain directly to mid-neck.[10] Presentation with lymph nodes in the low neck (level IV, supraclavicular fossa) is associated with a primary site below the clavicles.[11] Approximately 50% of cases present with a single lymph node, whereas 10% to 20% may have bilateral involvement.[12–14]

Three-dimensional anatomic head and neck imaging has consistently identified small primary tumors not appreciated on physical examination.[15,16] Positron emission tomography (PET) can further help identify small primaries not appreciated by anatomic imaging or physical examination.[17]

A chest radiograph is necessary before initiating therapy to evaluate for distant metastases. More advanced imaging can be obtained at the discretion of the treating physician. Metastases below the clavicle are uncommon, but may be detected incidentally by PET scans undertaken to identify a primary site.

Tissue Confirmation and Tumor Markers

Fine-needle aspiration (FNA) of the presenting lymph node is the preferred method for obtaining a tissue diagnosis. A nondiagnostic FNA with a clinical suspicion of SCCUP should be performed again, perhaps with ultrasound guidance. If necessary to assign diagnosis, open biopsy should be performed only by a surgeon prepared to undertake definitive surgical management (completion neck dissection) as part of the care at that setting.[2] Open biopsy as an isolated procedure to confirm the diagnosis is discouraged because of the possibility for tumor spillage and the disruption of fascial planes that act as a natural barrier to tumor spread.[18]

Testing of the neck nodes for Epstein-Bar virus (EBV) and HPV can focus diagnostic and therapeutic interventions for SCCUP.[2] The presence of EBV detected via in situ hybridization in metastatic lymph nodes has been associated with a nasopharyngeal primary.[8] A positive p16 stain is most commonly associated with HPV-associated oropharynx tumors,[19] although practitioners must be mindful that cancers from other head and neck sites may stain for p16.[20,21] A considerable number of unknown primary cases reported in modern literature are HPV-associated (**Table 1**).

Panendoscopy and Biopsy

If no potential primary site has been identified by physical examination or if imaging does not disclose a primary site, then an examination under anesthesia (EUA) should be performed. This may include a nasopharyngeal survey; esophagoscopy (especially for a level IV/supraclavicular lymph node); tonsillectomy; and direct laryngoscopy with directed biopsies of the nasopharynx, base of tongue, supraglottic larynx, and piriform sinus. Historically, the yield of panendoscopy yield was high.[22] Although the primary tumor identification at EUA is less frequent in modern series,[15] endoscopy and biopsy are essential parts of the evaluation because of the high rate of false-negative imaging examinations.

In addition to the typical targets for biopsy listed previously, and regardless of imaging findings, directed biopsies should sample all areas of mucosal irregularity or easy bleeding seen on endoscopy.

Role of Lingual or Palatine Tonsillectomy

The palatine tonsils often conceal an "occult" primary, and thus an ipsilateral palatine tonsillectomy has become a standard component of the initial evaluation of SCCUP.[23] Whether an ipsilateral or bilateral tonsillectomy is required is unclear. Although a small but measurable group of patients prove to have a contralateral occult primary,[24] patients spared a contralateral tonsillectomy do not seem to have an increased rate of mucosal relapse or progression.

Recently, advancements in transoral surgery (TOS) have allowed head and neck surgeons to perform a lingual tonsillectomy through the open mouth, frequently demonstrating a T1 tumor (**Table 2**).[25–29] It is uncertain whether the extraordinarily high rates of primary identification with TOS will demonstrably affect outcomes.

INITIAL TREATMENT

Most patients with SCCUP are treated with multimodality therapy. Similar to oropharynx cancer, multimodality therapy is most commonly either resection followed by adjuvant radiation (±chemotherapy) or primary chemoradiation (±post-therapy

Table 1
Human papilloma virus association of squamous cell carcinoma of an unknown primary (SCCUP)

Author, Year	n	Years	p16+, %
Keller et al,[4] 2013	35	1990–2010	74
Demiroz et al,[45] 2014	17	1994–2008	59
Nagel et al,[25] 2014	52	1996–2011	78 86 True unknown primary
Desai et al,[52] 2009	41	2000–2007	27
Graboyes et al,[28] 2014	71	2001–2012	92[a]
Compton et al,[53] 2011	25	2002–2009	28
Durmus et al,[26] 2014	22	2008–2012	95[a]

[a] Most patients in these 2 series had a small oropharyngeal primary found with transoral techniques and therefore do not represent true SCCUP. The information gained by including them is uncertain.

Table 2
Transoral surgical techniques to identify the primary cancer

Author, Year	n	Years	Prior EUA (Tonsillectomy), %	Prior CT or MRI, %	Prior PET/CT, %	Transoral Surgery Yield (in Either Tonsil or BOT), %
Durmus et al,[26] 2014	11[a]	2008–2012	100 (0)	100	100	63
Nagel et al,[25] 2014	36	2002–2011	100 (0)	—	—	86
Mehta et al,[27] 2013	10	2009–2011	100 (100)	100	100	100 (all in BOT)
Graboyes et al,[28] 2014	65	2001–2012	100 (0)	100	65	89
Patel et al,[29] 2013	18[a]	2010–2013	100 (13)	81 CT 6 MRI	57	72

Abbreviations: BOT, base of tongue; CT, computed tomography; EUA, examination under anesthesia; PET, positron emission tomography.
[a] Reporting in this table limited to the patients without examination/imaging highly suspicious for primary tumor before lingual ± palatine tonsillectomy.

neck dissection). Similar to known-primary mucosal cancer of the head and neck,[30] patients with SCCUP do well with either approach and institutional patterns of care often determine treatment. Efficacy data seem to be similar, so an evaluation of the toxicity of both treatment paradigms is warranted.

Surgery

Primary surgical treatment for SCCUP is a neck dissection. The extent of the neck dissection is determined by the disease presentation. Management with surgery alone for SCCUP requires the accurate identification of patients at low risk for both mucosal emergence and neck failure. Data reporting the outcomes of this management technique are sparse because of the relatively limited group of patients for whom it is appropriate.

The largest series of surgery alone reports the outcomes of 104 patients from 1948 to 1968.[14] During this time, 52 patients were treated with primary radiation (RT) and 28 were treated with surgery plus postoperative RT. In general, the patients treated by surgery alone had a lower disease burden in the neck. "Almost all" patients had an examination with biopsies under general anesthesia and none had cross-sectional imaging. The mucosal failure rate was 20%. The neck failure rate was 13% for patients with Nx/N1 necks and 32% for patients with N2/N3 necks. Other series[3,31–34] substantiate that both mucosal progression and contralateral neck failure are uncommon in selected patients, even in the absence of RT (**Table 3**). The most common sites of recurrence reported for SCCUP, even in the absence of pretreatment imaging, transoral diagnostic techniques, and RT, are in the ipsilateral neck and distantly. The notable exception to this is a Danish experience that demonstrates high rates of mucosal emergence and neck recurrence. Because the stated policy of the Danish health system during the study period was to approach head and neck cancer with primary RT, it seems likely that these results were referable to undetermined selection bias.

As a result of the low relapse rates in select patients with T0N1 SCCUP, it is generally accepted that surgery alone is sufficient for this presentation.[31] Historically, T0N1 squamous cancer of the head and neck has been a rare entity (6 patients total in the largest series referenced previously).

Radiation Therapy ± Neck Dissection

Most patients with SCCUP receive RT. Most also undergo a neck dissection. Retrospective series rarely indicate whether the neck dissection was performed before or

Table 3
Primary surgery alone for squamous cell carcinoma of an unknown primary

Author, Year	n	Years	NX/N1, %	Prior EUA (w Biopsy), %	Prior CT or MRI, %	Prior PET, %	Mucosal Emergence, %	Ipsilateral Neck Failure, %	Contralateral Neck Failure, %	Distant Failure, %
Jesse et al,[14] 1973	104	1948–1968	43	Almost all (usually)	0	0	20	24	16	—
Coster[31]	24	1965–1987	54	46 (not specified)	0	0	4	25	8	4
Wang[32]	57	1953–1988	>50	All (all)	All patients from 1982–1988	0	11	12	—	13
Coker[33]	26	1949–1976	35	69 (not specified)	0	0	12	8	4	16
Grau et al,[3] 2000	23	1975–1995	43	94 (55)	30 CT 7 MRI	1	54	42	42	—
Iganej[34]	29	1969–1994	17	100 (all after "late 1970s")	0	0	4	25	8	10

Abbreviations: CT, computed tomography; EUA, examination under anesthesia; PET, positron emission tomography. Values of mucosal emergence, contralateral/ipsilateral neck failure, and distant failure reflect crude reporting.

after RT as a component of combined modality therapy. There is no suggestion that the timing of the neck dissection informs disease-free survival.

Historically, SCCUP was treated with a 3-field technique.[35] All mucosal sites and both sides of the neck were treated. This was supplanted by larynx-sparing techniques, without a subsequent increase in mucosal failures in the blocked larynx/hypopharynx.[36] Today, salivary preservation intensity-modulated RT has become the most common radiation technique for SCCUP.[37] This affords considerable flexibility to the radiation oncologist when determining which tissues receive radiation.

Unilateral Versus Bilateral Neck Radiation

In most retrospective series involving RT for SCCUP (both definitive and adjuvant), a small proportion of patients receive unilateral treatment. Because the percentage of patients managed unilaterally is almost always smaller than those treated bilaterally (**Table 4**), it seems that unilateral therapy represents a departure from common practice. Despite this, mucosal emergence and contralateral neck recurrence are rare with unilateral treatment.[3,13,38–42]

The single prospective randomized study of SCCUP was EORTC 22205, a phase III trial comparing comprehensive bilateral neck and mucosal RT to 50 Gy (followed by a 10 Gy boost to the ipsilateral neck) and ipsilateral neck RT to 60 Gy alone. Planned accrual was 600 patients. The trial closed after 2 years because of poor accrual and no results have been reported.

Routine bilateral neck RT produces gratifying oncologic results (**Table 5**).[3,4,10,37,41–49] Mucosal emergence occurs in fewer than 10%. Contralateral neck failure is extremely rare. In modern series, the most common source of recurrence is distant metastatic disease.

Mucosal Sites

The oropharynx is the most common location to find an occult primary, and hence the oropharynx should be treated with radiation if the mucosa is to be treated. In view of the small but known incidence of bilateral tonsil cancer[24] and emerging transoral investigations demonstrating primary tumors in the contralateral base of tongue, it is standard to treat the bilateral mucosa.

Treatment of the nasopharynx is less common, and a number of practitioners omit the nasopharynx from the treatment field in selected patients, particularly those with p16+ nodal disease. Early experience suggests that treatment with this technique of non-Asian patients with p16+/EBV– neck nodes does not result in increased mucosal failure.[49] However, treatment to the ipsilateral retrostyloid space and the retropharyngeal nodes (recently termed level VII[50]) with an intensity-modulated technique generally results in considerable dose delivery to the nasopharynx regardless of whether or not it is included in the clinical target volume. Hence, the impact of nasopharyngeal avoidance may be small.

The previous paragraphs are applicable to SCCUP with cancer limited to level II or with a predominance of disease in level II and smaller-volume disease in level III. This is by far the most common presentation of SCCUP (estimated to be 70%–80%). By contrast, SCCUP presenting without involvement of level II is much more likely to have a mucosal primary in the supraglottic larynx or hypopharynx, in which case larynx-sparing RT would not be appropriate.

Radiation Dose

RT dose to the neck follows treatment paradigms for known-primary cancer: 66 to 70 Gy for gross disease, 60 to 66 Gy for adjuvant therapy to high-risk areas, and

Table 4
Unilateral neck radiation for squamous cell carcinoma of an unknown primary

Author, Year	Years	n[a]	Prior EUA (with Biopsy), %	Prior CT or MRI, %	Prior PET, %	Chemo RT, %	Neck Dissection, %	Mucosal Emergence, %	Ipsilateral Neck Failure, %	Contralateral Neck Failure, %	Distant Failure,[b] %
Glyyne-Jones[38]	1954–1986	34 (87)	94 (94)	0	0	0	7	6[c]	24	2	18
Marcial-Vega[39]	1965–1987	19 (72)	97 (89)	6	0	0	36 ExBx: 7	5[c]	—	—	31
Weir[40]	1970–1986	85 (144)	92 (68)	67 (Plain film and CT)	0	0	0 ExBx: 49	7[c]	46	3	8
Reddy[41]	1974–1989	16 (52)	All	All had CT after 1978	0	0	60 ExBx: 15	44[d]	19[d]	44[d]	15[d]
Grau et al,[3] 2000	1975–1995	26 (352)	94 (55)	30 CT 7 MRI	1	0	15	12[c]	Not reported LRC: 43	4	7
Sinnathamby et al,[13] 1997	1983–1992	48 (69)	84 (not specified)	55 CT	0	0	39 ExBx: 23	13[d]	29	4	6
Perkins[42]	1989–2008	21 (21)	100 (100)	100	50	IND: 9 CRT: 22	80 ExBx: 7.5	9.5	0	5[d]	22[d]

Abbreviations: ChemoRT, concurrent chemoradiation; CRT, concurrent chemotherapy; CT, computed tomography; EUA, examination under anesthesia; ExBx, excisional biopsy; IND, induction chemotherapy; LRC, local-regional control; PET, positron emission tomography.

[a] The number listed is the number of patients noted to receive unilateral neck RT. The number in parentheses is the total number of patients noted in the citation.

[b] For the entire series.

[c] Head and neck only.

[d] Actuarial value reported in the citation. Otherwise, values of mucosal emergence, contralateral/ipsilateral neck failure, and distant failure reflect crude reporting.

Table 5
Bilateral neck radiation

Author, Year	n[a]	Years	Prior EUA (with Biopsy), %	Prior CT or MRI, %	Prior PET, %	Chemo RT, %	Neck Dissection, %	Mucosal Emergence, %	Ipsilateral Neck Failure, %	Contralateral Neck Failure, %	Distant Failure,[b] %
Wallace[44]	179	1964–2006	87 (—)	74 CT 8 MRI	9	1 IND 5 CRT	61	8 actuarial rate at 5 y	19 actuarial rate at 5 y	8 actuarial rate at 5 y	14 actuarial rate at 5 y
Colletier[43]	136 (120)	1968–1992	96 (83)	45	0	0	71 29 ExBx	8 actuarial rate at 5 y	8	1	15 actuarial rate at 5 y
Reddy[41]	36	1974–1989	All	All after 1978	0	0	63	8	31	14	15
Grau et al,[3] 2000	224	1975–1995	94 (55)	30 CT 7 MRI	1	0	9 45 ExBx	8[c]	Not Reported LRC: 48	2	7
Perkins[42]	25	1989–2008	100 (100)	100 CT or MRI	36	28	68 8 ExBx	4	0	0	22
Ligey et al,[10] 2009	36	1990–2007	— (19)	Use of CT 'Varied' 2 MRI	17	6 IND 39 CRT	83	6	19	19	30
Keller et al,[4] 2013	35	1990–2010	100 (100)	100 CT or MRI	40	11	89 11 ExBx	3	0	0	8

Demiroz[45]	41	1994–2009	100 (100)	100 CT or MRI	66	61	54 ExBx:29	5	5	0	19.50
Frank[37]	52 (46)	1998–2005	100 (—)	100 CT or MRI	50	15 IND 12 CRT	50 27 ExBx	2 actuarial rate at 5 y	4	2	8.3 actuarial rate at 5 y
Klem[46]	21	2000–2005	—	100 CT and/or MRI	95	67	62 14 ExBx	0	10	0	10
Chen[47]	60	2001–2009	100 (100)	100 CT	32	53	70 5 ExBx	3	5	2	16 actuarial rate at 2 y
Sher[48]	24	2004–2009	100 (100)	100 CT	100	29 IND 100 CRT	25 33 ExBx	0	0	0	4
Mourad[49]	68	1998–2010	All	—	—	56	44 6 ExBx	2	3	0	0

Values reported for mucosal emergence, ipsilateral/contralateral neck failure, and distant failure reflect crude reporting unless otherwise specified.

Abbreviations: ChemoRT, concurrent chemoradiation; CRT, Concurrent chemotherapy; CT, computed tomography; EUA, examination under anesthesia; ExBx, Excisional biopsy; IND, induction chemotherapy; LRC, local-regional control; PET, positron emission tomography.

a In 2 series, a small number of patients were treated unilaterally. The number in parentheses represents the total number of patients treated bilaterally. Outcomes of those treated unilaterally were not reported separately from those treated bilaterally. This table is based on all patients treated (as reported in the citations).

b In all instances, distant metastases are reported as a single number in these citations, regardless of different treatment techniques.

c Head and neck only.

45 to 54 Gy to elective areas of the neck. RT dose to the mucosa is nuanced. Many institutions appear to treat the mucosa to a subclinical dose similar to what was considered standard in the failed EORTC trial (eg, 50 Gy in 25 fractions or 54 Gy in 30 fractions). The underlying assumption is that an area with no gross disease, but risk of harboring subclinical tumor, merits treatment with a subclinical dose of RT, regardless of whether it resides in the neck or the mucosa.[37] Other institutions prefer to increase the dose to the (ipsilateral) oropharynx to 60 to 64 Gy. The rationale for this is the knowledge that the ipsilateral oropharynx is the most likely location of the primary tumor.[25] Considering the good prognosis with this disease, and the paucity of mucosal failure regardless of elective RT dose, intensifying dose to the oropharynx seems unnecessary.

Chemotherapy

Although not included in prospective trials demonstrating the benefit of concurrent chemotherapy for locally advanced head and neck cancer, the ipsilateral neck failure rate of greater than 20% (see **Table 2**) suggests that intensification of therapy could be beneficial. Modern series using a variety of chemoradiation regimens demonstrate excellent tumor control.[48,51] Although some data sets do not demonstrate a benefit from concurrent systemic therapy,[47] the current approach is to deliver chemoradiation for the N2-N3 SCCUP when managed with primary RT.

SUMMARY

SCCUP is a rare diagnosis of exclusion. Although not included on prospective trials of "known-primary" head and neck cancer, application of the general principles of head and neck oncology to SCCUP generally results in a gratifying control rate.

The treatment of SCCUP has changed considerably in the past 70 years, and will likely continue to change secondary to the improving ability to identify small primary tumors and better tailor the implementation of multimodality therapy.

REFERENCES

1. Martin H, Morfit HM. Cervical lymph node metastasis as the first symptom of cancer. Surg Gynecol Obstet 1944;78:133–59.
2. National Comprehensive Cancer Network. Head and neck cancers V2. 2014. Available at: http://www.nccn.org/professionals/physician_gls/pdf/head-and-neck.pdf. Accessed June 24, 2014.
3. Grau C, Johansen LV, Jakobsen J, et al. Cervical lymph node metastases from unknown primary tumours. Results from a national survey by the Danish Society for Head and Neck Oncology. Radiother Oncol 2000;55:121–9.
4. Keller LM, Galloway TJ, Holdbrook T, et al. p16 status, pathologic and clinical characteristics, biomolecular signature, and long term outcomes in unknown primary carcinomas of the head and neck. Head Neck 2013;36(12):1677–84.
5. Galloway TJ, Davis KS, Burtness B, et al. Association and the Increasing incidence of unknown primary head and neck squamous cell carcinoma. ASCO/ASTRO Multidisciplinary Head and Neck Cancer Symposium. February 20-22. Scottsdale (AZ), 2014.
6. Vaamonde P, Martin Martin C, del Rio Valeiras M, et al. A study of cervical metastases from unknown primary tumor. Acta Otorrinolaringol Esp 2002;53:601–6 [in Spanish].
7. Strojan P, Anicin A. Combined surgery and postoperative radiotherapy for cervical lymph node metastases from an unknown primary tumour. Radiother Oncol 1998;49:33–40.

8. Lee WY, Hsiao JR, Jin YT, et al. Epstein-Barr virus detection in neck metastases by in-situ hybridization in fine-needle aspiration cytologic studies: an aid for differentiating the primary site. Head Neck 2000;22:336–40.

9. Giridharan W, Hughes J, Fenton JE, et al. Lymph node metastases in the lower neck. Clin Otolaryngol Allied Sci 2003;28:221–6.

10. Ligey A, Gentil J, Crehange G, et al. Impact of target volumes and radiation technique on loco-regional control and survival for patients with unilateral cervical lymph node metastases from an unknown primary. Radiother Oncol 2009;93:483–7.

11. Koivunen P, Laranne J, Virtaniemi J, et al. Cervical metastasis of unknown origin: a series of 72 patients. Acta Otolaryngol 2002;122:569–74.

12. Erkal HS, Mendenhall WM, Amdur RJ, et al. Squamous cell carcinomas metastatic to cervical lymph nodes from an unknown head and neck mucosal site treated with radiation therapy with palliative intent. Radiother Oncol 2001;59:319–21.

13. Sinnathamby K, Peters LJ, Laidlaw C, et al. The occult head and neck primary: to treat or not to treat? Clin Oncol (R Coll Radiol) 1997;9:322–9.

14. Jesse RH, Perez CA, Fletcher GH. Cervical lymph node metastasis: unknown primary cancer. Cancer 1973;31:854–9.

15. Mendenhall WM, Mancuso AA, Parsons JT, et al. Diagnostic evaluation of squamous cell carcinoma metastatic to cervical lymph nodes from an unknown head and neck primary site. Head Neck 1998;20:739–44.

16. Muraki AS, Mancuso AA, Harnsberger HR. Metastatic cervical adenopathy from tumors of unknown origin: the role of CT. Radiology 1984;152:749–53.

17. Johansen J, Buus S, Loft A, et al. Prospective study of 18FDG-PET in the detection and management of patients with lymph node metastases to the neck from an unknown primary tumor. Results from the DAHANCA-13 study. Head Neck 2008;30:471–8.

18. Schiff BA, Mutyala S, Smith RV. Ch. 12: metastatic cancer to the neck from an unknown primary site. In: Louis B, Harrison MD, Roy B, et al, editors. Head and neck cancer: a multidisciplinary approach. 3rd edition. Philadelphia: Wolters Kluwer Helath/Lipincott, Williams & Wilkins; 2009. p. 232–49.

19. Begum S, Gillison ML, Nicol TL, et al. Detection of human papillomavirus-16 in fine-needle aspirates to determine tumor origin in patients with metastatic squamous cell carcinoma of the head and neck. Clin Cancer Res 2007;13:1186–91.

20. Chung CH, Zhang Q, Kong CS, et al. p16 protein expression and human papillomavirus status as prognostic biomarkers of nonoropharyngeal head and neck squamous cell carcinoma. J Clin Oncol 2014;32(35):3930–8.

21. Beadle BM, William WN Jr, McLemore MS, et al. p16 expression in cutaneous squamous carcinomas with neck metastases: a potential pitfall in identifying unknown primaries of the head and neck. Head Neck 2013;35:1527–33.

22. Jones AS, Cook JA, Phillips DE, et al. Squamous carcinoma presenting as an enlarged cervical lymph node. Cancer 1993;72:1756–61.

23. Jereczek-Fossa BA, Jassem J, Orecchia R. Cervical lymph node metastases of squamous cell carcinoma from an unknown primary. Cancer Treat Rev 2004;30:153–64.

24. Koch WM, Bhatti N, Williams MF, et al. Oncologic rationale for bilateral tonsillectomy in head and neck squamous cell carcinoma of unknown primary source. Otolaryngol Head Neck Surg 2001;124:331–3.

25. Nagel TH, Hinni ML, Hayden RE, et al. Transoral laser microsurgery for the unknown primary: role for lingual tonsillectomy. Head Neck 2014;36:942–6.

26. Durmus K, Rangarajan SV, Old MO, et al. Transoral robotic approach to carcinoma of unknown primary. Head Neck 2014;36:848–52.
27. Mehta V, Johnson P, Tassler A, et al. A new paradigm for the diagnosis and management of unknown primary tumors of the head and neck: a role for transoral robotic surgery. Laryngoscope 2013;123:146–51.
28. Graboyes EM, Sinha P, Thorstad WL, et al. Management of human papillomavirus-related unknown primaries of the head and neck with a transoral surgical approach. Head Neck 2014. [Epub ahead of print].
29. Patel SA, Magnuson JS, Holsinger FC, et al. Robotic surgery for primary head and neck squamous cell carcinoma of unknown site. JAMA Otolaryngol Head Neck Surg 2013;139:1203–11.
30. Parsons JT, Mendenhall WM, Stringer SP, et al. Squamous cell carcinoma of the oropharynx: surgery, radiation therapy, or both. Cancer 2002;94:2967–80.
31. Coster JR, Foote RL, Olsen KD, et al. Cervical nodal metastasis of squamous cell carcinoma of unknown origin: indications for withholding radiation therapy. Int J Radiat Oncol Biol Phys 1992;23:743–9.
32. Wang RC, Goepfert H, Barber AE, et al. Unknown primary squamous cell carcinoma metastatic to the neck. Arch Otolaryngol Head Neck Surg 1990;116:1388–93.
33. Coker DD, Casterline PF, Chambers RG, et al. Metastases to lymph nodes of the head and neck from an unknown primary site. Am J Surg 1977;134:517–22.
34. Iganej S, Kagan R, Anderson P, et al. Metastatic squamous cell carcinoma of the neck from an unknown primary: management options and patterns of relapse. Head Neck 2002;24:236–46.
35. Million RR, Cassisi NJ, Mancuso AA. The unknown primary. In: Million RR, Cassisi NJ, editors. Management of head and neck cancer: a multidisciplinary approach. 2nd edition. Philadelphia: J.B. Lipincott; 1994. p. 311–20.
36. Barker CA, Morris CG, Mendenhall WM. Larynx-sparing radiotherapy for squamous cell carcinoma from an unknown head and neck primary site. Am J Clin Oncol 2005;28:445–8.
37. Frank SJ, Rosenthal DI, Petsuksiri J, et al. Intensity-modulated radiotherapy for cervical node squamous cell carcinoma metastases from unknown head-and-neck primary site: M. D. Anderson Cancer Center outcomes and patterns of failure. Int J Radiat Oncol Biol Phys 2010;78:1005–10.
38. Glynne-Jones RG, Anand AK, Young TE, et al. Metastatic carcinoma in the cervical lymph nodes from an occult primary: a conservative approach to the role of radiotherapy. Int J Radiat Oncol Biol Phys 1990;18:289–94.
39. Marcial-Vega VA, Cardenes H, Perez CA, et al. Cervical metastases from unknown primaries: radiotherapeutic management and appearance of subsequent primaries. Int J Radiat Oncol Biol Phys 1990;19:919–28.
40. Weir L, Keane T, Cummings B, et al. Radiation treatment of cervical lymph node metastases from an unknown primary: an analysis of outcome by treatment volume and other prognostic factors. Radiother Oncol 1995;35:206–11.
41. Reddy SP, Marks JE. Metastatic carcinoma in the cervical lymph nodes from an unknown primary site: results of bilateral neck plus mucosal irradiation vs. ipsilateral neck irradiation. Int J Radiat Oncol Biol Phys 1997;37:797–802.
42. Perkins SM, Spencer CR, Chernock RD, et al. Radiotherapeutic management of cervical lymph node metastases from an unknown primary site. Arch Otolaryngol Head Neck Surg 2012;138:656–61.
43. Colletier PJ, Garden AS, Morrison WH, et al. Postoperative radiation for squamous cell carcinoma metastatic to cervical lymph nodes from an unknown primary site: outcomes and patterns of failure. Head Neck 1998;20:674–81.

44. Wallace A, Richards GM, Harari PM, et al. Head and neck squamous cell carcinoma from an unknown primary site. Am J Otolaryngol 2011;32:286–90.
45. Demiroz C, Vainshtein JM, Koukourakis GV, et al. Head and neck squamous cell carcinoma of unknown primary: neck dissection and radiotherapy or definitive radiotherapy. Head Neck 2014;36:1589–95.
46. Klem ML, Mechalakos JG, Wolden SL, et al. Intensity-modulated radiotherapy for head and neck cancer of unknown primary: toxicity and preliminary efficacy. Int J Radiat Oncol Biol Phys 2008;70:1100–7.
47. Chen AM, Farwell DG, Lau DH, et al. Radiation therapy in the management of head-and-neck cancer of unknown primary origin: how does the addition of concurrent chemotherapy affect the therapeutic ratio? Int J Radiat Oncol Biol Phys 2011;81:346–52.
48. Sher DJ, Balboni TA, Haddad RI, et al. Efficacy and toxicity of chemoradiotherapy using intensity-modulated radiotherapy for unknown primary of head and neck. Int J Radiat Oncol Biol Phys 2011;80:1405–11.
49. Mourad WF, Hu KS, Shasha D, et al. Initial experience with oropharynx-targeted radiation therapy for metastatic squamous cell carcinoma of unknown primary of the head and neck. Anticancer Res 2014;34:243–8.
50. Gregoire V, Ang K, Budach W, et al. Delineation of the neck node levels for head and neck tumors: a 2013 update. DAHANCA, EORTC, HKNPCSG, NCIC CTG, NCRI, RTOG, TROG consensus guidelines. Radiother Oncol 2014;110:172–81.
51. Shehadeh NJ, Ensley JF, Kucuk O, et al. Benefit of postoperative chemoradiotherapy for patients with unknown primary squamous cell carcinoma of the head and neck. Head Neck 2006;28:1090–8.
52. Desai PC, Jaglal MV, Gopal P, et al. Human papillomavirus in metastatic squamous carcinoma from unknown primaries in the head and neck: a retrospective 7 year study. Exp Mol Pathol 2009;87:94–8.
53. Compton AM, Moore-Medlin T, Herman-Ferdinandez L, et al. Human papillomavirus in metastatic lymph nodes from unknown primary head and neck squamous cell carcinoma. Otolaryngol Head Neck Surg 2011;145:51–7.

Cutaneous Malignancy of the Head and Neck

Wojciech K. Mydlarz, MD, Randal S. Weber, MD, Michael E. Kupferman, MD*

KEYWORDS

- Head and neck • Nonmelanoma skin cancer • Melanoma
- Squamous cell carcinoma (SCC) • Basal cell carcinoma (BCC)
- Wide local excision (WLE) • Sentinel lymph node biopsy • Radiation therapy

KEY POINTS

- Nonmelanoma skin cancer (NMSC) is the most common malignancy in the United States, and surgical resection is curative in 95% of patients when treated early.
- Understanding the complex anatomy and lymphatic drainage patterns when managing melanoma is key because involvement of the regional nodes has the strongest impact on survival.
- Advanced and aggressive tumors merit comprehensive physical examination, radiographic and histopathology evaluation, and treatment by a multidisciplinary team of cutaneous oncology experts.
- Surgical resection with clear margins is essential for the oncologic control of disease.
- Advanced and aggressive lesions demand multimodality treatment entailing surgical resection, staging of the regional lymph node basins, and adjuvant radiation therapy to maximize locoregional control.

INTRODUCTION

Cutaneous malignancy represents a worldwide public health problem, with a rapidly rising incidence, decreasing age at presentation, and significant health care costs.[1–6] Head and neck skin cancers encompass a broad range of histologies, the most commonly encountered entities being basal cell carcinoma (BCC), squamous cell carcinoma (SCC), and melanoma. Many health care providers diagnose and treat skin cancer, from providers at rural primary care clinics to those at urban dermatologic surgery practices and large tertiary care head and neck cancer centers. Some of these tumors prove to be diagnostic and treatment challenges, with associated increased morbidity and mortality.[7]

The authors have nothing to disclose.
Department of Head and Neck Surgery, The University of Texas M. D. Anderson Cancer Center, 1515 Holcombe Boulevard, Houston, TX 77030, USA
* Corresponding author. Department of Head and Neck Surgery, The University of Texas M. D. Anderson Cancer Center, 1515 Holcombe Boulevard, Unit 1445, Houston, TX 77030.
E-mail address: mekupfer@mdanderson.org

Surg Oncol Clin N Am 24 (2015) 593–613
http://dx.doi.org/10.1016/j.soc.2015.03.010
1055-3207/15/$ – see front matter © 2015 Elsevier Inc. All rights reserved.

Most cutaneous malignancies, BCCs, and SCCs can effectively be treated through a variety of means when diagnosed early enough. Some NMSCs and melanoma spread to regional lymph nodes, can be aggressive, and recur locally. Aggressive and more advanced lesions demand multimodality treatment entailing surgical resection, staging of the regional lymph node basins, and radiation therapy, as the survival from aggressive disease remains poor because of locoregional recurrences and distant metastasis. Potentially advanced and aggressive tumors merit more comprehensive evaluation and treatment by a multidisciplinary team of experts in cutaneous oncology. This article reviews the management of skin cancer of the head and neck, including BCC, SCC, and melanoma.

EPIDEMIOLOGY

Cutaneous BCC and SCC are the most commonly diagnosed NMSCs in the United States and account for over 1 million new cancers annually.[1,3,5,6,8,9] Approximately 70% to 80% of all skin malignancies are BCCs, whereas 15% are SCCs. The remaining 5% are primarily melanoma and other uncommon entities, particularly adnexal tumors and Merkel cell carcinomas.[1,8,9] The clinical behavior of BCC is distinct from that of SCC. BCC is locally aggressive with a low propensity for metastasis; SCC may display aggressive biological behavior, characterized by perineural invasion and potential for regional metastasis.[8,9]

Although melanoma represents less than 5% of the cases, it is responsible for more than 75% of skin-cancer-related deaths.[3] In the United States, each year about 70,200 patients are diagnosed with melanoma and 8800 die of this disease. The incidence of melanoma has risen dramatically over the past several decades, with an increase of greater than 200% in the age-adjusted incidence from 1975 to 2008.[10–15] This increase is manifested across all age groups and primary tumor thicknesses. The mortality rate has also increased approximately 60% over time, primarily because of increased mortality in patients aged 65 years or older, particularly among men.[10,14,15] However, many patients who die of melanoma are young and healthy, so melanoma is among the cancers with the highest life years lost per fatality.[16,17]

RISK FACTORS

Sun exposure is the single greatest risk factor for the development of NMSC. Both the duration and intensity of UV radiation (UVR) exposure, primarily UV-A (320–400 nm) and UV-B (290–320 nm) radiations, contribute to DNA damage at the cellular level of the epidermis.[8,9,18,19] Thus, these cancers usually arise in sun-exposed areas and progress from premalignant actinic lesions to invasive carcinomas. Similarly, individuals with a history of facial or neck irradiation are at an increased risk for the development of skin cancer.[8,9,20]

For melanoma, there is also strong evidence that increased exposure to UVR plays a role.[6,21] Multiple studies support a causative role for UVR in cutaneous melanoma.[10] A history of sunburns from natural UVR and the use of tanning beds (artificial UVR) are risk factors for melanoma. Public surveys have reported increasing prevalence of both behaviors among US adults.[22] Intermittent sun damage/exposure has consistently been identified as a risk factor, whereas some studies suggest that long-term sun exposure is associated with a decrease in the risk of melanoma.[23] Other risk factors for cutaneous melanoma include a family history of the disease, multiple nevi, dysplastic nevi, freckled or fair skin, blue or green eyes, and red hair.[22,24]

It is increasingly recognized that patients who have undergone organ transplant have a 30-fold increased risk of developing cutaneous SCC and 10-fold increased risk of developing BCC.[9,25,26] The role of the human papillomavirus in skin carcinogenesis is under investigation.[27,28] Other than sun avoidance and the use of topical sunblock with a sun protection factor exceeding 30, no preventative treatments are available.[5,8,9]

NONMELANOMA SKIN CANCER
Clinical Evaluation

A complete history and physical examination is paramount in the accurate assessment of the patient with NMSC.[8,9,29] An enlarging or ulcerating skin lesion should be deemed to be a skin cancer until proven otherwise and should prompt immediate dermatologic attention for biopsy. Patients commonly report a remote history of a previously resected cutaneous malignancy, which may explain new-onset neck adenopathy, facial paresthesias, or a facial nerve paralysis. Complaints that suggest perineural invasion include facial weakness, formication (the sensation of insects crawling on the skin), hypesthesia, dysesthesia, and paresthesia.[30] A recurrent lesion may present as a slow-growing subcutaneous mass that invades the deep facial or neck musculature.

A complete dermatologic examination is necessary for the patient with NMSC. Numerous premalignant lesions may be present, and judicious biopsies should be performed. The clinician should pay particular attention to the identification of second primary tumors.[9,31,32] The dimensions of the primary tumor and its involvement with adjacent structures must be assessed. In the temporal and scalp regions, the cranial periosteum is a reliable barrier to bony invasion, which can be determined by the mobility of the lesion over the underlying deep tissue planes. Preauricular tumors may extend into the parotid gland or the external auditory canal, whereas cancers of the midface may extend along embryonic fusion planes to the nasal cavity or orbit. Other problematic areas are the nasolabial fold, the glabella, and the postauricular crease.[9,32]

The clinician should have a high index of suspicion for perineural invasion in the patient with SCC, and a thorough evaluation of the sensory and motor nerves may elicit objective evidence of nerve invasion. This evidence can sometimes be obtained through preoperative imaging such as computed tomography (CT) or MRI.[33,34]

BCC rarely spreads to the cervical lymphatics, whereas regional spread is common in patients with SCC. Overall, 25% of patients with advanced SCC ultimately develop parotid or neck metastases.[8,9] Lesions of the face and scalp that are anterior to an imaginary line drawn through the external auditory canal in the coronal plane frequently metastasize to the parotid bed. The posterior triangle and nuchal lymphatics may be involved by cutaneous lesions posterior to the anatomic plane, whereas submental and submandibular metastases arise from midface and lower lip lesions.[8,9]

High-resolution axial and coronal imaging is necessary for the complete staging of disease in the patient with NMSC. CT is generally preferred over MRI for evaluating the primary tumor, the status of the lymph nodes, and the presence of bony invasion.[35,36] MRI is better for the detection of perineural spread, dural invasion, and orbital disease (**Fig. 1**).[33,34] Patients with bulky lymph node metastasis should also be evaluated for distant metastasis with a CT scan of the chest. Ultrasonography of the neck and parotid bed is effective for the evaluation of the regional lymphatic basins. This technique can be combined with a fine-needle aspiration for the pathologic confirmation of neck node metastasis.[34,37] The role of fludeoxyglucose PET has not been fully elucidated, but this modality may have a role in the detection of deep soft tissue disease recurrence or distant metastasis in the previously treated patient.[38,39]

Histologic confirmation of all lesions is necessary in the treatment of NMSC because they may harbor aggressive pathologic features such as perineural or lymphovascular spread.

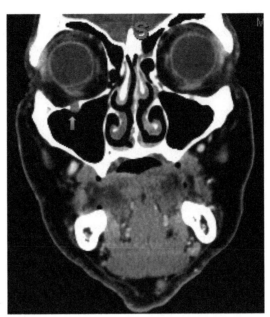

Fig. 1. Perineural spread. Coronal section of a contrast-enhanced CT scan of the head and neck depicting perineural spread along the right inferior orbital nerve. Note the abnormal thickening of the nerve within the infraorbital canal (*arrow*).

Staging

The American Joint Committee on Cancer's (AJCC's) (seventh edition) TNM staging system is currently used for staging BCCs and SCCs (**Tables 1** and **2**). Eyelid carcinoma has its own specific classification and staging system (**Tables 3** and **4**).

Pathology

Most NMSCs are BCCs, which arise from the basal layer of the cutaneous epithelium (**Fig. 2**). The 3 most common histologic subtypes of BCC, ranging from least to most aggressive, are (1) nodular, (2) superficial multifocal, and (3) infiltrative.[8,9,40,41] The nodular subtype accounts for 75% of all BCCs and is characterized by a raised, pearly lesion that is well circumscribed. The superficial subtype (10%) presents as an erythematous scaly plaque. The aggressive or infiltrative BCC (previously referred to as morpheaform BCC) has a propensity for subcutaneous invasion with fingerlike projections of tumor that extend into the surrounding soft tissues. Clinically, the lesion appears as a raised yellow plaque with indistinct borders.[40,41] Other less common histopathologic subtypes include basosquamous carcinoma and pigmented BCC.[8,9]

SCC accounts for 15% all skin cancers and is thought to arise from the spinous layer of the skin epithelium (see **Fig. 2**). Clinically, SCCs are ulcerative lesions that may arise in an actinic keratosis, a previous scar, or sun-exposed areas.[29,31] Squamous variants include adenosquamous carcinoma, spindle cell carcinoma, and clear cell tumors. In some cases, immunohistochemistry is necessary to establish the exact pathologic diagnosis.[29] These tumors display aggressive histopathologic behavior, with perineural invasion present in more than 15% of patients. Lymphovascular invasion is also common, with metastases to cervical lymphatics in 5% to 10% of patients. As expected, patients with SCC are at higher risk for distant metastasis and adverse prognosis than are those with BCC.[8,9,29]

Table 1
Classification of cutaneous SCC and other cutaneous carcinomas (excluding eyelid carcinoma)

Primary Tumor (T)	
Tx	Primary tumor cannot be assessed
T0	No evidence of primary tumor
Tis	Carcinoma in situ
T1	Tumor $\leq$2 cm in greatest dimension with <2 high-risk features[a]
T2	Tumor >2 cm in greatest dimension, or Tumor any size with $\geq$2 high-risk features[a]
T3	Tumor with invasion of maxilla, mandible, orbit, or temporal bone
T4	Tumor with invasion of skeleton (axial or appendicular) or perineural invasion of skull base

High-Risk Features for Primary Tumor (T)[a]	
Depth/invasion	>2 mm thickness (Breslow thickness) Clark level $\geq$IV Perineural invasion
Anatomic	Primary site ear
Location	Primary site hair-bearing lip
Differentiation	Poorly differentiated or undifferentiated

Regional Lymph Nodes (N)	
Nx	Regional lymph nodes cannot be assessed
N0	No regional lymph nodes
N1	Metastasis in a single ipsilateral lymph node, $\leq$3 cm in greatest dimension
N2a	Metastasis in a single ipsilateral lymph node, >3 cm but $\leq$6 cm in greatest dimension
N2b	Metastases in multiple ipsilateral lymph nodes, $\leq$6 cm in greatest dimension
N2c	Metastases in bilateral or contralateral lymph nodes, $\leq$6 cm in greatest dimension
N3	Metastasis in a lymph node, >6 cm in greatest dimension

Distant Metastasis (M)	
M0	No distant metastasis
M1	Distant metastasis present

[a] High risk tumor features which are listed and explained under High-Risk Features for Primary Tumor (T).

Table 2
Stage/prognostic groups for cutaneous SCC and other cutaneous carcinomas (excluding eyelid carcinoma)

Stage Groupings			
Stage 0	Tis	N0	M0
Stage I	T1	N0	M0
Stage II	T2	N0	M0
Stage III	T3	N0	M0
	T1-T3	N1	M0
Stage IV	T1-T3	N2	M0
	Any T	N3	M0
	T4	Any N	M0
	Any T	Any N	M1

Table 3
Classification of eyelid carcinoma

Primary Tumor (T)

Tx	Primary tumor cannot be assessed
T0	No evidence of primary tumor
Tis	Carcinoma in situ
T1	Tumor ≤5 mm in greatest dimension, or Not invading the tarsal plate or eyelid margin
T2a	Tumor >5 mm but not >10 mm in greatest dimension, or Any tumor that invades the tarsal plate or eyelid margin
T2b	Tumor >10 mm but not >20 mm in greatest dimension, or Tumor that involves full-thickness eyelid
T3a	Tumor >20 mm in greatest dimension, or Any tumor that invades adjacent ocular or orbital structures, or Any tumor with perineural invasion
T3b	Complete tumor resection requires enucleation, exenteration, or bone resection
T4	Tumor is not resectable because of extensive invasion of ocular, orbital, or craniofacial structures, or brain

Regional Lymph Nodes (N)

Nx	Regional lymph nodes cannot be assessed
cN0	No regional lymph node metastasis based on clinical evaluation or imaging
pN0	No regional lymph node metastasis based on lymph node biopsy
N1	Regional lymph node metastasis

Distant Metastasis (M)

M0	No distant metastasis
M1	Distant metastasis present

Treatment

Surgery

Primary tumor Surgical resection is the mainstay of treatment of NMSC. A variety of surgical options are available for local treatment of lesions that are smaller than 1 cm. Electrodessication or cryotherapy should not be used, because margin analysis is not

Table 4
Stage/prognostic groups for eyelid carcinoma

Stage Groupings			
Stage 0	Tis	N0	M0
Stage IA	T1	N0	M0
Stage IB	T2a	N0	M0
Stage IC	T2b	N0	M0
Stage II	T3a	N0	M0
Stage IIIA	T3b	N0	M0
Stage IIIB	T1-3b	N1	M0
Stage IIIC	T4	Any N	M0
Stage IV	Any T	Any N	M1

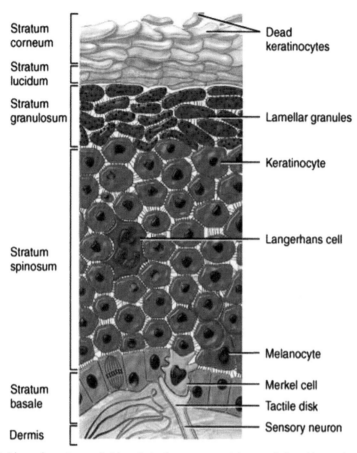

Stratum corneum	Dead keratinocytes
Stratum lucidum	
Stratum granulosum	Lamellar granules
	Keratinocyte
	Langerhans cell
Stratum spinosum	
	Melanocyte
Stratum basale	Merkel cell
	Tactile disk
Dermis	Sensory neuron

Fig. 2. Epidermal anatomy. Epidermis is the outermost layer of the skin and contains 5 specialized layers.

possible. Wide local excision and Mohs surgery are equally effective and offer at least 95% cure rate with minimal morbidity.[42,43] Margins of 0.5 cm are usually sufficient for 1-cm lesions. Tumors that are larger than 1 cm in greatest dimension should be resected with 1-cm margins circumferentially. In every case margin assessment is critical to ensure complete tumor removal.[42,43]

Larger lesions that are deeply invasive require a more generous surgical margin of at least 1 to 2 cm, which may necessitate a complex reconstruction. The deep and lateral margins of the tumor must be cleared histopathologically at the time of resection, particularly when immediate reconstruction is contemplated.[42,44] Frozen section analysis of the adjacent tissue margins is mandatory before reconstruction is undertaken. Close cooperation between the surgeon and the pathologist is necessary to permit intraoperative assessment of all critical margins. The extent of surgical resection is dictated by the clinical and radiographic evaluation, and the patient should be prepared for bony, cartilaginous, neural, or soft tissue resection.[9] For tumors arising on the ear or preauricular skin, deep invasion may require parotidectomy to clear the tumor margins and safely preserve the facial nerve.[37] For tumors fixed to or invading the skull, preoperative consultation with a neurosurgeon is necessary if the resection requires a craniectomy. Surgical resection and reconstruction of the eyelids typically requires input from an experienced oculoplastic surgeon.

Large (>4 cm) deeply invasive BCCs and SCCs are best treated with resection and histologic confirmation of margin clearance. These tumors may require parotidectomy with or without preservation of the facial nerve, amputation of the auricle, and even maxillectomy or mandibulectomy.[9,37] Antegrade and retrograde resection of the facial or trigeminal nerves requires oncologic surgical experience to ensure complete tumor removal. Mohs surgery has a clear role in the following scenarios: (1) tumors extending along embryonic fusion planes, (2) lesions of the eyelid or periorbital region, (3) localized BCC and SCC, and (4) when maximum tissue conservation is important. The long-term results after Mohs surgery for these lesions are favorable, although close surveillance for the development of recurrence is necessary.[45,46]

Regional nodes As less than 1% of all BCC metastasize, regional progression is generally not an issue in this disease.[40,41] SCC, however, has an overall 5% rate of spread to the neck. The following risk factors have been identified that portend lymphatic metastasis: (1) tumor size greater than 5 cm (2) perineural invasion, and (3) deep soft tissue invasion. Elective dissection of the neck is generally not indicated, except when parotid metastases are identified.[47,48] Most patients with these aggressive lesions require postoperative radiation, and thus the neck may be included in the radiation fields for elective neck treatment.[44] When clinical or radiographic metastases are evident, a therapeutic neck dissection is warranted.

The type of neck dissection performed is predicated on the location and extent of metastasis. The parotid gland is the lymphatic watershed for cutaneous malignancies arising on the ear, anterior scalp, forehead, upper and lower eyelid, and preauricular skin.[37] Efferent lymphatics from the parotid drain to the upper jugular lymph nodes and the superficial lymph node that lies adjacent to the upper external jugular vein. When a parotid metastasis is due to a tumor in one of the locations described, coexistent metastasis to the upper cervical nodes is present in 20% to 30% of patients.[37,47] The appropriate lymphadenectomy would include parotidectomy and dissection of the lymph nodes in levels I–IV. Nodes in level V should be dissected if clinically involved or if lesion arises in a postauricular location. In most instances, a neck dissection can be performed while sparing nonlymphatic structures such as the sternocleidomastoid muscle, internal jugular vein, and the spinal accessory nerve.[9,48]

Radiotherapy

Primary tumor Primary radiation for BCC and SCC is primarily reserved for patients who are not surgical candidates. Other clinical situations in which primary radiation therapy may be considered are lesions that involve cosmetically or functionally important anatomic regions, such as the eyelid or the lip.[8,9]

Adjuvant radiation External beam radiotherapy is used as a postsurgical adjuvant for patients with high-risk NMSC (**Box 1**). In a few patients who have marginally resectable tumors involving the face or neck, preoperative radiotherapy can be used to decrease the tumor size and permit resection. However, an operation followed by postoperative radiation therapy (PORT) is preferred for patients with recurrent tumors, perineural invasion, lymph node metastasis, extracapsular lymph node disease, positive margins, deep soft tissue or bony invasion, tumors larger than 4 cm, and unfavorable or aggressive histologies.[44,48] Treatment decisions in this regard should be made in the context of a multidisciplinary team.[9]

Box 1
Indications for radiotherapy
Perineural invasion
Lymphatic or parotid metastasis
Recurrent lesions
Bone invasion
Extracapsular spread
Unfavorable histologies
Large tumors (>4 cm)

Chemotherapy

Several defined genetic mutations have been isolated to the hedgehog pathway in BCC, which plays a key role in embryogenesis but is then usually inactive in adult skin.[49] Systemic therapy for BCC changed substantially with the development of hedgehog inhibitors as unique targeted agents in these tumors. These drugs in advanced stages showed striking regression and apparent clearing of large erosive preexisting tumors, but discontinuation of treatment usually leads to tumor regrowth and progression.[50,51] For SCC, chemotherapy is of limited value and is used for unresectable disease or for palliation. The use of EGFR inhibitors met with limited success.[52,53] Adjuvant chemoradiotherapy may be used (an approach that has been extrapolated from experiences with mucosal SCC of the head and neck). Generally, a platinum-based regimen is administered, although the clinical benefit in this subset of patients is not truly defined. Topical cytotoxic agents such as 5-fluorouracil can be useful for premalignant lesions.[8,9]

Prognosis

The outcomes for patients with BCC are favorable, with 5-year survival rates greater than 95%, even with large lesions.[8,9,40,41] For SCC, 95% of patients are cured with surgical resection alone. For large tumors, perineural invasion, and lymphatic metastasis, long-term survival decreases to approximately 70%.[9,32,54]

MELANOMA
Clinical Evaluation

Presentation

Most patients with cutaneous melanoma of the head and neck present in an early stage. A pigmented lesion may have been present for many years, but only substantial change in its clinical appearance prompts a biopsy. The classic mnemonic "ABCDE" of pigmented lesions represents an important reminder of the warning signs of melanoma because the vast majority of melanomas (>70%) arise in a preexisting mole. These signs include *a*symmetry, *b*order irregularity, *c*olor variegation, *d*iameter greater than 6 mm, and *e*volution.

Anatomy

Melanomas of the head and neck most commonly present on the face, the area that receives the highest lifetime cumulative dosages of UV light. The scalp and ears are the next most common sites of presentation, followed by the neck skin. Of utmost importance in the management of head and neck melanoma is a sophisticated understanding of the surgical anatomy of the lymphatics, because the status of the regional nodes has the strongest impact on survival. Sentinel lymph node biopsy (SLNB) in the head and neck may be challenging because of their relationship to the cranial nerves and the erratic lymphatic drainage patterns.[55] Lesions of the scalp that are anterior to a line drawn along the coronal plane through the tragus often drain to the parotid, submental, or anterior cervical lymph nodes.[56] Melanomas posterior to this line often drain to either the suboccipital, retroauricular, or posterior triangle cervical lymphatics.[57]

Pathology

Most cutaneous melanomas fall into one of the following subtypes: superficial spreading melanoma (SSM), nodular melanoma (NM), lentigo maligna melanoma (LMM), and acral lentiginous melanoma (ALM). A rarer but clinically relevant subtype in the head and neck is desmoplastic melanoma (DM).[9]

SSM, the most common subtype (∼70%), generally arises on skin with intermittent sun exposure. NM (∼15%) is characterized by vertical growth without a prior radial growth phase. NM is often highly aggressive, and clinically appears as raised nodules. LMMs (∼10%) appear as flat brown macules, often with hypopigmented areas. LMMs are associated with chronic sun exposure and are typically located on the head, neck, and arms. ALM (∼5%) is the least common subtype among Caucasians, but represents 30% to 70% of the melanomas diagnosed in African Americans and Hispanics. ALM occurs on the palms or soles, or underneath the nail plate, where exposure to UVR is relatively limited. DM occurs in areas with chronic sun exposure, particularly of the head and neck. DMs are usually detected in elderly patients and are highly invasive, often presenting as lesions with significant (>5 mm) thickness. DMs often invade along neural tracks, which can result in significant symptoms.

Diagnostic evaluation and staging

The evaluation of a suspected head and neck melanoma entails biopsy, which may be performed as either an excisional or incisional procedure, depending on the anatomic location and size of the lesion. An excisional biopsy with 1 to 2 mm margins is preferred, allowing adequate pathologic analysis of the entire specimen for staging, without disrupting the lymphatics should an SLNB be necessary. An excisional biopsy does not suffice for surgical management of a melanoma; appropriate surgical margins should be taken in a separate procedure. An incisional or punch biopsy may be performed for large lesions and for those in cosmetically critical areas, such as the nose, eyelid, or ear. In these situations, a complete excision may require significant reconstruction and rotational flaps, which are best performed after definitive resection has been completed. The general principles of biopsy for a suspected melanoma include representative lesion sampling, adequate depth, and proper specimen orientation. Shave biopsies may not provide adequate representation of the depth of the lesion when performed for a pigmented lesion. AJCC's classification and staging for melanoma (seventh edition) is more complex than that for NMSC and is included in **Tables 5** and **6**.

Evaluation of stage 0–II melanoma The diagnostic evaluation of melanomas of the head and neck outlined in **Fig. 3** is based on the current National Comprehensive Cancer Network (NCCN) guidelines.[58] In patients with stage 0–II melanoma, histologic analysis of the primary tumor is the major diagnostic study; for patients with thin melanomas without high-risk features, a thorough history and physical examination may suffice. For those with ulcerated lesions, imaging of the head and neck may be beneficial, because this subset of patients is at a higher risk of harboring lymph node metastasis.

Table 5
Melanoma TNM classification

Primary Tumor (T)		
T	Thickness (mm)	Ulceration/Mitoses
Tx	Primary tumor cannot be assessed	N/A
T0	No evidence of primary tumor	N/A
Tis	Melanoma in situ	N/A
T1	≤1.00	a. w/o ulceration and mitosis <1/mm^2 b. w/ ulceration or mitosis ≥1/mm^2
T2	1.01–2.00	a. w/o ulceration b. w/ ulceration
T3	2.01–4.00	a. w/o ulceration b. w/ ulceration
T4	>4.00	a. w/o ulceration b. w/ ulceration
Regional Lymph Nodes (N)		
N	Number of Metastatic Nodes	Nodal Metastatic Burden
Nx	Lymph nodes cannot be assessed	N/A
N0	0	N/A
N1	1	a. Micrometastases b. Macrometastases
N2	2–3	a. Micrometastases b. Macrometastases c. In-transit met(s)/satellite(s) w/o metastatic node(s)
N3	>4, or matted nodes, or in-transit met(s)/satellite(s) w/ metastatic node(s)	N/A
Distant Metastasis (M)		
M	Site	Serum LDH
M0	No distant metastasis	N/A
M1a	Distant skin, or subcutaneous, or nodal mets	Normal
M1b	Lung metastases	Normal
M1c	All other visceral metastases Any distant metastases	Normal Elevated

Abbreviations: LDH, lactate dehydrogenase; met, metastasis; N/A, not applicable; w/, with; w/o, without.

Evaluation of stage III–IV Patients harboring nodal metastasis, whether occult or clinical, should undergo staging studies to exclude the presence of distant metastasis. These studies may include CT of the chest, abdomen, and pelvis; an MRI of the brain; and determination of serum lactate dehydrogenase levels. The role of PET-CT for the evaluation of stage III melanoma has not been defined.

Role of sentinel lymph node biopsy The status of lymph nodes is the most powerful prognostic factor for patients with head and neck melanoma; proper staging of the lymphatics is one of the major management criteria for patients with melanoma of

Table 6
Stage/prognostic groups for melanoma

	Clinical Staging				Pathologic Staging		
Stage 0	Tis	N0	M0	Stage 0	Tis	N0	M0
Stage IA	T1a	N0	M0	Stage IA	T1a	N0	M0
Stage IB	T1b-2a	N0	M0	Stage IB	T1b-2a	N0	M0
Stage IIA	T2b-3a	N0	M0	Stage IIA	T2b-3a	N0	M0
Stage IIB	T3b-4a	N0	M0	Stage IIB	T3b-4a	N0	M0
Stage IIC	T4b	N0	M0	Stage IIC	T4b	N0	M0
Stage III	Any T	≥N1	M0	Stage IIIA	T1-4a	N1a-N2a	M0
				Stage IIIB	T1-4b	N1a-2a	M0
					T1-4a	N1b-2b	M0
					T1-4a	N2c	M0
				Stage IIIC	T1-4b	N1b	M0
					T1-4b	N2b	M0
					T1-4b	N2c	M0
					Any T	N3	M0
Stage IV	Any T	Any N	M1	Stage IV	Any T	Any N	M1

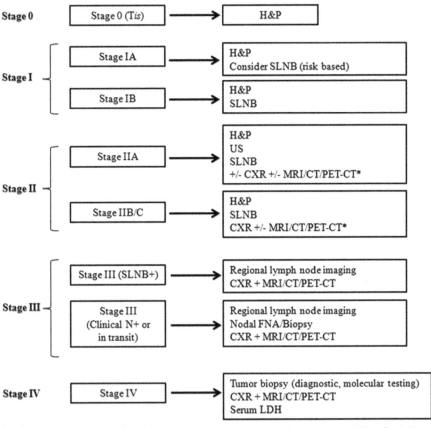

Fig. 3. Diagnostic evaluation of cutaneous melanoma by clinical stage. CXR, chest X-ray; FNA, fine-needle aspiration; H&P, History and physical exam; LDH, lactate dehydrogenase; N+, presence of cervical lymph node metastasis; US, ultrasonography. * Based on physician preference for anatomic imaging modality to be used for evaluation.

the head and neck.[59] SLNB has been established as the preferred staging modality to assess nodal involvement in patients with intermediate-thickness melanomas and selected thin and thick lesions. This approach is based on the principle that melanoma metastasizes in an orderly manner to the first-echelon-draining lymphatic basin.[60] In the evaluation and staging of the patient with melanoma, SLNB offers the following: (1) increased sensitivity to detect regional metastases, (2) limited morbidity compared with elective nodal dissection, (3) identification of patients who may benefit from further therapies such as a neck dissection or systemic adjuvant therapy, and (4) potential halting of the regional progression of disease. Initially met with skepticism, SLNB is now the established approach for determining the presence of occult metastasis.[61] While early studies suggested that head and neck sites were associated with higher regional failure rates after a negative result of SLNB,[62] more recent results suggest a regional failure rate of 4% to 8% after a negative result of SLNB (comparable to that for other anatomic sites).[63–65] SLNB for cutaneous melanomas of the head and neck has a negative predictive value close to 98% and a false-negative rate of 5%.[66,67]

The benefits from SLNB have been established in both retrospective studies and prospective multicenter trials.[68,69] For most patients with lesions less than 1 mm thick, and thus at less than a 5% risk of metastasis, an SLNB may not identify enough nodal disease to justify the morbidity and expense. This risk of nodal involvement increases with increasing thickness of the lesion, and those with melanomas measuring 2 to 4 mm have approximately 30% to 40% nodal positivity, rising to nearly 50% for patients with lesions greater than 4 mm. Patients without sentinel lymph node metastases have a substantially better survival compared with those whose sentinel node contains cancer, even when only micrometastases are present.[70] The number of positive sentinel nodes and the size of the metastatic foci directly correlate with the risk of nonsentinel node metastases.[70–72] Thus, the status of the sentinel lymph nodes plays an important role in establishing the need for adjuvant therapy for patients with malignant melanoma.[73]

One area of substantial controversy is the role of SLNB for patients with thin melanomas. Studies support that those with melanomas less than 1 mm thickness with risk factors such as mitotic figures greater than $1/mm^2$, the presence of ulceration, or tumors greater than 0.7 mm thickness may benefit from SLNB.[74] The likelihood of identifying a positive sentinel node for all anatomic sites is in the range of 5% to 7%, although this rate is unclear in the head and neck. Consideration of performing an SLNB in this group must be placed in the context of the potential morbidity of cranial nerve injury and the cosmetic issues associated with surgical incisions in the face and neck region. Therefore, the decision to perform an SLNB for patients with thin head and neck melanomas should be made on an individualized basis.

Sentinel nodes are often close to the facial and the spinal accessory nerves, and an iatrogenic injury is a major surgical complication. For melanomas in face and temporal scalp region, drainage to the parotid is common, requiring dissection in proximity to the facial nerve. Thus, an understanding of its anatomy is of utmost importance. Initial concerns surrounding removal of sentinel lymph node from the parotid gland proved unfounded, and lymphadenectomy within the gland can be safely performed by an experienced surgeon without injury to the facial nerve.[66,75–80]

Treatment

Surgery is the principal treatment of malignant melanoma, with local excision of the primary tumor and operative resection of the involved lymphatic basins. Radiation therapy is offered to selected patients, and systemic therapies are indicated for selected patients with stage II melanoma, and most with stages III and IV melanomas. General treatment algorithms are outlined in **Fig. 4.**

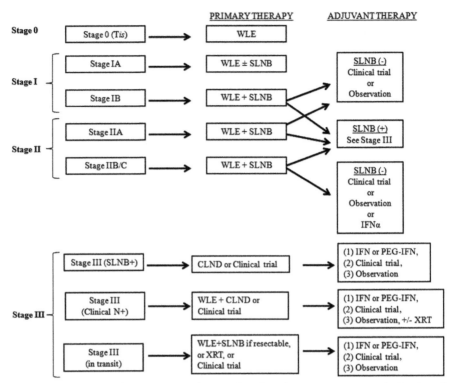

Fig. 4. Management of cutaneous melanoma by clinical stage. CLND, completion lymph node dissection; IFN, interferon; N+, presence of cervical lymph node metastasis; PEG-INF, pegylated interferon; WLE, wide local excision; XRT, radiation therapy.

Stage 0–II

Surgery Although debate has persisted regarding the extent of surgical resection for malignant melanoma, randomized trials have demonstrated that for thin (<1 mm Breslow thickness) melanomas, margins of 1 cm are sufficient for local control.[81] For intermediate thickness lesions, margins of 1 to 2 cm are adequate to prevent local recurrences, while margins of 0.5 cm are sufficient for melanoma in situ.[82] These management principles have been validated in randomized trials in the United States and internationally.[81–83] The current NCCN guidelines (**Table 7**) describe the standard approach for margin control in cutaneous melanoma. In the head and neck, the recommended margins are not always practical because of functional and cosmetic constraints. The excision should include the subcutaneous fat and underlying fascia of the neck, scalp, or face. The routine resection of sensory nerves and facial nerve branches is unnecessary. On the scalp, the pericranium can be left intact, whereas on the ear

Table 7	
Recommended primary tumor surgical margins for cutaneous melanoma	
Depth of Invasion	**Recommended Surgical Margins (cm)**
In situ	0.5
≤2 mm	1.0
≥2.01 mm	2.0

and nose, resections should include the perichondrium because of the thinness of the skin in these regions.

Radiation In general, adjuvant radiation therapy is not indicated for stage 0–II melanomas, although it may be used selectively. For example, DMs have a high propensity for perineural spread and thus have a high risk of local recurrence at the primary tumor site that can be reduced with PORT.[84] Primary tumors that exhibit extensive lymphovascular invasion are also at high risk for local and in-transit recurrence, and patients may benefit from PORT. PORT may also be used in the setting of close or positive margins in areas that are not amenable to more extensive or repeat resection. For patients with extensive areas of melanoma in situ or lentigo maligna, where surgical resection would lead to profound functional or cosmetic sequelae, local radiation is a reasonable treatment option.[85] Primary radiation is not the standard of care.

Stage III melanoma
Surgery Surgery is the mainstay of treatment for patients with regionally metastatic melanoma of the head and neck. Wide excision of the primary tumor to clear margins should be performed, as described above, with reconstruction dictated by the size and location of the defect. Clinically apparent nodal disease mandates a complete lymphadenectomy of the involved stations. For tumors involving the face, neck, and anterior scalp (as defined by the sagittal plane through the external auditory canals), a modified radical neck dissection to remove nodes at levels I–V, with preservation of the spinal accessory nerve, sternocleidomastoid muscle, and internal jugular vein, should typically be performed. The decision to perform a superficial parotidectomy, with preservation of the facial nerve, should be based on the anatomic location of the tumor and the SLNB findings. In general, patients with disease in the parotid bed should undergo parotidectomy and neck dissection. Patients with regional metastasis and a lesion with first-echelon drainage to the parotid gland (eg, anterior lateral scalp melanoma and lateral cheek melanoma) should be considered for parotidectomy even if the gland does not harbor gross metastatic disease. A posterolateral neck dissection, with removal of nodes at levels II–V as well as suboccipital and retroauricular nodes, is necessary for patients with metastasis from a posterior scalp or posterior neck melanoma.

Radiotherapy The indications for adjuvant radiotherapy in stage III disease are based primarily on the risk of regional recurrences after complete nodal dissection. For regionally metastatic melanoma of the head and neck, adjuvant radiation should be considered for patients with (1) extracapsular extension of disease, (2) nodal stage at least N2 (≥2 lymph nodes), (3) nodes larger than 2 cm, and (4) extensive dermal metastasis or satellitosis.[86–89]

Stage IV melanoma
A discussion of the management of metastatic melanoma is beyond the scope of this article; systemic treatment is appropriate. Surgery generally has a limited role for patients with stage IV disease. The benefits for surgical extirpation of local or regional disease in the face of distant metastases are palliative and include (1) limiting the morbidity of continued tumor growth into local structures, (2) reducing nodal burden to lessen great vessel and muscular invasion, and (3) potentially decreasing the source of future metastatic foci. In the head and neck, uncontrolled tumor growth can lead to a substantial decrement in quality of life, and thus locoregional control of clinical disease should be offered when appropriate. Systemic therapies are the primary therapeutic modality for patients with stage IV disease (**Table 8**).

Table 8
Systemic therapy for cutaneous melanoma

Approach	Targets	Agents	Comments
Chemotherapy	DNA replication	Temozolomide, dacarbazine	N/A
Immune therapy	Immune stimulation	Interferon	N/A
Biochemotherapy	Immune stimulation	IL-2 + chemotherapy	N/A
Targeted therapy	BRAF	Vemurafenib	Tumors must harbor BRAF mutation
Immune checkpoint	CTLA4	Ipilimumab	Antibody-based therapy
Immune checkpoint	PD1/PD-L1	Nivolumab	N/A

Abbreviations: IL, interleukin; N/A, not applicable.

Prognosis

Melanoma comprises only about 5% of all cutaneous malignancies, but it is responsible for over 75% of skin-cancer-related deaths.[1,15,90] Significantly, melanomas of the head and neck have a worse prognosis than those from the trunk or extremities. This finding is true for patients with and without regional metastases.[72,91]

Metastasis to a regional lymph node is the single most important prognostic factor in early-stage melanoma, hence the importance of performing SLNB and if its result is positive, regional lymphadenectomy, because this may confer a survival benefit. Regional disease is a predictor of recurrence as well as melanoma-specific death.[72,92] The most predictive independent factors for survival of patients with stage III disease (see **Table 6**) include the number of nodes involved with tumor, tumor burden, and presence or absence of primary tumor ulceration.[70] Five-year survival rates vary widely from 70% for patients with thin melanomas with micrometastases to a single lymph node to 39% for patients with 4 or more involved nodes.[92]

With distant metastatic disease, survival can vary by metastatic site. Involvement of skin, subcutaneous tissue, or distant lymph nodes has a 1-year survival of around 60%. Lung metastasis results in a 1-year survival of about 50%, and metastases to other organs decrease the survival to about 30%.

SUMMARY

NMSCs and melanoma skin cancers are the most common cancer in the United States. Most NMSCs and early-stage melanomas are highly curable if treatment guidelines are closely followed. Thorough clinical and radiographic evaluation is necessary for advanced, recurrent or aggressive lesions, especially advanced-stage melanomas. The more aggressive and recurrent tumors should be evaluated and managed in a multidisciplinary manner to help ensure best patient functional and survival outcomes. Surgical resection to achieve clear margins affords the best chance for cure, and a neck dissection is performed for clinically positive disease. SLNB is a critical tool in the evaluation and staging of melanoma and should be performed when indicated. Radiation therapy is reserved for aggressive lesions after tumor resection and for regional metastases in melanoma. Although NMSCs have a favorable prognosis, patients with large tumors, perineural invasion, or lymphatic metastasis are at risk for recurrences and adverse outcomes. Melanoma survival is the lowest of all common skin cancers and a reflection of the potential for regional and distant metastases. At present, prevention and screening programs to identify early melanoma represent the best chance to improve survival.

REFERENCES

1. Surveillance, epidemiology and end results. 2011. Available at: http://www.seer. cancer.gov/. Accessed November 1, 2014.
2. Chen JG, Fleischer AB Jr, Smith ED, et al. Cost of nonmelanoma skin cancer treatment in the United States. Dermatol Surg 2001;27(12):1035–8.
3. Skin cancer facts. 2012. Available at: http://www.skincancer.org/skin-cancer-facts. Accessed November 1, 2014.
4. Housman TS, Feldman SR, Williford PM, et al. Skin cancer is among the most costly of all cancers to treat for the Medicare population. J Am Acad Dermatol 2003;48(3):425–9.
5. Robinson JK. Sun exposure, sun protection, and vitamin D. JAMA 2005;294(12): 1541–3.
6. Robinson JK, Rigel DS, Amonette RA. Trends in sun exposure knowledge, attitudes, and behaviors: 1986 to 1996. J Am Acad Dermatol 1997;37(2 Pt 1):179–86.
7. Housman TS, Williford PM, Feldman SR, et al. Nonmelanoma skin cancer: an episode of care management approach. Dermatol Surg 2003;29(7):700–11.
8. Weber RS, Miller MJ, Goepfert H. Basal and squamous cell skin cancers of the head and neck. Baltimore (MD): Williams & Wilkins; 1996.
9. Weber RS, Moore BA. Cutaneous malignancy of the head and neck: a multidisciplinary approach. San Diego (CA): Plural Publishing; 2011.
10. Kanavy HE, Gerstenblith MR. Ultraviolet radiation and melanoma. Semin Cutan Med Surg 2011;30(4):222–8.
11. Howe HL, Wingo PA, Thun MJ, et al. Annual Report to the Nation on the Status of Cancer (1973 Through 1998), Featuring Cancers With Recent Increasing Trends. J Natl Cancer Inst 2001;93(11):824–42.
12. Hall HI, Miller DR, Rogers JD, et al. Update on the incidence and mortality from melanoma in the United States. J Am Acad Dermatol 1999;40(1):35–42.
13. Lee JA. Trends in melanoma incidence and mortality. Clin Dermatol 1992;10(1): 9–13.
14. Hollestein LM, van den Akker SA, Nijsten T, et al. Trends of cutaneous melanoma in the Netherlands: increasing incidence rates among all Breslow thickness categories and rising mortality rates since 1989. Ann Oncol 2012;23(2):524–30.
15. Jemal A, Saraiya M, Patel P, et al. Recent trends in cutaneous melanoma incidence and death rates in the United States, 1992-2006. J Am Acad Dermatol 2011;65(5 Suppl 1):17–25.e13.
16. Burnet NG, Jefferies SJ, Benson RJ, et al. Years of life lost (YLL) from cancer is an important measure of population burden—and should be considered when allocating research funds. Br J Cancer 2005;92(2):241–5.
17. Ekwueme DU, Guy GP Jr, Li C, et al. The health burden and economic costs of cutaneous melanoma mortality by race/ethnicity–United States, 2000 to 2006. J Am Acad Dermatol 2011;65(5 Suppl 1):S133–43.
18. Urbach F. Welcome and introduction: evidence and epidemiology of ultraviolet-induced cancers in man. Natl Cancer Inst Monogr 1978;(50):5–10.
19. Wang LE, Xiong P, Strom SS, et al. In vitro sensitivity to ultraviolet B light and skin cancer risk: a case-control analysis. J Natl Cancer Inst 2005;97(24):1822–31.
20. Lichter MD, Karagas MR, Mott LA, et al. Therapeutic ionizing radiation and the incidence of basal cell carcinoma and squamous cell carcinoma. The New Hampshire Skin Cancer Study Group. Arch Dermatol 2000;136(8):1007–11.
21. Gilchrest BA, Eller MS, Geller AC, et al. The pathogenesis of melanoma induced by ultraviolet radiation. N Engl J Med 1999;340(17):1341–8.

22. Gandini S, Sera F, Cattaruzza MS, et al. Meta-analysis of risk factors for cutaneous melanoma: I. Common and atypical naevi. Eur J Cancer 2005;41(1):28–44.

23. Caini S, Gandini S, Sera F, et al. Meta-analysis of risk factors for cutaneous melanoma according to anatomical site and clinico-pathological variant. Eur J Cancer 2009;45(17):3054–63.

24. Gandini S, Sera F, Cattaruzza MS, et al. Meta-analysis of risk factors for cutaneous melanoma: III. Family history, actinic damage and phenotypic factors. Eur J Cancer 2005;41(14):2040–59.

25. Berg D, Otley CC. Skin cancer in organ transplant recipients: epidemiology, pathogenesis, and management. J Am Acad Dermatol 2002;47(1):1–17 [quiz: 18–20].

26. Kovach BT, Stasko T. Skin cancer after transplantation. Transplant Rev 2009; 23(3):178–89.

27. Accardi R, Gheit T. Cutaneous HPV and skin cancer. Presse Med 2014;43(12 Pt 2):e435–43.

28. Karagas MR, Nelson HH, Sehr P, et al. Human papillomavirus infection and incidence of squamous cell and basal cell carcinomas of the skin. J Natl Cancer Inst 2006;98(6):389–95.

29. Cassarino DS, Derienzo DP, Barr RJ. Cutaneous squamous cell carcinoma: a comprehensive clinicopathologic classification–part two. J Cutan Pathol 2006; 33(4):261–79.

30. Goepfert H, Dichtel WJ, Medina JE, et al. Perineural invasion in squamous cell skin carcinoma of the head and neck. Am J Surg 1984;148(4):542–7.

31. Bhawan J. Squamous cell carcinoma in situ in skin: what does it mean? J Cutan Pathol 2007;34(12):953–5.

32. Rudolph R, Zelac DE. Squamous cell carcinoma of the skin. Plast Reconstr Surg 2004;114(6):82e–94e.

33. Ginsberg LE. MR imaging of perineural tumor spread. Neuroimaging Clin N Am 2004;14(4):663–77.

34. Nakamura T, Sumi M. Nodal imaging in the neck: recent advances in US, CT and MR imaging of metastatic nodes. Eur Radiol 2007;17(5):1235–41.

35. Castelijns JA, van den Brekel MW. Imaging of lymphadenopathy in the neck. Eur Radiol 2002;12(4):727–38.

36. Gor DM, Langer JE, Loevner LA. Imaging of cervical lymph nodes in head and neck cancer: the basics. Radiol Clin North Am 2006;44(1):101–10, viii.

37. Lai SY, Weinstein GS, Chalian AA, et al. Parotidectomy in the treatment of aggressive cutaneous malignancies. Arch Otolaryngol Head Neck Surg 2002;128(5): 521–6.

38. Hillner BE, Siegel BA, Liu D, et al. Impact of positron emission tomography/ computed tomography and positron emission tomography (PET) alone on expected management of patients with cancer: initial results from the National Oncologic PET Registry. J Clin Oncol 2008;26(13):2155–61.

39. Hillner BE, Siegel BA, Shields AF, et al. Relationship between cancer type and impact of PET and PET/CT on intended management: findings of the national oncologic PET registry. J Nucl Med 2008;49(12):1928–35.

40. Crowson AN. Basal cell carcinoma: biology, morphology and clinical implications. Mod Pathol 2006;19(Suppl 2):S127–47.

41. Lear W, Dahlke E, Murray CA. Basal cell carcinoma: review of epidemiology, pathogenesis, and associated risk factors. J Cutan Med Surg 2007;11(1):19–30.

42. Choo R, Woo T, Assaad D, et al. What is the microscopic tumor extent beyond clinically delineated gross tumor boundary in nonmelanoma skin cancers? Int J Radiat Oncol Biol Phys 2005;62(4):1096–9.

43. Veness MJ. Treatment recommendations in patients diagnosed with high-risk cutaneous squamous cell carcinoma. Australas Radiol 2005;49(5):365–76.
44. Veness MJ, Palme CE, Smith M, et al. Cutaneous head and neck squamous cell carcinoma metastatic to cervical lymph nodes (nonparotid): a better outcome with surgery and adjuvant radiotherapy. Laryngoscope 2003;113(10):1827–33.
45. Kallini JR, Hamed N, Khachemoune A. Squamous cell carcinoma of the skin: epidemiology, classification, management, and novel trends. Int J Dermatol 2015;54(2):130–40.
46. Narayanan K, Hadid OH, Barnes EA. Mohs micrographic surgery versus surgical excision for periocular basal cell carcinoma. Cochrane Database Syst Rev 2014;(12):CD007041.
47. Chu A, Osguthorpe JD. Nonmelanoma cutaneous malignancy with regional metastasis. Otolaryngol Head Neck Surg 2003;128(5):663–73.
48. Moore BA, Weber RS, Prieto V, et al. Lymph node metastases from cutaneous squamous cell carcinoma of the head and neck. Laryngoscope 2005;115(9):1561–7.
49. Rubin LL, de Sauvage FJ. Targeting the Hedgehog pathway in cancer. Nat Rev Drug Discov 2006;5(12):1026–33.
50. Mohan SV, Chang AL. Precision medicine and precision therapeutics: hedgehog signaling pathway, basal cell carcinoma and beyond. Semin Cutan Med Surg 2014;33(2):68–71.
51. Wong SY, Dlugosz AA. Basal cell carcinoma, Hedgehog signaling, and targeted therapeutics: the long and winding road. J Invest Dermatol 2014;134(e1):E18–22.
52. Galer CE, Corey CL, Wang Z, et al. Dual inhibition of epidermal growth factor receptor and insulin-like growth factor receptor I: reduction of angiogenesis and tumor growth in cutaneous squamous cell carcinoma. Head Neck 2011;33(2):189–98.
53. Lewis CM, Glisson BS, Feng L, et al. A phase II study of gefitinib for aggressive cutaneous squamous cell carcinoma of the head and neck. Clin Cancer Res 2012;18(5):1435–46.
54. Clayman GL, Lee JJ, Holsinger FC, et al. Mortality risk from squamous cell skin cancer. J Clin Oncol 2005;23(4):759–65.
55. O'Brien CJ, Uren RF, Thompson JF, et al. Prediction of potential metastatic sites in cutaneous head and neck melanoma using lymphoscintigraphy. Am J Surg 1995;170(5):461–6.
56. Shah JP, Kraus DH, Dubner S, et al. Patterns of regional lymph node metastases from cutaneous melanomas of the head and neck. Am J Surg 1991;162(4):320–3.
57. Pathak I, O'Brien CJ, Petersen-Schaeffer K, et al. Do nodal metastases from cutaneous melanoma of the head and neck follow a clinically predictable pattern? Head Neck 2001;23(9):785–90.
58. Coit DG, Andtbacka R, Bichakjian CK, et al. Melanoma. J Natl Compr Canc Netw 2009;7(3):250–75.
59. Gershenwald JE, Thompson W, Mansfield PF, et al. Multi-institutional melanoma lymphatic mapping experience: the prognostic value of sentinel lymph node status in 612 stage I or II melanoma patients. J Clin Oncol 1999;17(3):976–83.
60. Morton DL, Wen D-R, Wong JH, et al. Technical details of intraoperative lymphatic mapping for early stage melanoma. Arch Surg 1992;127(4):392–9.
61. Morton DL, Essner R, Kirkwood JM, et al. Malignant melanoma. In: Kufe DW, Bast RC, Hait WN, et al, editors. Cancer medicine, vol. 7. Hamilton (Canada): BC Decker Inc; 2006. p. 1644–62.
62. Carlson GW, Page AJ, Cohen C, et al. Regional recurrence after negative sentinel lymph node biopsy for melanoma. Ann Surg 2008;248(3):378–86.

63. Schmalbach CE, Nussenbaum B, Rees RS, et al. Reliability of sentinel lymph node mapping with biopsy for head and neck cutaneous melanoma. Arch Otolaryngol Head Neck Surg 2003;129(1):61–5.

64. Miller MW, Vetto JT, Monroe MM, et al. False-negative sentinel lymph node biopsy in head and neck melanoma. Otolaryngol Head Neck Surg 2011; 145(4):606–11.

65. Murali R, Haydu LE, Quinn MJ, et al. Sentinel lymph node biopsy in patients with thin primary cutaneous melanoma. Ann Surg 2012;255(1):128–33.

66. Erman AB, Collar RM, Griffith KA, et al. Sentinel lymph node biopsy is accurate and prognostic in head and neck melanoma. Cancer 2012;118(4):1040–7.

67. Saltman BE, Ganly I, Patel SG, et al. Prognostic implication of sentinel lymph node biopsy in cutaneous head and neck melanoma. Head Neck 2010;32(12): 1686–92.

68. Ross MI, Gershenwald JE. Evidence-based treatment of early-stage melanoma. J Surg Oncol 2011;104(4):341–53.

69. Gershenwald JEM, Ross MIM. Sentinel-lymph-node biopsy for cutaneous melanoma. N Engl J Med 2011;364(18):1738–45.

70. Balch CM, Gershenwald JE, Soong SJ, et al. Final version of 2009 AJCC melanoma staging and classification. J Clin Oncol 2009;27(36):6199–206.

71. Balch CM, Buzaid AC, Soong SJ, et al. Final version of the American Joint Committee on Cancer staging system for cutaneous melanoma. J Clin Oncol 2001; 19(16):3635–48.

72. Balch CM, Soong SJ, Gershenwald JE, et al. Prognostic factors analysis of 17,600 melanoma patients: validation of the American Joint Committee on Cancer Melanoma Staging System. J Clin Oncol 2001;19(16):3622–34.

73. Morton DL, Cochran AJ, Thompson JF, et al. Sentinel node biopsy for early-stage melanoma: accuracy and morbidity in MSLT-I, an international multicenter trial. Ann Surg 2005;242(3):302–11 [discussion: 311–3].

74. Andtbacka RH, Gershenwald JE. Role of sentinel lymph node biopsy in patients with thin melanoma. J Natl Compr Canc Netw 2009;7(3):308–17.

75. Loree TR, Tomljanovich PI, Cheney RT, et al. Intraparotid sentinel lymph node biopsy for head and neck melanoma. Laryngoscope 2006;116(8):1461–4.

76. Ariyan S, Ariyan C, Farber LR, et al. Reliability of identification of 655 sentinel lymph nodes in 263 consecutive patients with malignant melanoma. J Am Coll Surg 2004;198(6):924–32.

77. Gibbs JF, Huang PP, Zhang PJ, et al. Accuracy of pathologic techniques for the diagnosis of metastatic melanoma in sentinel lymph nodes. Ann Surg Oncol 1999;6(7):699–704.

78. Koopal SA, Tiebosch AT, Albertus Piers D, et al. Frozen section analysis of sentinel lymph nodes in melanoma patients. Cancer 2000;89(8):1720–5.

79. Stojadinovic A, Allen PJ, Clary BM, et al. Value of frozen-section analysis of sentinel lymph nodes for primary cutaneous malignant melanoma. Ann Surg 2002;235(1):92–8.

80. Prieto VG. Sentinel lymph nodes in cutaneous melanoma: handling, examination, and clinical repercussion. Arch Pathol Lab Med 2010;134(12):1764–9.

81. Veronesi U, Cascinelli N, Adamus J, et al. Thin stage I primary cutaneous malignant melanoma. Comparison of excision with margins of 1 or 3 cm. N Engl J Med 1988;318(18):1159–62.

82. Balch CM, Soong SJ, Smith T, et al. Long-term results of a prospective surgical trial comparing 2 cm vs. 4 cm excision margins for 740 patients with 1-4 mm melanomas. Ann Surg Oncol 2001;8(2):101–8.

83. Balch CM, Urist MM, Karakousis CP, et al. Efficacy of 2-cm surgical margins for intermediate-thickness melanomas (1 to 4 mm) results of a multi-institutional randomized surgical trial. Ann Surg 1993;218(3):262–9.
84. Chen JY, Hruby G, Scolyer RA, et al. Desmoplastic neurotropic melanoma. Cancer 2008;113(10):2770–8.
85. Farshad A, Burg G, Panizzon R, et al. A retrospective study of 150 patients with lentigo maligna and lentigo maligna melanoma and the efficacy of radiotherapy using Grenz or soft X-rays. Br J Dermatol 2002;146(6):1042–6.
86. Burmeister BH, Mark Smithers B, Burmeister E, et al. A prospective phase II study of adjuvant postoperative radiation therapy following nodal surgery in malignant melanoma–Trans Tasman Radiation Oncology Group (TROG) Study 96.06. Radiother Oncol 2006;81(2):136–42.
87. Agrawal S, Kane JM, Guadagnolo BA, et al. The benefits of adjuvant radiation therapy after therapeutic lymphadenectomy for clinically advanced, high-risk, lymph node-metastatic melanoma. Cancer 2009;115(24):5836–44.
88. Bonnen MD, Ballo MT, Myers JN, et al. Elective radiotherapy provides regional control for patients with cutaneous melanoma of the head and neck. Cancer 2004;100(2):383–9.
89. Henderson MA, Burmeister B, Thompson JF, et al. Adjuvant radiotherapy and regional lymph node field control in melanoma patients after lymphadenectomy: results of an intergroup randomized trial (ANZMTG 01.02/TROG 02.01). J Clin Oncol 2009;27(18s):LBA9084.
90. Jemal A, Siegel R, Ward E, et al. Cancer statistics, 2009. CA Cancer J Clin 2009; 59(4):225–49.
91. Paek SC, Griffith KA, Johnson TM, et al. The impact of factors beyond Breslow depth on predicting sentinel lymph node positivity in melanoma. Cancer 2007; 109(1):100–8.
92. Morton DL, Thompson JF, Cochran AJ, et al. Sentinel-node biopsy or nodal observation in melanoma. N Engl J Med 2006;355(13):1307–17.

Cancers of Major Salivary Glands

Aru Panwar, MD[a],*, Jessica A. Kozel, MD[b], William M. Lydiatt, MD[c]

KEYWORDS

- Salivary glands • Cancer • Malignancy • Neoplasm

KEY POINTS

- Major salivary gland malignancies are a rare but histologically diverse group of entities.
- Establishing the diagnosis of a malignant salivary neoplasm may be challenging because of the often minimally symptomatic nature of disease, and limitations of imaging modalities and cytology.
- Treatment is centered on surgical therapy and adjuvant radiation in selected scenarios.
- Systemic therapy with chemotherapeutic agents and monoclonal antibodies lacks evidence in support of its routine use.

Salivary gland malignancies are rare tumors with an estimated population incidence of 1.2 per 100,000.[1] These tumors constitute about 5% of all head and neck malignancies and tend to occur most frequently among men.[2,3] Most salivary gland tumors arise in the parotid gland. Although benign neoplasms outnumber malignant tumors, most malignant salivary gland tumors involve the parotid gland; typically in the superficial lobe. The other major salivary glands, the submandibular and sublingual glands, have a higher proportion of malignant versus benign tumors, but these constitute a minority of all primary salivary malignancies.[4]

The cause for malignant salivary gland tumors has not been clearly defined. Ionizing radiation may play a role in development of these malignancies.[4–7] Tobacco and alcohol use have not been reliably proven to be causative in salivary gland malignancies.[8] Similarly, exposure to wireless phones has not been associated with these tumors.[9–11]

HISTOLOGIC CLASSIFICATION AND STAGING

Salivary gland malignancies represent a cohort of varied histopathologic subtypes, and the revised World Health Organization (WHO) classification identifies 23 separate

Disclosures: The authors have nothing to disclose.
[a] Division of Head and Neck Surgery, University of Nebraska Medical Center, 600 S, 42nd Street, Omaha, NE 68198, USA; [b] Department of Pathology and Microbiology, University of Nebraska Medical Center, Omaha, NE, USA; [c] Division of Head and Neck Surgery, Nebraska Methodist Hospital, 8303 Dodge Street, Omaha, NE 68114, USA
* Corresponding author. 981225 Nebraska Medical Center, Omaha, NE 68198-1225.
E-mail address: aru.panwar@unmc.edu

primary salivary gland malignant tumors (**Box 1**).[12] In addition, several tumors may show a spectrum of histologic grades that have disparate clinical profiles relating to their local aggression, risk for regional and distant metastases, and overall prognosis. The diverse nature and clinical behavior of these tumors pose unique difficulties in generating uniformity in staging and prognostic information.

The current staging system offered by the American Joint Committee on Cancer (AJCC) accounts for characteristics of the primary tumor (T stage), regional lymph node status (N stage), and presence or absence or distant metastases (M stage).[13] However, the staging system does not factor the histologic grading of tumors, and fails to distinguish more indolent forms of disease from aggressive variants (**Table 1**). Thus, staging information should not be the sole determinant of the management offered,

---

Box 1
WHO classification of salivary gland malignancies

Acinic cell carcinoma

Mucoepidermoid carcinoma

Adenoid cystic carcinoma

Polymorphous low-grade adenocarcinoma

Epithelial-myoepithelial carcinoma

Clear cell carcinoma, not otherwise specified

Basal cell adenocarcinoma

Sebaceous carcinoma

Sebaceous lymphadenocarcinoma

Cystadenocarcinoma

Low-grade cribriform cystadenocarcinoma

Mucinous adenocarcinoma

Oncocytic carcinoma

Salivary duct carcinoma

Adenocarcinoma, not otherwise specified

Myoepithelial carcinoma

Carcinoma ex pleomorphic adenoma

Carcinosarcoma

Metastasizing pleomorphic adenoma

Squamous cell carcinoma

Small cell carcinoma

Large cell carcinoma

Lymphoepithelial carcinoma

Sialoblastoma

From Eveson JW, Auclair PL, Gnepp DR. Tumors of the salivary glands: introduction. In: Barnes L, Eveson JW, Reichert P, et al, editors. Pathology and genetics of head and neck tumors. Lyon (France): World Health Organization Classification of Tumors; IARC Press; 2005. p. 210, with permission.

Table 1
AJCC staging for salivary gland cancers

Primary Tumor (T)

TX	Primary tumor cannot be assessed
T0	No evidence of primary tumor
T1	Tumor 2 cm or less in greatest dimension without extraparenchymal extension
T2	Tumor more than 2 cm but not more than 4 cm in greatest dimension without extraparenchymal extension
T3	Tumor more than 4 cm and/or tumor having extraparenchymal extension
T4a	Moderately advanced disease Tumor invades skin, mandible, ear canal, and/or facial nerve
T4b	Very advanced disease Tumor invades skull base and/or pterygoid plates and/or encases carotid artery

Regional Lymph Nodes (N)

NX	Regional lymph nodes cannot be assessed
N0	No regional lymph node metastasis
N1	Metastasis in a single ipsilateral lymph node, 3 cm or less in greatest dimension
N2	Metastasis in a single ipsilateral lymph node, more than 3 cm but not more than 6 cm in greatest dimension; or in multiple ipsilateral lymph nodes, none more than 6 cm in greatest dimension; or in bilateral or contralateral lymph nodes, none more than 6 cm in greatest dimension
N2a	Metastasis in a single ipsilateral lymph node, more than 3 cm but not more than 6 cm in greatest dimension
N2b	Metastasis in multiple ipsilateral lymph nodes, none more than 6 cm in greatest dimension
N2c	Metastasis in bilateral or contralateral lymph nodes, none more than 6 cm in greatest dimension
N3	Metastasis in a lymph node, more than 6 cm in greatest dimension

Distant Metastasis (M)

M0	No distant metastasis
M1	Distant metastasis

Anatomic Stage/Prognostic Groups

Stage I	T1	N0	M0
Stage II	T2	N0	M0
Stage III	T3	N0	M0
	T1	N1	M0
	T2	N1	M0
	T3	N1	M0
Stage IVA	T4a	N0	M0
	T4a	N1	M0
	T1	N2	M0
	T2	N2	M0
	T3	N2	M0
	T4a	N2	M0
Stage IVB	T4b	Any N	M0
	Any T	N3	M0
Stage IVC	Any T	Any N	M1

Used with the permission of the American Joint Committee on Cancer (AJCC), Chicago, Illinois. The original source for this material is the AJCC Cancer Staging Manual, Seventh Edition (2010) published by Springer Science and Business Media LLC, www.springer.com.

and histologic information and other variables should be considered before assignment of treatment options and prognostication.[14–16]

PRESENTATION AND WORK-UP

Patients with major salivary gland tumors often present with an asymptomatic mass. Findings such as rapid increase in size of the mass, pain, and local soft tissue invasion suggest malignancy. In addition, facial nerve or other cranial neuropathy and presence of clinically evident regional adenopathy are strong predictors of a malignant process.[17] Most patients have no specific clinical symptoms and the establishment of a malignant diagnosis requires additional investigations and/or invasive procedures.

Individuals presenting with a neoplasm of a major salivary gland should undergo a detailed history and physical examination. Historical features such as pain, trismus, skin changes, paresthesias, rapid growth, facial weakness, or other cranial neuropathies suggest a malignant neoplasm.[17] Patients should be asked about history of skin malignancies, lymphoproliferative disorders, and autoimmune processes that may suggest a systemic secondary malignancy involving salivary tissue.

A comprehensive head and neck examination should include evaluation of the primary site (size of primary neoplasm, mobility of the mass, characteristics of overlying skin and soft tissue, and any extension to deep/parapharyngeal space), functional assessment of cranial nerves, and pathologic adenopathy in the draining nodal basins. Mucosal and cutaneous surfaces should be inspected for alternative sources of malignancy.

Imaging modalities should be directed at answering clinical questions and shaping the diagnostic and therapeutic pathways. The typical modalities used include ultrasonography, contrast-enhanced computed tomography (CT) scan, magnetic resonance imaging (MRI), and PET.

Ultrasonography is useful for anatomic and morphologic characterization of salivary gland tumors in the absence of deep parapharyngeal extension. In addition, it can assess regional nodes and assist guided aspiration biopsy where indicated.[18] Ultrasonography is cost-effective and is often available in the outpatient clinical setting as an extension of the physical examination. Sonographic distinction of malignant neoplasms from benign masses may be possible, and malignancy should be suspected when features such as prominent heterogeneity in internal echo patterns, unclear borders, and increased internal vascular flow are seen.[19–21] However, accuracy is diminished in small and low-grade malignant tumors.[22,23] Other limitations of ultrasonography include its inability to identify and evaluate the parapharyngeal space, skull base, mandible, and perineural spread of tumor.[18]

Cross-sectional imaging modalities, including CT scan and MRI, provide accurate localization and assessment of the extent of the tumor. These modalities assess nodal status and may provide clinically relevant information relating to neurotropic spread of tumor. MRI is considered the investigation of choice when a malignant neoplasm of a major salivary gland is suspected. Malignant tumors in the parotid are often less intense on T2-weighted images compared with benign counterparts.[24,25] Other features on MRI that may point to a malignant tumor include ill-defined margins, infiltration of surrounding soft tissue, diffuse growth pattern, and pathologic lymphadenopathy.[24]

PET-CT scans may not be useful in the initial assessment of salivary gland tumors for a variety of reasons, including inherent inability to distinguish between malignant and benign tumors, because many benign tumors accumulate fluorodeoxyglucose similarly to salivary malignancies.[26] Moreover, PET-CT is cost intensive, and routine use is not advisable in the increasingly cost-sensitive health care environment.

However, there is some evidence that, compared with conventional CT scans, PET-CT may provide a more accurate prediction of disease extent associated with a known high-grade salivary gland malignancy.[27] It may also have some additional value in identification of locoregionally recurrent and metastatic disease.[28]

Fine-needle aspiration (FNA) is variably incorporated by physicians in the management of major salivary gland neoplasms. The controversy relating to the utility of FNA is rooted in the histologic diversity shown by salivary gland malignancies. Several members of this morphologically complex group of malignancies may display close resemblance to histologically distinct entities.[29] Although FNA has shown high sensitivity and specificity in several studies, these results may not be reproduced in community settings where experience with salivary cytology may be limited.[29–32] Additional concerns about the ability of FNA to distinguish between benign and malignant salivary neoplasms persist. Despite reliable overall sensitivity and specificity of FNA, Colella and colleagues[32] found that the final histopathology was discordant from the FNA results in more than 20% of salivary gland malignancies. Another study recognized that FNA might miss the malignant nature of salivary mass in 40% of cases investigated.[33] In contrast, false-positives may lead to unnecessary interventions.[34]

FNA could be significant in providing preoperative information distinguishing high-grade malignancies from low-grade malignant and nonmalignant disorders. This information may be critical in alteration of intraoperative management of high-grade malignancies, which differs from others in potential use of elective nodal dissection.[29,35] However, Zbaren and colleagues[36] found that tumor grade could be predicted with accuracy in one-third of parotid carcinomas subjected to FNA; another study noted high sensitivity, specificity, and diagnostic accuracy (94%, 99%, and 99%, respectively) in identifying high-grade malignancy.[35] This information contributed to additional imaging or change in extent of surgery in most of the included patient cohort. Because of controversies related to routine use of FNA in major salivary neoplasms and its limitations, some investigators propose the use of image-guided core needle biopsies as an alternative strategy with acceptable safety.[37,38]

SELECTED HISTOLOGIC SUBTYPES OF MAJOR SALIVARY GLAND MALIGNANCIES
Mucoepidermoid Carcinoma

Mucoepidermoid carcinoma (MEC) is the most common malignant neoplasm of the major salivary glands.[3,7,39–42] It represents nearly one-third of all malignancies involving the major salivary glands.[3,40–42] MEC occurs most commonly in women in their third to seventh decades of life. Parotid gland is most frequently involved, followed by submandibular and sublingual gland in that order.

On histology, MEC is composed of mucin-secreting cells, intermediate cells, and epidermoid cells. Tumors vary in the proportion of cell types, degree of cellular maturation, and frequency of mitoses and neurovascular invasion, and degree of necrosis. In addition, tumor foci may show variable degrees of solid and cystic morphology.[39] Mucoepidermoid carcinomas can therefore be classified as low-grade, intermediate-grade, or high-grade tumors.[7] This differentiation is relevant to prediction of oncologic behavior, and affects choice and extent of therapy. A variety of grading systems, including 2 tiered (low and high grade) and 3 tiered (low, intermediate, and high grade), have been proposed; however, no system is universally accepted and they have traditionally been cumbersome to use.[39]

Clinical presentation of MEC depends on histologic grade. Low-grade and intermediate-grade tumors often present as slow-growing, solitary masses with a lack of symptoms. In contrast, high-grade tumors may progress rapidly and may present with symptoms including pain, nerve deficits, and local soft tissue invasion.

Because of the indolent nature of low-grade and intermediate-grade tumors, surgical resection of the primary site with negative margins may be considered sufficient.[43] Overall, survival at 5 years approaches 80% to 90%.[44–47] In contrast, high-grade histology in mucoepidermoid carcinoma is an independent factor predictive of poor overall survival (40%–50% at 5 years), and for increased risk for locoregional failure and distant metastases.[43–47] Recommended therapy for tumors with high-grade histology includes surgical resection with adjuvant radiation therapy. In patients with high-grade histology, elective nodal dissection may be considered at the time of primary surgical intervention. However, information about histologic grade of the tumor is seldom available preoperatively.

Other factors associated with poor outcome include advanced T stage, clinically evident nodal metastases, and identification of distant metastases at presentation.[48] Presence of perineural invasion implies high-grade histology and associated poor outcomes (**Fig. 1**).[43]

Adenoid Cystic Carcinoma

Adenoid cystic carcinoma is the second most common malignancy of the major salivary glands, and represents 10% to 22% of all malignant salivary gland tumors.[3,40–42] It accounts for 5% of all parotid and nearly 15% of submandibular gland malignancies.[7] There is a slight predilection toward women and most patients are in their fifth to seventh decades in life.[3] Most patients present without symptoms. Occasionally, a painful mass or neural deficits involving cranial nerves are seen. Clinically evident nodal disease is seen infrequently, although occult metastases to cervical lymph nodes may be present in as many as 24% of all patients.[49] Distant metastases may be seen in up to 20% of early stage tumors, and a third of affected patients overall.[50,51] Commonly involved sites of metastases include lung and bony structures. Metastatic foci generally show a slow but relentless course, but occasionally progression can be precipitous.

On histology, adenoid cystic carcinoma presents as an unencapsulated, infiltrative neoplasm with varied patterns of growth, which bear prognostic significance. Hyperchromatic basaloid cells are seen.[7] The cribriform or Swiss-cheese pattern is the most commonly encountered pattern, with pseudocysts that are contiguous with stromal

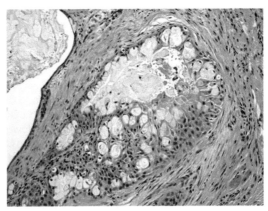

Fig. 1. Mucoepidermoid carcinoma showing cystic change with epidermoid, mucous, and intermediate cell types (hematoxylin-eosin stain [HE], 100× magnification).

tissue and abluminal basaloid cells. Alternative patterns include solid and tubular variants. The solid type is least common and shows solid nests of neoplastic cells. It is generally more aggressive than other variants and shows higher propensity for distant metastases.[50,52–54] Tubular variants are associated with the best prognosis overall. Tumors generally show more than 1 growth pattern and the predominant component should dictate the final classification. A high incidence of perineural invasion is associated with all patterns of growth.

Adenoid cystic carcinoma often behaves in an indolent manner. A Surveillance, Epidemiology, and End Results (SEER) program database identified the overall survival rates at 5, 10, and 15 years to be 90%, 80%, and 70%, respectively.[55,56] Initial stage at presentation is considered to be the strongest predictor of overall clinical behavior.[57] Other factors that predict poor outcome are presence of neural invasion and female gender.[58]

Treatment includes surgery and adjuvant radiation therapy. Elective nodal dissection may identify occult nodal metastases in one-quarter of clinically node-negative patients, but does not seem to affect overall survival.[49] Adjuvant radiation may reduce the risk for local failure and improve disease-free survival (**Fig. 2**).[59]

Acinic Cell Carcinoma

Acinic cell carcinoma constitutes nearly 8% to 14% of all malignant salivary gland neoplasms.[3,40–42] The parotid gland is the most commonly involved major salivary gland, and a small subset of patients present with bilateral tumors.[60] A slight predilection for women is noted.[3] The tumor usually presents as a slow-growing solitary mass. Neural deficits, pain, regional nodal metastases, and soft tissue involvement are less frequent.

Characteristically, these tumors display cells with granular, metachromatic cytoplasm, recapitulating that seen in the serous acinar cells of salivary glands. Varied tumor growth patterns may be seen, including solid, microcystic, papillary cystic, and follicular. However, individual growth patterns do not bear prognostic significance.[7]

Acinic cell carcinomas behave indolently. A SEER database review noted overall survival rates of 97%, 93%, and 89% at 5, 10, and 15 years, respectively.[61] Distant metastases are associated with poor long-term prognosis. Treatment involves surgical resection. Radiation therapy is generally not used for primary disease management (**Fig. 3**).

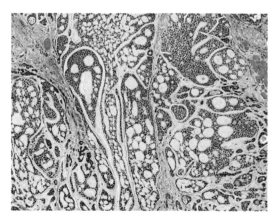

Fig. 2. Adenoid cystic carcinoma with angulated, hyperchromatic basaloid cells in a cribriform Swiss-cheese pattern (HE, 100× magnification).

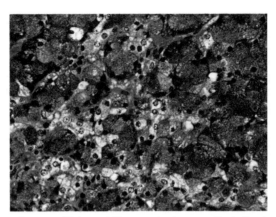

Fig. 3. Acinic cell carcinoma with basophilic granular tumor cells similar to serous acinar cells (HE, 400× magnification).

Malignant Mixed Tumors of Salivary Glands

Malignant mixed tumors of salivary glands include entities such as carcinoma ex pleomorphic adenoma (CEPA), intracapsular carcinoma ex pleomorphic adenoma, carcinosarcoma, and metastasizing pleomorphic adenoma.

CEPA is the most common variant, and the parotid gland is involved more often than the other major salivary glands.[62] Typically, it presents in a preexisting pleomorphic adenoma with accelerated growth and new-onset pain and/or neuropathy. Pathology reveals residual histologic evidence of pleomorphic adenoma with a carcinomatous component with enlarged cells, marked nuclear pleomorphism, prominent nucleoli, increased mitotic activity, and necrosis. These tumors characteristically lack evidence of coexistent mesenchymal malignancy.[7] The incidence of malignant transformation of a preexisting pleomorphic adenoma is estimated to be around 10% over a 15-year period.[7,12] Nodal metastasis may be an early finding and predicts poor overall survival.[63] Tumor grade, evidence of metastatic disease, capsular and neural invasion, and surgical margin status are other prognostic variables of significance.[64] Adjuvant radiation following surgery (including primary site and nodal basins) may contribute to improved local control rates.[63] Overall survival at 5 years is poor at 40%, and is comparably worse than other high-grade salivary malignancies.[65–67]

Intracapsular carcinoma ex pleomorphic adenoma shows cytologic evidence of malignancy confined within the capsule of a preexisting pleomorphic adenoma. In general, prognosis is better than that of invasive variants and treatment involves surgical excision of the primary site.

Carcinosarcoma shows both epithelial and mesenchymal malignant components. These rare tumors are associated with frequent recurrences, distant metastases, and poor overall survival. Treatment requires surgery and adjuvant radiation therapy. Metastasizing pleomorphic adenomas show histologic features of benign pleomorphic adenoma, but present with distant metastases and multiply recurrent tumors locally. Treatment requires surgical resection of involved sites (local, regional, and distant) when possible. Prognosis is favorable despite metastases (**Fig. 4**).[7]

Salivary Duct Carcinoma

Salivary duct carcinoma is an uncommon tumor of the major salivary glands.[68] It arises from the excretory ducts of the salivary glands. On histology, it bears close resemblance to ductal carcinoma of breast, with intraductal and infiltrating tumor showing

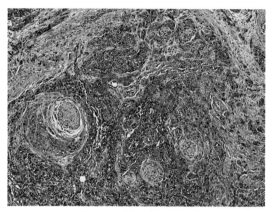

Fig. 4. High-grade carcinoma ex pleomorphic adenoma with extensive perineural invasion (other areas showed the histomorphology of bland pleomorphic adenoma) (HE, 100× magnification).

cell nest formation, nodules, and comedo-type necrosis.[7,69] Patients often present with a neoplastic mass involving the salivary gland, cranial neuropathies, and cervical nodal metastases. Most tumors arise de novo, but some may develop in the setting of a malignant mixed tumor. Parotid gland is the most common major salivary gland involved.[70]

Tumor biology is aggressive and treatment requires surgery for primary site and nodal basins, when preoperative cytology indicates the presence of a high-grade malignancy.[69,70] Adjuvant therapy is indicated and overall 5-year survival is modest at 40%.[70]

Salivary duct carcinoma may present with amplification of the HER-2 gene. Overexpression of HER-2 protein has been associated with poor prognosis.[71] In contrast with ductal carcinoma of the breast, salivary duct carcinoma shows significant intratumoral heterogeneity in protein expression of HER-2.[68] Monoclonal antibodies such as trastuzumab have been of interest in the management of these tumors.[72] Although some investigators have reported limited improvement in outcomes in adjuvant and palliative settings, data supporting routine use of these agents for systemic therapy in salivary duct carcinoma are still lacking (**Fig. 5**).[73]

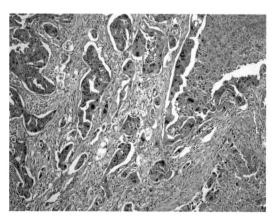

Fig. 5. Salivary duct carcinoma with areas of comedo necrosis and ductlike infiltrating tumor nests (similar to that seen in ductal carcinoma of the breast) (HE, 100× magnification).

Primary Squamous Cell Carcinoma

Major salivary glands can be affected by squamous cell carcinoma in varied settings including metastases from head and neck or distant sites, direct extension from adjacent head and neck primary neoplasms, and rarely by a primary squamous cell carcinoma arising from metaplastic ductal epithelium.[74] The diagnosis of a primary squamous cell carcinoma requires exclusion of clinical evidence or history of alternative primary sources, and differentiation from high-grade histologic components of other tumor types such as mucoepidermoid carcinoma.[74,75]

These tumors are more common in men than in women and usually present asymptomatically as masses or with pain, facial paralysis, or cervical nodal enlargement.[76] Tumor histology involves epidermoid cells with keratin pearl formation and intercellular bridges.[7]

These aggressive tumors are managed with radical surgery and adjuvant radiation.[76–78] Outcomes remain poor with frequent locoregional failure and overall survival that approaches 50% at 5 years.[76–79]

Mammary Analog Secretory Carcinoma

Mammary analog secretory carcinoma is a new entity with some similarities with its breast counterparts in terms of morphology and cytogenetics. This malignancy often affects men and the most common salivary gland affected is the parotid gland. Cervical nodal involvement is common.[80] Histology can be confused with that of oncocytic salivary neoplasms such as Warthin tumor, acinic cell carcinoma, and mucoepidermoid carcinoma. However, a unique translocation between chromosome 12 and 15, resulting in fusion of ETV6 and NTRK3 genes with resultant activated tyrosine kinase enzyme, is characteristic of this tumor.[80]

Lymphoma

Non-Hodgkin lymphoma (NHL) may involve the parotid gland, often secondary to more diffuse disease. However, isolated neoplastic lymphoproliferative changes may be observed in major salivary glands in the setting of nodal or glandular epithelium–based NHL. De novo salivary gland lymphomas usually present as large B-cell lymphomas. In addition, low-grade B-cell lymphomas involving the mucosa-associated lymphoid tissue, called extranodal marginal zone B-cell lymphomas, arise in the background of preexisting lymphoepithelial sialadenitis.[81] Patients with autoimmune disorders such as Sjögren disease may have a 20-fold to 40-fold higher risk of developing lymphoma of a major salivary gland.[7,82,83]

Most patients with primary salivary gland lymphomas present as having stage I or stage II disease.[84] Most patients present with an asymptomatic salivary gland mass and management may involve a variable combination of surgery, radiation, and systemic therapy. Prognosis is usually favorable, especially in the setting of localized disease.[85]

Secondary Tumors of Salivary Glands

Major salivary glands can be involved by locally invasive neoplasms that arise from the cutaneous or mucosal surfaces of the head and neck. In addition, regional nodal metastases may present because of involvement of the intraparotid lymph nodes by epithelial malignancies and melanoma. Distant metastases to the major salivary glands may also arise from malignancies that originate in the lung, kidney, and breast tissue, and other sites.

The incidence of nonmelanoma skin malignancies is increasing, and cutaneous malignancies located in the head and neck region (especially the scalp, temple, and pinna) often lead to intraparotid nodal metastases.[86] Identification of intraparotid nodal metastases is associated with a high incidence of clinically apparent and occult neck nodal involvement, and serves as an independent indicator for poor prognosis.[87,88] Anatomic studies suggest that most parotid lymph nodes are located in the superficial lobe of the gland.[89,90] Therefore, treatment usually involves a superficial parotidectomy, selective neck dissection (based on location of primary malignancy), and adjuvant radiation therapy.[91–93] Deep lobe resection is recommended when clinical findings suggest the presence of nodal metastases in the deep lobe of the parotid.

Sentinel lymph node biopsy has been validated as a reliable and safe technique in management of head and neck melanomas.[94–96] Lymphatic drainage in the head and neck region follows a complex pattern. However, sentinel lymph nodes may be localized to the parotid gland in up to one-quarter of all head and neck melanomas.[96] Although some surgeons use a superficial parotidectomy, in many cases biopsy of intraparotid sentinel lymph nodes can be performed safely with a parotid-sparing approach.[97,98]

TREATMENT
Salivary Gland Surgery

Salivary gland resection is central to therapy for malignant salivary gland tumors that are locoregionally confined. In the absence of clinically evident regional or distant metastasis, and other features that suggest invasiveness, the diagnosis of a malignancy may remain elusive until after surgical intervention.

Superficial parotidectomy is indicated for tumors limited to the lateral lobe of the parotid gland. Tumors that originate in or extend to the deep parotid lobe, and parapharyngeal space tumors, may require resection of the deep lobe of the parotid gland or a total parotidectomy. A modified Blair incision is preferred to provide broad exposure of the surgical field. Careful identification of anatomic landmarks, including the tragal pointer, the tympanomastoid suture, and the posterior belly of the digastric muscle helps in localization of the facial nerve and the pes anserinus. In rare circumstances, tumor location and extent may necessitate retrograde dissection of facial nerve branches or a mastoidectomy to identify the intratemporal course of the nerve. Facial nerve monitoring may be instituted based on surgeon preference.[99] When preoperative assessment indicates an intact facial nerve, efforts should be made to preserve the nerve as long as gross tumor excision can be achieved. Although a deviation from classic oncologic principles, it avoids the morbidity associated with iatrogenic facial nerve deficits. With appropriate adjuvant radiation, acceptable local control can be achieved.[100] Facial nerve section and cable nerve grafts may be used when gross tumor encasement or infiltration or loss of nerve function is established preoperatively.

When resecting a submandibular gland, care must be exercised in preserving the marginal mandibular, hypoglossal, and lingual nerves. Similarly, cannulation and preservation of the submandibular duct and lingual nerve should be attempted when excising the sublingual gland via a transoral approach.

Local invasion may dictate wide clearance of affected skin, soft tissue, or bony structures, and may require consideration for complex reconstruction using local tissue rearrangement or free tissue transfer.

Management of Regional Lymph Nodes

Clinically apparent cervical nodal metastases are managed with comprehensive neck dissection. However, occult nodal metastases may be present in 14% to 33% of patients.[36,101,102] Management of clinically node-negative necks has been debated. Predicting which patients may benefit from an elective neck dissection is challenging.[103] Increasing age, advanced T stage, high-grade histology, and presence of salivary duct carcinoma is associated with higher incidence of occult nodal involvement.[104]

Evidence suggests that elective neck dissection may be superior to observation in ensuring disease-free survival in primary parotid malignancies.[36] An alternative management strategy uses elective neck irradiation following surgical resection of the primary tumor. In high-grade malignant tumors, elective neck irradiation may have a trend toward superior regional control and cause specific survival.[105,106] Single-modality treatment should be used for the management of neck nodes when feasible.

Radiation Therapy

Adjuvant radiation therapy is indicated for patients with advanced tumor stage and high-grade histology. Additional factors to consider in planning adjuvant radiation therapy include positive margins not amenable to surgery, nodal metastases, and perineural invasion.

A recent SEER database review concluded that adjuvant radiation therapy afforded a significant survival benefit for high-grade and/or locally advanced major salivary gland carcinoma.[107] In another study evaluating the outcomes of patients with squamous cell carcinoma of the parotid gland, surgery combined with adjuvant radiation offered a survival advantage compared with radiation alone.[44] In addition, radiation therapy reduces risk for regional failure.[36,106]

Radiation therapy is used as the primary treatment modality in patients with unresectable or macroscopically residual tumor. Fast neutron therapy has been explored as an alternative to photon therapy, and a phase III trial indicated superior locoregional control with neutron therapy. However, this was associated with severe treatment-related toxicities and did not affect overall survival.[108,109] In other studies, photon-based therapy compares favorably with neutron therapy outcomes.[110] Enthusiasm for neutron therapy has been tempered by concerns about the long-term toxicity and limited availability of centers with ability to treat with neutrons.[111] There has been recent interest in carbon ion therapy, which has similar relative biological effectiveness to neutrons. In a phase II trial, 5-year local control rates of 73% were achieved for patients with adenoid cystic carcinoma and adenocarcinoma with unresectable disease, and a milder late toxicity profile was observed.[112]

Chemotherapy and Molecular Agents

Use of systemic therapy has been explored for patients with unresectable locally advanced disease or patients with distant metastases. Several single-agent or multi-agent chemotherapy regimens including platinum and Taxol have been used.[113–115] However, response to therapy is only modest and ranges between 15% to 50%, and overall impact on survival remains unclear.[114–116] The lack of measurable tumor response may be associated with the indolent nature of many salivary malignancies. In the absence of proven benefit, possible comorbidity related to chemotherapy, and fairly asymptomatic presentation, patients with unresectable or metastatic salivary malignancies may do well without institution of systemic therapy.

Increased expression of epidermal growth factor receptors (EGFRs), including HER-2, in several salivary gland tumors has prompted interest in the use of targeted therapy. Although overexpression of EGFR proteins is common, it is not always associated with EGFR gene amplification.[117] Phase 2 trials of the EGFR monoclonal antibody cetuximab revealed disease stability in half of the study population. However, most patients who were evaluated had adenoid cystic carcinoma, which is expected to follow an indolent course, thus complicating the interpretation of these data.[118] Another oral agent with anti-EGFR activity, gefitinib, failed to show any objective evidence of tumor response to therapy.[119] Increased HER-2 protein expression in salivary duct carcinoma is associated with intratumoral heterogeneity, which likely plays a role in the variable response to anti–HER-2 therapy.[68] Other targets for molecular therapy include c-kit and vascular endothelial growth factor. Clear data to support use of monoclonal antibodies against these targets in salivary gland malignancies are unavailable.[115,120,121]

Identification of fusion oncogenes may become clinically significant in tumors such as adenoid cystic carcinoma and mucoepidermoid carcinoma.[122] The ETV6-NTRK3 fusion oncogene is critical in differentiation of mammary analog secretory carcinoma from other histologic entities.[80]

SUMMARY

Major salivary gland malignancies are a rare but histologically diverse group of entities. Establishing the diagnosis of a malignant salivary neoplasm may be challenging because of the often minimally symptomatic nature of the disease, and limitations of imaging modalities and cytology. Treatment is centered on surgical therapy and adjuvant radiation in selected scenarios. Systemic therapy with chemotherapeutic agents and monoclonal antibodies lacks evidence in support of its routine use.

REFERENCES

1. Center for Disease Control Statistics. United States cancer statistics [Internet]. 2014. Available at: apps.nccd.cdc.gov/uscs/cancersbyraceandethnicity.aspx. Accessed December 20, 2014.
2. Speight PM, Barrett AW. Salivary gland tumours. Oral Dis 2002;8(5):229–40.
3. Boukheris H, Curtis RE, Land CE, et al. Incidence of carcinoma of the major salivary glands according to the WHO classification, 1992 to 2006: a population-based study in the United States. Cancer Epidemiol Biomarkers Prev 2009; 18(11):2899–906.
4. Shah J, Patel S, Singh B. Salivary glands. In: Shah J, Patel S, Singh B, editors. Head and neck surgery and oncology. 3rd edition. Philadelphia: Elsevier; 2007. p. 526–69.
5. van der Laan BF, Baris G, Gregor RT, et al. Radiation-induced tumours of the head and neck. J Laryngol Otol 1995;109(4):346–9.
6. Scanlon EF, Sener SF. Head and neck neoplasia following irradiation for benign conditions. Head Neck Surg 1981;4(2):139–45.
7. Wenig BM. Section 4: major and minor salivary glands. Neoplasms of the salivary glands. In: Wenig BM, editor. Atlas of head and neck pathology. 2nd edition. Philadelphia: Elsevier; 2008. p. 582–702.
8. Sadetzki S, Oberman B, Mandelzweig L, et al. Smoking and risk of parotid gland tumors: a nationwide case-control study. Cancer 2008;112(9):1974–82.
9. de Souza FT, Correia-Silva JF, Ferreira EF, et al. Cell phone use and parotid salivary gland alterations: no molecular evidence. Cancer Epidemiol Biomarkers Prev 2014;23(7):1428–31.
10. Repacholi MH, Lerchl A, Roosli M, et al. Systematic review of wireless phone use and brain cancer and other head tumors. Bioelectromagnetics 2012;33(3): 187–206.

11. Soderqvist F, Carlberg M, Hardell L. Use of wireless phones and the risk of salivary gland tumours: a case-control study. Eur J Cancer Prev 2012;21(6): 576–9.

12. Eveson JW, Auclair PL, Gnepp DR. Tumors of the salivary glands: introduction. In: Barnes L, Eveson JW, Reichert P, et al, editors. Pathology and genetics of head and neck tumors. Lyon (France): World Health Organization Classification of Tumors; IARC Press; 2005. p. 212–7.

13. Major salivary glands (parotid, submandibular, and sublingual). In: Edge SB, Byrd DR, Compton CC, editors. AJCC cancer staging manual. 7th edition. New York: Springer; 2010. p. 79–82.

14. Speight PM, Barrett AW. Prognostic factors in malignant tumours of the salivary glands. Br J Oral Maxillofac Surg 2009;47(8):587–93.

15. Bjorndal K, Krogdahl A, Therkildsen MH, et al. Salivary gland carcinoma in Denmark 1990–2005: outcome and prognostic factors. Results of the Danish Head and Neck Cancer Group (DAHANCA). Oral Oncol 2012;48(2):179–85.

16. Ali S, Palmer FL, Yu C, et al. Postoperative nomograms predictive of survival after surgical management of malignant tumors of the major salivary glands. Ann Surg Oncol 2014;21(2):637–42.

17. Stodulski D, Mikaszewski B, Stankiewicz C. Signs and symptoms of parotid gland carcinoma and their prognostic value. Int J Oral Maxillofac Surg 2012; 41(7):801–6.

18. Katz P, Hartl DM, Guerre A. Clinical ultrasound of the salivary glands. Otolaryngol Clin North Am 2009;42(6):973–1000 [Table of Contents].

19. Shimizu M, Ussmuller J, Hartwein J, et al. Statistical study for sonographic differential diagnosis of tumorous lesions in the parotid gland. Oral Surg Oral Med Oral Pathol Oral Radiol Endod 1999;88(2):226–33.

20. Shimizu M, Ussmuller J, Hartwein J, et al. A comparative study of sonographic and histopathologic findings of tumorous lesions in the parotid gland. Oral Surg Oral Med Oral Pathol Oral Radiol Endod 1999;88(6):723–37.

21. Schick S, Steiner E, Gahleitner A, et al. Differentiation of benign and malignant tumors of the parotid gland: value of pulsed Doppler and color Doppler sonography. Eur Radiol 1998;8(8):1462–7.

22. Klein K, Turk R, Gritzmann N, et al. The value of sonography in salivary gland tumors. HNO 1989;37(2):71–5 [in German].

23. Koischwitz D, Gritzmann N. Ultrasound of the neck. Radiol Clin North Am 2000; 38(5):1029–45.

24. Christe A, Waldherr C, Hallett R, et al. MR imaging of parotid tumors: typical lesion characteristics in MR imaging improve discrimination between benign and malignant disease. AJNR Am J Neuroradiol 2011;32(7):1202–7.

25. Celebi I, Mahmutoglu AS, Ucgul A, et al. Quantitative diffusion-weighted magnetic resonance imaging in the evaluation of parotid gland masses: a study with histopathological correlation. Clin Imaging 2013;37(2):232–8.

26. Toriihara A, Nakamura S, Kubota K, et al. Can dual-time-point 18F-FDG PET/CT differentiate malignant salivary gland tumors from benign tumors? AJR Am J Roentgenol 2013;201(3):639–44.

27. Jeong HS, Chung MK, Son YI, et al. Role of 18F-FDG PET/CT in management of high-grade salivary gland malignancies. J Nucl Med 2007;48(8):1237–44.

28. Cermik TF, Mavi A, Acikgoz G, et al. FDG PET in detecting primary and recurrent malignant salivary gland tumors. Clin Nucl Med 2007;32(4):286–91.

29. Westra WH. Diagnostic difficulties in the classification and grading of salivary gland tumors. Int J Radiat Oncol Biol Phys 2007;69(2 Suppl):S49–51.

30. Carrillo JF, Ramirez R, Flores L, et al. Diagnostic accuracy of fine needle aspiration biopsy in preoperative diagnosis of patients with parotid gland masses. J Surg Oncol 2009;100(2):133–8.
31. Tryggvason G, Gailey MP, Hulstein SL, et al. Accuracy of fine-needle aspiration and imaging in the preoperative workup of salivary gland mass lesions treated surgically. Laryngoscope 2013;123(1):158–63.
32. Colella G, Cannavale R, Flamminio F, et al. Fine-needle aspiration cytology of salivary gland lesions: a systematic review. J Oral Maxillofac Surg 2010;68(9): 2146–53.
33. Das DK, Petkar MA, Al-Mane NM, et al. Role of fine needle aspiration cytology in the diagnosis of swellings in the salivary gland regions: a study of 712 cases. Med Princ Pract 2004;13(2):95–106.
34. Mallon DH, Kostalas M, MacPherson FJ, et al. The diagnostic value of fine needle aspiration in parotid lumps. Ann R Coll Surg Engl 2013;95(4):258–62.
35. Kim BY, Hyeon J, Ryu G, et al. Diagnostic accuracy of fine needle aspiration cytology for high-grade salivary gland tumors. Ann Surg Oncol 2013;20(7): 2380–7.
36. Zbaren P, Schupbach J, Nuyens M, et al. Elective neck dissection versus observation in primary parotid carcinoma. Otolaryngol Head Neck Surg 2005;132(3): 387–91.
37. Huang YC, Wu CT, Lin G, et al. Comparison of ultrasonographically guided fine-needle aspiration and core needle biopsy in the diagnosis of parotid masses. J Clin Ultrasound 2012;40(4):189–94.
38. Witt BL, Schmidt RL. Ultrasound-guided core needle biopsy of salivary gland lesions: a systematic review and meta-analysis. Laryngoscope 2014;124(3): 695–700.
39. Seethala RR. An update on grading of salivary gland carcinomas. Head Neck Pathol 2009;3(1):69–77.
40. Bradley PJ, McGurk M. Incidence of salivary gland neoplasms in a defined UK population. Br J Oral Maxillofac Surg 2013;51(5):399–403.
41. Jones AV, Craig GT, Speight PM, et al. The range and demographics of salivary gland tumours diagnosed in a UK population. Oral Oncol 2008;44(4):407–17.
42. Spitz MR, Batsakis JG. Major salivary gland carcinoma. Descriptive epidemiology and survival of 498 patients. Arch Otolaryngol 1984;110(1):45–9.
43. McHugh CH, Roberts DB, El-Naggar AK, et al. Prognostic factors in mucoepidermoid carcinoma of the salivary glands. Cancer 2012;118(16):3928–36.
44. Chen AM, Lau VH, Farwell DG, et al. Mucoepidermoid carcinoma of the parotid gland treated by surgery and postoperative radiation therapy: clinicopathologic correlates of outcome. Laryngoscope 2013;123(12):3049–55.
45. Brandwein MS, Ivanov K, Wallace DI, et al. Mucoepidermoid carcinoma: a clinicopathologic study of 80 patients with special reference to histological grading. Am J Surg Pathol 2001;25(7):835–45.
46. Auclair PL, Goode RK, Ellis GL. Mucoepidermoid carcinoma of intraoral salivary glands. Evaluation and application of grading criteria in 143 cases. Cancer 1992;69(8):2021–30.
47. Goode RK, Auclair PL, Ellis GL. Mucoepidermoid carcinoma of the major salivary glands: clinical and histopathologic analysis of 234 cases with evaluation of grading criteria. Cancer 1998;82(7):1217–24.
48. Emerick KS, Fabian RL, Deschler DG. Clinical presentation, management, and outcome of high-grade mucoepidermoid carcinoma of the parotid gland. Otolaryngol Head Neck Surg 2007;136(5):783–7.

49. Amit M, Na'ara S, Sharma K, et al. Elective neck dissection in patients with head and neck adenoid cystic carcinoma: an international collaborative study. Ann Surg Oncol 2015;22(4):1353–9.

50. Bhayani MK, Yener M, El-Naggar A, et al. Prognosis and risk factors for early-stage adenoid cystic carcinoma of the major salivary glands. Cancer 2012; 118(11):2872–8.

51. Gao M, Hao Y, Huang MX, et al. Clinicopathological study of distant metastases of salivary adenoid cystic carcinoma. Int J Oral Maxillofac Surg 2013;42(8):923–8.

52. Perzin KH, Gullane P, Clairmont AC. Adenoid cystic carcinomas arising in salivary glands: a correlation of histologic features and clinical course. Cancer 1978;42(1):265–82.

53. Spiro RH, Huvos AG, Strong EW. Adenoid cystic carcinoma of salivary origin. A clinicopathologic study of 242 cases. Am J Surg 1974;128(4):512–20.

54. van Weert S, van der Waal I, Witte BI, et al. Histopathological grading of adenoid cystic carcinoma of the head and neck: analysis of currently used grading systems and proposal for a simplified grading scheme. Oral Oncol 2015;51(1): 71–6.

55. Ellington CL, Goodman M, Kono SA, et al. Adenoid cystic carcinoma of the head and neck: incidence and survival trends based on 1973–2007 Surveillance, Epidemiology, and End Results data. Cancer 2012;118(18):4444–51.

56. Lee SY, Kim BH, Choi EC. Nineteen-year oncologic outcomes and the benefit of elective neck dissection in salivary gland adenoid cystic carcinoma. Head Neck 2014;36(12):1796–801.

57. Spiro RH, Huvos AG. Stage means more than grade in adenoid cystic carcinoma. Am J Surg 1992;164(6):623–8.

58. Marcinow A, Ozer E, Teknos T, et al. Clinicopathologic predictors of recurrence and overall survival in adenoid cystic carcinoma of the head and neck: a single institutional experience at a tertiary care center. Head Neck 2014;36(12):1705–11.

59. Shen C, Xu T, Huang C, et al. Treatment outcomes and prognostic features in adenoid cystic carcinoma originated from the head and neck. Oral Oncol 2012;48(5):445–9.

60. Levin JM, Robinson DW, Lin F. Acinic cell carcinoma: collective review, including bilateral cases. Arch Surg 1975;110(1):64–8.

61. Patel NR, Sanghvi S, Khan MN, et al. Demographic trends and disease-specific survival in salivary acinic cell carcinoma: an analysis of 1129 cases. Laryngoscope 2014;124(1):172–8.

62. Gnepp DR. Malignant mixed tumors of the salivary glands: a review. Pathol Annu 1993;(28 Pt 1):279–328.

63. Chen AM, Garcia J, Bucci MK, et al. The role of postoperative radiation therapy in carcinoma ex pleomorphic adenoma of the parotid gland. Int J Radiat Oncol Biol Phys 2007;67(1):138–43.

64. Zhao J, Wang J, Yu C, et al. Prognostic factors affecting the clinical outcome of carcinoma ex pleomorphic adenoma in the major salivary gland. World J Surg Oncol 2013;11(1):180.

65. Olsen KD, Lewis JE. Carcinoma ex pleomorphic adenoma: a clinicopathologic review. Head Neck 2001;23(9):705–12.

66. Nouraei SA, Hope KL, Kelly CG, et al. Carcinoma ex benign pleomorphic adenoma of the parotid gland. Plast Reconstr Surg 2005;116(5):1206–13.

67. Lim CM, Hobson C, Kim S, et al. Clinical outcome of patients with carcinoma ex pleomorphic adenoma of the parotid gland: a comparative study from a single tertiary center. Head Neck 2015;37(4):543–7.

68. Kondo Y, Kikuchi T, Esteban JC, et al. Intratumoral heterogeneity of HER2 protein and amplification of HER2 gene in salivary duct carcinoma. Pathol Int 2014; 64(9):453–9.

69. Wee DT, Thomas AA, Bradley PJ. Salivary duct carcinoma: what is already known, and can we improve survival? J Laryngol Otol 2012;126(Suppl 2): S2–7.

70. Salovaara E, Hakala O, Back L, et al. Management and outcome of salivary duct carcinoma in major salivary glands. Eur Arch Otorhinolaryngol 2013;270(1): 281–5.

71. Lee JS, Kwon OJ, Park JJ, et al. Salivary duct carcinoma of the parotid gland: is adjuvant HER-2-targeted therapy required? J Oral Maxillofac Surg 2014;72(5): 1023–31.

72. Perissinotti AJ, Lee Pierce M, Pace MB, et al. The role of trastuzumab in the management of salivary ductal carcinomas. Anticancer Res 2013;33(6): 2587–91.

73. Limaye SA, Posner MR, Krane JF, et al. Trastuzumab for the treatment of salivary duct carcinoma. Oncologist 2013;18(3):294–300.

74. Taxy JB. Squamous carcinoma in a major salivary gland: a review of the diagnostic considerations. Arch Pathol Lab Med 2001;125(6):740–5.

75. Batsakis JG. Primary squamous cell carcinomas of major salivary glands. Ann Otol Rhinol Laryngol 1983;92(1 Pt 1):97–8.

76. Gaughan RK, Olsen KD, Lewis JE. Primary squamous cell carcinoma of the parotid gland. Arch Otolaryngol Head Neck Surg 1992;118(8):798–801.

77. Akhtar K, Ray PS, Sherwani R, et al. Primary squamous cell carcinoma of the parotid gland: a rare entity. BMJ Case Rep 2013;15. pii:bcr2013009467.

78. Chen MM, Roman SA, Sosa JA, et al. Prognostic factors for squamous cell cancer of the parotid gland: an analysis of 2104 patients. Head Neck 2015;37(1): 1–7.

79. Shemen LJ, Huvos AG, Spiro RH. Squamous cell carcinoma of salivary gland origin. Head Neck Surg 1987;9(4):235–40.

80. Samulski TD, LiVolsi VA, Baloch Z. The cytopathologic features of mammary analog secretory carcinoma and its mimics. Cytojournal 2014;11:24.

81. Paliga A, Farmer J, Bence-Bruckler I, et al. Salivary gland lymphoproliferative disorders: a Canadian tertiary center experience. Head Neck Pathol 2013; 7(4):381–8.

82. Voulgarelis M, Dafni UG, Isenberg DA, et al. Malignant lymphoma in primary Sjogren's syndrome: a multicenter, retrospective, clinical study by the European Concerted Action on Sjogren's Syndrome. Arthritis Rheum 1999;42(8): 1765–72.

83. Jonsson MV, Theander E, Jonsson R. Predictors for the development of non-Hodgkin lymphoma in primary Sjogren's syndrome. Presse Med 2012;41(9 Pt 2):e511–6.

84. Anacak Y, Miller RC, Constantinou N, et al. Primary mucosa-associated lymphoid tissue lymphoma of the salivary glands: a multicenter Rare Cancer Network study. Int J Radiat Oncol Biol Phys 2012;82(1):315–20.

85. Vazquez A, Khan MN, Sanghvi S, et al. Extranodal marginal zone lymphoma of mucosa-associated lymphoid tissue of the salivary glands: a population-based study from 1994 to 2009. Head Neck 2015;37(1):18–22.

86. Gurney B, Newlands C. Management of regional metastatic disease in head and neck cutaneous malignancy. 1. Cutaneous squamous cell carcinoma. Br J Oral Maxillofac Surg 2014;52(4):294–300.

87. O'Brien CJ, McNeil EB, McMahon JD, et al. Incidence of cervical node involvement in metastatic cutaneous malignancy involving the parotid gland. Head Neck 2001;23(9):744–8.
88. Ch'ng S, Maitra A, Lea R, et al. Parotid metastasis–an independent prognostic factor for head and neck cutaneous squamous cell carcinoma. J Plast Reconstr Aesthet Surg 2006;59(12):1288–93.
89. Marks NJ. The anatomy of the lymph nodes of the parotid gland. Clin Otolaryngol Allied Sci 1984;9(5):271–5.
90. McKean ME, Lee K, McGregor IA. The distribution of lymph nodes in and around the parotid gland: an anatomical study. Br J Plast Surg 1985;38(1):1–5.
91. Yilmaz M, Eskiizmir G, Friedman O. Cutaneous squamous cell carcinoma of the head and neck: management of the parotid and neck. Facial Plast Surg Clin North Am 2012;20(4):473–81.
92. Hinerman RW, Indelicato DJ, Amdur RJ, et al. Cutaneous squamous cell carcinoma metastatic to parotid-area lymph nodes. Laryngoscope 2008;118(11):1989–96.
93. Ebrahimi A, Moncrieff MD, Clark JR, et al. Predicting the pattern of regional metastases from cutaneous squamous cell carcinoma of the head and neck based on location of the primary. Head Neck 2010;32(10):1288–94.
94. Picon AI, Coit DG, Shaha AR, et al. Sentinel lymph node biopsy for cutaneous head and neck melanoma: mapping the parotid gland. Ann Surg Oncol 2006. [Epub ahead of print]. http://dx.doi.org/10.1245/ASO.2006.03.051.
95. Loree TR, Tomljanovich PI, Cheney RT, et al. Intraparotid sentinel lymph node biopsy for head and neck melanoma. Laryngoscope 2006;116(8):1461–4.
96. Schmalbach CE, Nussenbaum B, Rees RS, et al. Reliability of sentinel lymph node mapping with biopsy for head and neck cutaneous melanoma. Arch Otolaryngol Head Neck Surg 2003;129(1):61–5.
97. Samra S, Sawh-Martinez R, Tom L, et al. A targeted approach to sentinel lymph node biopsies in the parotid region for head and neck melanomas. Ann Plast Surg 2012;69(4):415–7.
98. Sawh-Martinez R, Douglas S, Pavri S, et al. Management of head and neck melanoma: results of a national survey. Ann Plast Surg 2014;73(Suppl 2):S175–7.
99. Andersen PE. Superficial parotidectomy. In: Cohen JI, Clayman GL, editors. Atlas of head and neck surgery. 1st edition. Philadelphia: Elsevier; 2011. p. 227–35.
100. Pfister DG, Spencer S, Brizel DM, et al. Head and neck cancers, version 2.2014. Clinical practice guidelines in oncology. J Natl Compr Canc Netw 2014;12(10):1454–87.
101. Valstar MH, van den Brekel MW, Smeele LE. Interpretation of treatment outcome in the clinically node-negative neck in primary parotid carcinoma: a systematic review of the literature. Head Neck 2010;32(10):1402–11.
102. Stenner M, Molls C, Luers JC, et al. Occurrence of lymph node metastasis in early-stage parotid gland cancer. Eur Arch Otorhinolaryngol 2012;269(2):643–8.
103. Nobis CP, Rohleder NH, Wolff KD, et al. Head and neck salivary gland carcinomas–elective neck dissection, yes or no? J Oral Maxillofac Surg 2014;72(1):205–10.
104. Ettl T, Gosau M, Brockhoff G, et al. Predictors of cervical lymph node metastasis in salivary gland cancer. Head Neck 2014;36(4):517–23.
105. Herman MP, Werning JW, Morris CG, et al. Elective neck management for high-grade salivary gland carcinoma. Am J Otolaryngol 2013;34(3):205–8.

106. Chen AM, Garcia J, Lee NY, et al. Patterns of nodal relapse after surgery and postoperative radiation therapy for carcinomas of the major and minor salivary glands: what is the role of elective neck irradiation? Int J Radiat Oncol Biol Phys 2007;67(4):988–94.

107. Mahmood U, Koshy M, Goloubeva O, et al. Adjuvant radiation therapy for high-grade and/or locally advanced major salivary gland tumors. Arch Otolaryngol Head Neck Surg 2011;137(10):1025–30.

108. Laramore GE, Krall JM, Griffin TW, et al. Neutron versus photon irradiation for unresectable salivary gland tumors: final report of an RTOG-MRC randomized clinical trial. Radiation Therapy Oncology Group. Medical Research Council. Int J Radiat Oncol Biol Phys 1993;27(2):235–40.

109. Griffin TW, Pajak TF, Laramore GE, et al. Neutron vs photon irradiation of inoperable salivary gland tumors: results of an RTOG-MRC cooperative randomized study. Int J Radiat Oncol Biol Phys 1988;15(5):1085–90.

110. Spratt DE, Salgado LR, Riaz N, et al. Results of photon radiotherapy for unresectable salivary gland tumors: is neutron radiotherapy's local control superior? Radiol Oncol 2014;48(1):56–61.

111. Abratt RP. Neutron therapy and increased late complication rates. Radiother Oncol 2014;110(2):375.

112. Mizoe JE, Hasegawa A, Jingu K, et al. Results of carbon ion radiotherapy for head and neck cancer. Radiother Oncol 2012;103(1):32–7.

113. Ross PJ, Teoh EM, A'hern RP, et al. Epirubicin, cisplatin and protracted venous infusion 5-fluorouracil chemotherapy for advanced salivary adenoid cystic carcinoma. Clin Oncol (R Coll Radiol) 2009;21(4):311–4.

114. Gilbert J, Li Y, Pinto HA, et al. Phase II trial of Taxol in salivary gland malignancies (E1394): a trial of the Eastern Cooperative Oncology Group. Head Neck 2006;28(3):197–204.

115. Mehra R, Cohen RB. New agents in the treatment for malignancies of the salivary and thyroid glands. Hematol Oncol Clin North Am 2008;22(6):1279–95, xi.

116. Surakanti SG, Agulnik M. Salivary gland malignancies: the role for chemotherapy and molecular targeted agents. Semin Oncol 2008;35(3):309–19.

117. Clauditz TS, Gontarewicz A, Lebok P, et al. Epidermal growth factor receptor (EGFR) in salivary gland carcinomas: potentials as therapeutic target. Oral Oncol 2012;48(10):991–6.

118. Locati LD, Bossi P, Perrone F, et al. Cetuximab in recurrent and/or metastatic salivary gland carcinomas: a phase II study. Oral Oncol 2009;45(7):574–8.

119. Jakob JA, Kies MS, Glisson BS, et al. A phase II study of gefitinib in patients with advanced salivary gland cancers. Head Neck 2014. [Epub ahead of print].

120. Haddad R, Colevas AD, Krane JF, et al. Herceptin in patients with advanced or metastatic salivary gland carcinomas. A phase II study. Oral Oncol 2003;39(7): 724–7.

121. Glisson B, Colevas AD, Haddad R, et al. HER2 expression in salivary gland carcinomas: dependence on histological subtype. Clin Cancer Res 2004;10(3): 944–6.

122. Stenman G. Fusion oncogenes in salivary gland tumors: molecular and clinical consequences. Head Neck Pathol 2013;7(Suppl 1):S12–9.

Printed and bound by CPI Group (UK) Ltd, Croydon, CR0 4YY

03/10/2024

01040497-0006